Methodist Sports
Medicine Ctr.

Edited by

BERTRAM ZARINS, M.D.

Assistant Clinical Professor, Orthopaedic Surgery, Harvard University Medical School; Chief, Sports Medicine Unit, Massachusetts General Hospital; Team Physician, Boston Bruins Hockey Team and New England Patriots Football Team, Boston, Massachusetts; Chairman, Education Committee, United States Olympic Committee Sports Medicine Council

JAMES R. ANDREWS, M.D.

Clinical Associate Professor, Section of Sports Medicine, Division of Orthopaedics, Tulane University School of Medicine, New Orleans, Louisiana; Director of Orthopaedic Training, Hughston Orthopaedic Clinic, Columbus, Georgia

WILLIAM G. CARSON, Jr., M.D.

Orthopaedic Surgeon, Tampa Orthopaedic and Sports Medicine Group; Assistant Clinical Professor of Orthopaedics, University of South Florida, Tampa, Florida

INJURIES TO the THROWING ARM

BASED ON THE PROCEEDINGS
OF THE NATIONAL CONFERENCES
SPONSORED BY THE U.S.O.C.
SPORTS MEDICINE COUNCIL

1985

W. B. SAUNDERS COMPANY
Philadelphia/London/Toronto/Mexico City/
Rio de Janeiro/Sydney/Tokyo/Hong Kong

W. B. Saunders Company: West Washington Square
                          Philadelphia, PA   19105

Library of Congress Cataloging in Publication Data

Main entry under title:

Injuries to the throwing arm.

Includes index.

1. Arm—Wounds and injuries—Congresses.   2. Shoulder—
   Wounds and injuries—Congresses.   3. Baseball—Accidents
   and injuries—Congresses.   I. Zarins, Bertram.
   II. Andrews, James R. (James Rheuben), 1942–   .
   III. Carson, William G. (William George), 1952–   .
   IV. U.S.O.C. Sports Medicine Council. [DNLM:
   1. Arm Injuries—congresses.   2. Athletic Injuries—
   congresses.   3. Sports—congresses.   4. Sports
   Medicine—congresses. WE 805 I56]

RD557.I55 1985   617'.574   84–20236   Rev.

ISBN 0–7216–1416–7

Acquisition Editor: Barbara Cohen

Production Manager: Frank Polizzano

Compositor: W. B. Saunders Company Typesetting

Printer: W. B. Saunders Company Press

Injuries to the Throwing Arm   ISBN   0-7216-1416-7

Last digit is the print number: 9   8   7   6   5   4   3   2   1

CONTRIBUTORS

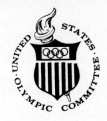

JOHN ALBRIGHT, M.D.

Professor of Orthopaedic Surgery, University of Iowa School of Medicine, Iowa City, Iowa; Director of the University of Iowa Sports Medicine Services; Staff Orthopaedic Surgeon and Chief, Sports Medicine Clinic, the University of Iowa Hospitals and Clinics, Iowa City, Iowa.

Shoulder Arthrotomography in the Evaluation of the Injured Throwing Arm

FRED L. ALLMAN, JR., M.D.

Director, Sports Medicine Clinic PC, Atlanta, Georgia; Vice Chairman, Medical Staff, Doctors Memorial Hospital, Atlanta, Georgia.

Impingement, Biceps, and Rotator Cuff Lesions

JAMES R. ANDREWS, M.D.

Clinical Associate Professor, Section of Sports Medicine, Division of Orthopaedics, Tulane University School of Medicine, New Orleans, Louisiana; Chief, Orthopaedic Surgery, St. Francis Hospital, Columbus, Georgia; Director of Orthopaedic Training, Hughston Orthopaedic Clinic, Columbus, Georgia.

Proper Pitching Technique; Physical Examination of the Shoulder in Throwing Athletes; Operative Arthroscopy of the Shoulder in the Throwing Athlete; Arthroscopy of the Elbow; Valgus Extension Overload in the Pitching Elbow.

GIDEON B. ARIEL, PH.D.

President, Coto Research Center, Trabuco Canyon, California.

Body Mechanics

CHAMP L. BAKER, JR., M.D.

Clinical Assistant Professor, Department of Orthopaedics, Tulane University, New Orleans, Louisiana; Director of Medical Education, Hughston Sports Medicine Hospital; Attending Physician, St. Francis Hospital, Doctors Hospital, Medical Center, Columbus, Georgia; Attending Physician, Cobb Hospital, Phoenix City, Alabama.

Neurovascular Syndromes

v

JAMES B. BENNETT, M.D.

Assistant Professor of Orthopedic Surgery, Chief Hand and Upper Extremity Section, Baylor College of Medicine, Houston, Texas.

Surgical Management of Acute and Chronic Elbow Problems

MICHAEL E. BERKELEY, M.D.

Instructor, Orthopedic Surgery, Baylor College of Medicine, Houston, Texas.

Surgical Management of Acute and Chronic Elbow Problems

T. A. BLACKBURN, M.Ed., R.P.T., A.T.C.

Adjunct Assistant Professor, Columbus College, Columbus, Georgia; Chief, Sports Physical Therapy, Rehabilitation Services of Columbus, Inc., Columbus, Georgia.

The Off-Season Program for the Throwing Arm

WILLIAM JAY BRYAN, M.D.

Assistant Professor, Division of Orthopedic Surgery, Baylor College of Medicine, Houston, Texas; Attending Physician, The Methodist Hospital, Houston, Texas; Team Physician, The Houston Astros.

Functional Anatomy of the Elbow; Examination of the Throwing Elbow

WILLIAM G. CARSON, Jr., M.D.

Assistant Clinical Professor of Orthopaedics, University of South Florida, Tampa, Florida; Orthopaedic Surgeon, Tampa Orthopaedic and Sports Medicine Group, Tampa, Florida.

Arthroscopy of the Shoulder: Normal Anatomy; Operative Arthroscopy of the Shoulder in the Throwing Athlete; Arthroscopy of the Elbow

DON FAULS, A.T.C.

Associate Professor and Head Athletic Trainer, Florida State University, Tallahassee, Florida.

General Training Techniques to Warm Up and Cool Down the Throwing Arm

GERALD A. M. FINERMAN, M.D.

Professor of Surgery/Orthopaedics, UCLA, Los Angeles, California; Attending Surgeon, UCLA, Los Angeles, California.

Water Polo Injuries to the Upper Extremity

JOE H. GIECK, Ed.D., A.T.C., R.P.T.

Curriculum Director, Head Athletic Trainer, Division of Sports Medicine and Athletic Training, Department of Athletics; Assistant Professor, School of Education; Assistant Professor, Orthopaedics and Rehabilitation, University of Virginia, Charlottesville, Virginia.

Throwing Injuries to the Shoulder

SCOTT D. GILLOGLY, M.D.

Captain, Medical Corps, United States Army; Clinical Instructor, Department of Surgery, Uniformed Services University of Health Sciences, Bethesda, Maryland; Chief Resident, Orthopaedic Service, Walter Reed Army Medical Center, Washington, D.C.

Physical Examination of the Shoulder in Throwing Athletes

CHARLES P. GREENE, ED.D., PH.D.

Head Baseball Coach and Professor of Physical Education, Miami-Dade Community College, South Campus, Miami, Florida.

The Curve Ball and the Elbow; Spring Training Conditioning for the Throwing Shoulder

ROBERT J. GREGOR, PH.D.

Associate Professor, Department of Kinesiology, UCLA, Los Angeles, California.

Water Polo Injuries to the Upper Extremity

JACK C. HUGHSTON, M.D.

Clinical Professor, Department of Orthopaedics, Tulane University School of Medicine, New Orleans, Louisiana; Adjunct Professor, Auburn University School of Veterinary Medicine, Auburn, Alabama; Chairman of the Board of Directors, Hughston Sports Medicine Hospital, Columbus, Georgia.

Functional Anatomy of the Shoulder

STEPHEN C. HUNTER, M.D.

Clinical Assistant Professor, Department of Orthopaedic Surgery, Section of Sports Medicine, Tulane University, New Orleans, Louisiana; Orthopaedic Surgeon, Hughston Sports Medicine Hospital, Columbus, Georgia.

Little Leaguer's Elbow

ROBERT K. KERLAN, M.D.

Associate Clinical Professor, Orthopaedic Surgery, University of Southern California School of Medicine, Los Angeles, California; Attending Staff, Centinela Hospital Medical Center, Inglewood, California.

The Treatment of Common Throwing Injuries to the Shoulder

GEORGES EL KHOURY, M.D.

Professor of Radiology and Orthopaedic Surgery; Head, Skeletal Radiology Section; Professor of Radiology and Orthopaedic Surgery, University of Iowa School of Medicine, Iowa City, Iowa; Staff Radiologist and Head of Skeletal Radiology Section, University of Iowa Hospitals and Clinics, Iowa City, Iowa.

Shoulder Arthrotomography in the Evaluation of the Injured Throwing Arm

ROBERT E. LEACH, M.D.

Professor and Chairman, Department of Orthopedics, Boston University School of Medicine, Boston, Massachusetts; Member, Sports Medicine Council, U.S. Olympic Committee.

The Impingement Syndrome; Tennis Serving Compared with Baseball Pitching

FRANK C. McCUE, III, M.D.

Alfred R. Shands Professor of Orthopaedic Surgery and Plastic Surgery of the Hand; Director, Division of Sports Medicine and Hand Surgery; Team Physician, Department of Athletics, University of Virginia, Charlottesville, Virginia.

Throwing Injuries to the Shoulder

THOMAS M. McLAUGHLIN, PH.D.

President, Biomechanics, Inc., Atlanta, Georgia.

Strength/Power Training for Baseball Pitchers

WILLIAM D. McLEOD, PH.D.

Adjunct Instructor, Department of Orthopaedics, Tulane University School of Medicine, New Orleans, Louisiana.

The Pitching Mechanism

LYLE A. NORWOOD, M.D.

Assistant Clinical Professor, Orthopaedics, Tulane University, New Orleans, Louisiana; Staff Physician, Hughston Sports Medicine Hospital, Columbus, Georgia.

Posterior Shoulder Instability

FRANK A. PETTRONE, M.D.

Associate Clinical Professor of Orthopedics, Georgetown University Medical School, Washington, D.C.; Attending Orthopedist, Arlington Hospital, Arlington, Virginia.

Shoulder Problems in Swimmers

JAMES C. PUFFER, M.D.

Assistant Professor, Division of Family Medicine, Associate Team Physician, Department of Intercollegiate Athletics, UCLA School of Medicine, Center for the Health Sciences, Los Angeles, California; Physician, USA Water Polo Team.

Water Polo Injuries to the Upper Extremity

JOHN S. ROLLINS, M.D.

San Jose, California

Water Polo Injuries to the Upper Extremity

CARTER R. ROWE, M.D.

Associate Clinical Professor Emeritus of Orthopaedic Surgery, Harvard Medical School, Boston, Massachusetts; Senior Orthopaedic Surgeon, Massachusetts General Hospital, Boston, Massachusetts.

Anterior Subluxation of the Throwing Shoulder

JOHN SAIN

Pitching Coach, Atlanta Braves.

Proper Pitching Techniques

KENNETH M. SINGER, M.D.

Clinical Instructor of Surgery, Division of Orthopedic Surgery and Rehabilitation, School of Medicine, University of Oregon Health Science Center; Sacred Heart Hospital, Eugene, Oregon.

Radiographic Evaluation of the Throwing Elbow

MARCUS J. STEWART, M.D.

Clinical Professor of Orthopaedic Surgery, University of Tennessee Center for the Health Sciences, Memphis, Tennessee; Chief, Department of Orthopaedics, Veterans Administration Hospital, Memphis, Tennessee.

The Acromioclavicular Joint in the Throwing Arm

ROBERT L. THORNBERRY, M.D.

Private Practice of Orthopedics, Tallahassee Community and Tallahassee Memorial Hospital, Tallahassee, Florida.

Neurovascular Syndromes

HUGH S. TULLOS, M.D.

Professor and Chief, Division of Orthopedic Surgery, Baylor College of Medicine, Houston, Texas; Chief, Department of Orthopedic Surgery, The Methodist Hospital, Houston, Texas.

Functional Anatomy of the Elbow; Examination of the Throwing Elbow

ROBERT E. WELLS, M.D.

Clinical Associate Professor of Orthopaedic Surgery, Emory University School of Medicine, Atlanta, Georgia; Chairman, Department of Orthopaedic Surgery, Piedmont Hospital, Atlanta, Georgia.

Suprascapular Nerve Entrapment

JAMES O. WEST, Ed.D.

Associate Athletic Director, Former Baseball Coach, University of Virginia, Charlottesville, Virginia.

Throwing Injuries to the Shoulder

WILLIAM C. WHITING, Ph.D.

Research Associate, Department of Kinesiology, UCLA, Los Angeles, California.

Water Polo Injuries to the Upper Extremity

FRANKLIN D. WILSON, M.D.

Clinical Assistant Professor, Indiana University, Indianapolis, Indiana; Director, Sports Medicine, Indiana University Medical Center, Community Hospital, Indianapolis, Indiana.

Valgus Extension Overload in the Pitching Elbow

G. WILLIAM WOODS, M.D.

Assistant Professor of Orthopedic Surgery, Baylor College of Medicine, Houston, Texas.

Surgical Management of Acute and Chronic Elbow Problems

BERTRAM ZARINS, M.D.

Assistant Clinical Professor of Orthopaedic Surgery, Harvard University Medical School, Boston, Massachusetts; Chief, Sports Medicine Unit, Massachusetts General Hospital, Boston, Massachusetts; Team Physician, Boston Bruins Hockey Team and New England Patriots Football Team, Boston, Massachusetts; Chairman, Education Committee, United States Olympic Committee Sports Medicine Council.

Arthroscopy of the Shoulder: Technique

FOREWORD

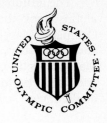

The United States Olympic Committee book *Injuries to the Throwing Arm* is an outgrowth of two sports medicine conferences of the same name held in Atlanta, Georgia, in February 1983 and in Tampa, Florida, in January 1984. The conferences were sponsored by the United States Olympic Committee Sports Medicine Council and the United States Baseball Federation. The speakers and the audience of these interdisciplinary meetings were composed of team physicians, orthopedic surgeons, athletic trainers, physical therapists, coaches, biomechanists, and athletes. *Injuries to the Throwing Arm* is a compilation of the material presented at these conferences, with chapters contributed by more than 30 authors. The editors believe this book represents the "state of the art" in knowledge of biomechanics, prevention, diagnosis, and treatment of common throwing injuries, conditioning programs, off-season training techniques, and rehabilitation of the injured athlete. Because of the interdisciplinary nature of this subject, certain sections of the book will be more or less applicable to the individual reader's needs.

Injuries to the Throwing Arm is divided into five sections:
1. The Thowing Motion
2. The Shoulder in the Throwing Athlete
3. The Elbow in the Throwing Athlete
4. Conditioning and Rehabilitation
5. The Throwing Motion in Other Sports

Although the past two decades have produced an explosion of scientific knowledge in medicine, progress in the management of injuries in throwing athletes has lagged behind. It is our hope that *Injuries to the Throwing Arm* will be a major contribution to this field of study and will become valuable to all who participate in the training, coaching, and medical care of the throwing athlete. It is only by a team effort and communication between players, coaches, trainers, biomechanists, and physicians that important advances can be made and the eventual goal of injury prevention will be reached.

The editors would like to acknowledge contributions to the production of this book that have been made by Barbara Cohen of W. B. Saunders Company, Mary Margaret Newsom of the United States Olympic Committee, and Claire Christiansen. They would also like to thank Joyce Carr of the Massachusetts General Hospital and Dale Baker of the Hughston Orthopaedic Clinic for organizational and technical assistance in producing the conferences.

BERTRAM ZARINS, M.D.
JAMES R. ANDREWS, M.D.
WILLIAM G. CARSON, JR., M.D.

INTRODUCTION

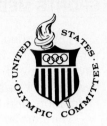

UNITED STATES OLYMPIC COMMITTEE

Injuries to the Throwing Arm, first as two major conferences of the USOC Sports Medicine Council and now as a major publication containing the substance of those conferences, reflects advantageously on the "new" United States Olympic Committee and its principal ingredients. The purpose of the conferences was to help bring quality medical attention to the needs of all of our nation's athletes. The sponsors of the conferences combined the interests and resources of the USOC and a national governing body (the generic term for the organizations approved to accept the responsibility for the development of the respective Olympic and Pan American sports). The persons who designed and administered the course (and prepared this book) were volunteers in the field who have expertise and were supported by USOC staff with expertise. The speakers (now authors) who created the conferences were state-of-the-art experts in their selected topics, who shared their knowledge as contributions for the cause.

The drafters of the Amateur Sports Act of 1978 had these achievements in mind when they successfully enabled the United States Olympic Committee to become a unifying force in the promotion both of amateur sport and of the health and satisfaction of the amateur athlete. It will only be through the organizational cooperation and altruistic professional alliances that we will keep the role of sport in perspective and the actions of sports experiences as beneficial as possible.

My congratulations are extended equally to the conference registrants who through their own pursuit of excellence furthered the goals of those who prepared the conferences and this book.

F. DON MILLER
Executive Director,
United States Olympic Committee, 1973–1985;
President, United States Olympic Foundation, 1985

SPORTS MEDICINE COUNCIL

The United States Olympic Committee Sports Medicine Council is proud to have worked with the United States Baseball Federation in the development of national conferences on *Injuries to the Throwing Arm*. In particular, I wish to thank Robert E. Smith, President of the Baseball Federation, and Richard W. Case, Executive Director, for their support.

The mutual goal is that these programs be organized and designed to make current concepts of prevention, treatment, and rehabilitation of injuries to the throwing arm available throughout the country. The conference series, however, presents only a beginning of the cooperative development and application of a comprehensive sports medicine program to benefit our nation's athletes.

It is worthwhile to recognize that the success of these conferences is further enhanced by the fact that they are being used as a model for the future expansion of sport medicine education for other governing bodies of the United States Olympic Committee.

On behalf of the President of the United States Olympic Committee, William E. Simon, and our Executive Director, Col. F. Don Miller, we thank Bertram Zarins, M.D., and all of the contributors who made the book *Injuries to the Throwing Arm* possible.

IRVING I. DARDIK, M.D., F.A.C.S.
Chairman, Sports Medicine Council

UNITED STATES BASEBALL FEDERATION

The United States Baseball Federation is pleased to have had the opportunity to team up with the United States Olympic Committee in the production of this sports medicine conference.

For some time we felt that the general public in America was confused somewhat by the relatively new field of sports medicine. We also believed that the general public held many misconceptions about the USOC and its sport-governing bodies, of which we are one.

Owing to baseball's popularity as both a participant and a spectator sport, we felt the conference would provide a bridge of interest and understanding between the world of sports medicine and the general public. A sports medicine seminar on *Injuries to the Throwing Arm* was planned to draw a wide variety of people and provide us with a forum to explain the nature of the USOC and the USBF, as well as the role of medicine in sports.

Our goal was to blend the knowledge of the orthopedic surgeons with the hands-on relationship coaches and trainers have with the athlete.

The sports medicine conference on *Injuries to the Throwing Arm* drew several hundred people and was successful enough to warrant a follow-up conference. Representatives of professional baseball have since approached us with interest in this type of seminar for their trainers and athletes. With a positive reaction from all sides, we feel our preliminary goals have been reached.

On the basis of this foundation of success, we look forward to other joint sports medicine conferences with the USOC and to future opportunities to teach and educate the public about sports medicine, the USOC, and the USBF through a common interest in baseball.

RICHARD W. CASE
Executive Director

CONTENTS

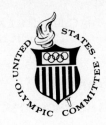

9

10

11

12

13

14

PART THREE

THE ELBOW IN THE THROWING ATHLETE

20

21

EXAMINATION OF THE THROWING ELBOW... 201
Hugh S. Tullos, M.D. / William Jay Bryan, M.D.

22

RADIOGRAPHIC EVALUATION OF THE THROWING ELBOW 211
Kenneth M. Singer, M.D.

23

ARTHROSCOPY OF THE ELBOW.. 221
William G. Carson, Jr., M.D. / James R. Andrews, M.D.

24

LITTLE LEAGUER'S ELBOW 228
Stephen C. Hunter, M.D.

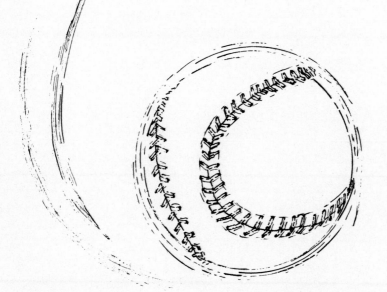

PART
ONE

THE
THROWING
MOTION

BODY MECHANICS

GIDEON ARIEL, Ph.D.

INTRODUCTION

In order to understand human motion, regardless of the task or sophistication of the action, the body must be perceived in its total complexity. The purpose of this chapter is to specify some of the different systems or mechanisms that should be considered in relation to the motion of the arm. Attention must be directed at multiple disciplines so that humans do not receive the same incorrect definitions as the blind men gave to the elephant.

The common denominator for all athletic activity is movement. There are three elementary requirements of movements. The first is muscle; the second, a signaling system that makes muscles contract in an orderly manner; and the third, the mechanical laws affecting all bodies on the Earth.

To begin with, not all muscles work in the same way. For example, the muscles of the human eye must operate with great speed and precision to quickly orient the eyeball and to focus on an object. The fine control needed in eye movement calls for a high *innervation ratio*. This is the ratio of the number of neurons with axons terminating on the outer membrane of muscle cells to the number of cells in the muscle. For the eye muscles, the innervation ratio is about one to three, which means that the axon terminals of a single motor neuron release their chemical transmitter to no more than three individual muscle cells.

In contrast to this high innervation ratio, the axon terminals of a single motor neuron for an arm muscle such as a biceps muscle may deliver their chemical transmitter to hundreds of muscle fibers. Therefore the muscle may have a low ratio of one to many hundreds. As a result, the output of the motor unit for an arm muscle is correspondingly coarse, particularly when compared with the fine precision needed in eye control.

Muscle motor units also differ in their susceptibility to fatigue.[1] At one extreme are *slow-twitch motor units*, which have great resistance to fatigue. Such units can remain active for long periods, but they generate relatively little muscle tension. At the opposite extreme are *fast-twitch motor units*, which can generate great peak muscle tension but fatigue rapidly.[2] Within a single human muscle the fibers of slow and fast motor units are intermixed.

In order to understand the importance of these contrasting motor unit properties to the organization of movement, how the motor units of a muscle are sequentially recruited in the course of a movement must be considered. In general, muscle tension is regulated in two ways. One is through control of the number of motor units recruited to act; the other is through control of the firing frequency of the recruited units. Slow-twitch units, which are resistant to fatigue and generate little tension, are the first to be recruited. The last motor units used are the fast-twitch units, which generate large peak tensions but are quickly fatigued.

Movement of the human body, then, is a series of separate and individual actions.[3] These actions begin with minute electrochemical processes that are incredibly fast yet extremely complicated. Human muscles are thin strands of fibers that can contract or relax because of these electrochemical reactions. The result is movement of the body with a fluidity that defies the capacity of even the sharpest eyes to distinguish the separate actions.

For instance, the simplest of human movements, such as crooking a finger or raising an eyebrow, involves complex neuromuscular happenings that cannot be duplicated by artificial means. The movements of the best manmade robot are still jerky when compared with the subtle flowing motions of a human.

BIOMECHANICS

Athletic performances consist of many and varied combinations of these chemical activities. The science that measures the resulting actions is *biomechanics*. The science of biomechanics consists, as its name suggests, of the *bio* and the *mechanics* parts. These two parts are coordinated by the mechanisms of neural control. Therefore, to properly evaluate the motion of the arm it becomes necessary to quantify the entire body and its coordinated link system.

The *biological component* of biomechanics is perhaps more properly placed within the section of biology known as physiology, which deals with the functioning of living organisms or their parts. The building frames of the human body are the bones, which are joined by connective tissues known as ligaments and tendons. Bones, however, have no power to move.

Like the frame of an automobile, bones provide the basic structure upon which the body rests. Muscles are comparable to the engine that supplies the power to move. It is the 600 muscles of the body that do the work. It is this relationship between levers, fulcrums, muscular power, and all of the inertial forces that are measured and quantified that constitutes the mechanical portion of biomechanics.

Muscles are made to contract by signals from the central nervous system. However, muscles do not respond unless they receive the appropriate stimulation, and they require a given signal every time they are expected to perform.[4] Muscular contraction causes the joint angles to change, in an isotonic movement, according to the coordination of the different amounts of tension produced in the individual fibers. Individual cadres of these muscles surround the various joints and control the segments so that the body's actions are like those of a mechanical link system moved by reciprocating engines. With this intricate arrangement of bones, muscles, and neural control all muscular activities take place.

In the 1700s Galvanni studied the movements of frog muscles and saw that they contracted when electrically stimulated. He deduced that electrical current must be involved in the normal muscle contraction process. While chemical-mechanical interaction operates muscles, an understanding of this biofeedback function that governs action requires an appreciation of *biocybernetics*, which is the study of control and communication.

THE CENTRAL NERVOUS SYSTEM

The central nervous system, originating in the brain, is a special activity center. Billions of cells engage in electrochemical operations that in conjunction with other body parts permit the individual to see, hear, reason, imagine, create, love, hate, move, and be aware of exactly which process he or she is involved in through the capacity to incorporate feedback into the operation.

The building block of the system is a specialized nerve cell known as a *neuron*. Bundles of neurons are organized into larger entities called *nerves*. These serve as gateways to speed a constant stream of information from the eyes, ears, nose, and other areas to the neurons of the brain, which evaluate the data in light of evolution and individual experience. Other kinds of nerves, with special cells known as *receptors*, monitor stimuli such as pain, cold, touch, pressure, and even blood and body chemistry. Another set of special neurons are known as *motor neurons*. Motor neurons within the brain and at the target sites control the movement of muscles and the secretions of glands. They not only trigger the chemicomechanical process of working muscles but also affect the action.[5]

For the body to regulate movement in athletic performance, it must "know" information about what it controls. In order to accomplish this, a servomechanism must be introduced. Many current concepts of the brain mechanisms of movement have evolved from the work of the British physiologist Sir Charles Sherrington. Early in the 20th century, Sherrington[6] investigated the function of the motor neuron in certain reflexive forms of motor activity. Sherrington's work led to today's concept of the "triggered movement" based on a "central program" involving a spinal rhythm generator.

Proprioceptors and Sensory Feedback

Many current investigations of the neurophysiology of locomotion are aimed at clarifying the interaction between what may be termed *central programs* from the brain and *sensory feedback* from outside the nervous system. Sherrington introduced the term *proprioception* to describe the organism's detection of stimuli by the receptors. Muscle proprioceptors are of two kinds. One kind senses elongation and the other, tension. The length receptors of muscles send fibers into the spinal cord to form synapses on motor neurons that terminate on the same muscles. Hence any increased length receptor activity that results from muscle elongation activates the motor neurons of the elongated muscle. This in turn gives rise to a muscular contraction that opposes elongation.

The tension receptors, the second kind of proprioceptor, sense force rather than elongation. Their activation leads to the inhibition of the associated motor neurons. Thus, when an increase in muscle tension activates these receptors their response acts on the associated motor neurons and gives rise to a reduction in force. Both the length receptors and the tension receptors therefore may be viewed as components of what an engineer would call a negative feedback control system. This particular system maintains its stability by resisting changes in muscle length and tension.

These control mechanisms in the muscles and tendons themselves are governed by higher level mechanisms in the brain.[7] In fact, the control of movement relies on hierarchical structure. The sensory information in the muscle itself processes local information and transmits net results to higher centers. Feedback enters the hierarchy at every level. At the lowest levels the feedback is unprocessed and hence fast-acting with a very short delay. At higher levels feedback data pass through more and more stages of an ascending sensory-processing organization. Feedback thus closes a real-time control loop at each level in the hierarchy. The lower level loops are simple and fast-acting. The higher level loops are more sophisticated and slower. The combination generates a lengthy sequence of behavior that is both goal-directed and appropriate to the environment.[8]

Such behavior appears to an external observer to be intentional or purposeful. The top-level input command is a goal or task, which is successively partitioned into subgoals or subtasks at each rung of the control organizational ladder until at the lowest level output signals drive the muscles and produce observable action. The success or failure of any particular task depends on whether or not the higher-level functions are capable of providing the correct information. This hierarchical control is necessary to direct the output to the lower level for successful performance in spite of perturbations and uncertainties in the environment.

Small perturbations can usually be corrected by low-level feedback loops. These involve relatively little sensory data processing and thus respond quickly. Larger disturbances, caused by changes in the environment, or perhaps related to performing a difficult activity, may overwhelm the lower-level feedback loops and require strategic changes at higher levels in order to maintain the system within the region of successful performance. Thus, a highly skilled and well-practiced performer such as a baseball pitcher or an archer can execute maneuvers with apparent ease.

Many such athletic activities seem to be performed with a minimum of physical and mental effort. These performances are often characterized as, "He moved effortlessly" or "She seemed to float without even thinking." What is really meant is that the athlete's lower-level corrections are so quick and precise that the performance does not deviate significantly from the ideal, and the system need not have access to higher-level loops for emergency changes in strategy.

On the other hand, a novice discus thrower may have great difficulty in even executing a successful performance. The beginner is continually forced to rely on higher-level intervention to prevent total failure. Even the slightest deviation from the planned or desired motion results in a poor throw. Because the responses are late and often misdirected, the performance is erractic and rarely resembles the ideal. However, practice allows the mistimed functions to synchronize into a more regular and, perhaps more importantly, a recognizable pattern. The system "learns" a movement pattern that becomes more and more precise with repetition. The degree and precision of these corrections and the method by which they are computed determine the rate of convergence of the learning process into an efficient and successful performance.

The control of muscular contraction in all activities, athletic or otherwise, is very sophisticated and elaborately programmed. One of the more skilled activities, the signing of one's name, serves as a good example. Whenever Mr. Smith signs his name it is consistent enough to be recognizable yet different enough so that no other person can accurately duplicate it. Even if Mr. Smith uses chalk and signs his name on a blackboard the signature appears the same, although he used different muscles than those normally employed in signing a check. In other words, the individuality remains.

Inherent in this complex handwriting movement and in all muscular activities there is a preprogrammed control mechanism. Optimal performance depends on the efficiency of the control and is little affected by the strength of the muscles or by the efficiency of the metabolism. Mounting evidence suggests that it is this neural control of the muscles in executing a skill rather than other, albeit necessary, factors that is most important.

Most people associate the brain primarily with the process of thinking. Yet research shows it to be first and foremost a control system. Thought is not the primary function of the brain; rather, it is an artifact that arises out of the complex computing mechanism required to generate and control extremely sophisticated behavior. Sometimes this ability to think causes inhibition in our control mechanism. This is obviously the case with athletes who fail to perform because of "mental" inhibition or what is commonly known on the athletic field as "choking"—in other words, "paralysis by analysis."

This control mechanism or biofeedback function in the body may be compared with the modern computer. However, within this greater system lies the single computer element in the brain, which is the cell. Each cell acts as a computer, and there are billions of them. The vast quantities of feedback information are analyzed and processed in innumerable computing centers that detect patterns, compare incoming data with stored expectations, and evaluate the results. One of the main differences between the brain and a computer is that the brain is capable of many computations in many different places simultaneously. The brain does not execute sequential programs of instructions as does a computer; rather, it executes many processes simultaneously.

These biofeedback functions are executed in two basic methods. In the first a signal is broken into many values, and these quantities can be added to other numbers. This is the way a computer adds signals. It is called *digital processing*. The other method is called *analog processing*, and the brain relies on this method for its fundamental computations. Analog computers perform operations by addition of continuous signal values. Each neuron in the brain is essentially an analog computer performing complex additions, integrations, differentiations, and nonlinear operations on input variables that can number from one to several hundred thousand.

The brain is a digital device only in that information is encoded for transmission from one neuron to another over long transmission lines, called *axons*, by pulse-frequency or pulse-phase modulation. When these pulse-encoded signals reach their destinations they are converted into analog voltages from the computations that take place in the dendrites and cell bodies of the receiving neurons.

The success of performance in a particular event, whether it is for explosive, endurance, or esthetic purposes, depends on the motor programming that initiates a proper biofeedback signal to the motor pool. Individual muscle fibers make a muscle contract and relax in an elaborate synchronization.[9] The arrangement permits them all to arrive at a peak of action simultaneously. But certain recruitment patterns characterize each event in a unique way. Synchronization of muscle firing is critical for optimizing many athletic performances. In the power events such as throwing the discus or in high jumping it is extremely important that the muscle actions be simultaneously activated to optimize the force. Lack of synchronization in the power events results in lesser force and poorer performance. On the other hand, in events of endurance such as long distance running or cross country skiing asynchronization is important, since fewer fibers are needed to maintain the action, thus permitting alternating fibers to rest. Some long distance runners may "overrecruit" muscle fibers and therefore fatigue sooner.[10] This emphasizes the importance of technique in achieving optimal performance. The question arises of how the brain adapts to the specific activity requirements. The answer lies in the great number of approximations that must form the correct signal.

The brain achieves its incredible precision and reliability through redundancy and statistical techniques. Many axons carry feedback and "feedforward" information concerning the value of the same variable, each encoded slightly differently. The statistical summation of these many imprecise and noisy information channels results in the reliable transmission of precise messages over long distances. In a similar way, a multiplicity of neurons may compute roughly the same input variables. Clusters of such computing devices provide statistical precision and reliability orders of magnitude greater than that achievable by any single neuron. The outputs of such clusters are transmitted and become inputs to other clusters, which perform additional analog computations.

CONTROL OF MUSCLE GROUPS

In addition to understanding the control of each fiber, attention must be given to groups of muscles. The muscles of all animals, including humans, usually come in pairs, one known as a *flexor* and the other as an *extensor*. When an arm bends at the elbow, one of the pairs of muscles contracts while the other relaxes. A motor neuron transmission initiates the contraction, while a lack of a motor neuron transmission to the other member of the pair allows the fibers of the muscle to remain in a relaxed state.

The importance of the motor control is not in the contraction of individual muscles but in the coordinated contraction and relaxation of many muscles. In making a fist or grasping an object, for example, a person cannot merely flex the fingers by contracting the flexor muscles in the forearm. The extensor muscles in the forearm must also be contracted to keep the finger's flexor muscles from flexing the wrist.

All of this complex motor control requires the participation of millions of neurons throughout the central nervous system. Consider the incredible job of the brain in the simple act of breathing, which demands the precise coordination of no less than 90 muscles. The work that must be done for something as complex as eye movement requires interaction between neurons concerned with optic muscles, sensors, and comprehension.

The fineness of control depends on the number of motor nerve units per muscle fiber. The more neurons there are, the finer is the ability to maneuver, as in the case of the muscles that operate the eye. When fewer motor nerve units are involved, the action becomes less refined.

Fast-Twitch and Slow-Twitch Fibers

Another important factor that must be controlled is the amount of tension in a muscle, which varies according to the length of the muscle.[11] The speed with which the muscle is brought into play is also an important factor. Slower movements, for instance, allow greater force development than do fast motions. Scientists have also discovered that muscle fibers can be classified as either slow-twitch or fast-twitch. However, additional data from the field of histology reveal subdivisions and a whole spectrum of fiber characteristics. Whether the individual is equipped with a preponderance of slow- or fast-twitch fibers or a more equal balance of both appears to be largely a matter of genetics. Further research is necessary to determine the degree of importance of fiber type in performance.

For example, biopsies of the tissue of world-class athlete indicate that those who excel in endurance events have a preponderance of slow-twitch fibers.[12] Perhaps 80 per cent of the muscles that are employed in their events are so characterized.

Sprinters, on the other hand, appear to have an extremely high proportion of fast-twitch fibers. Distance runners thrive on slow-twitch fibers, which by contracting more slowly consume less energy and do not fatigue as readily. The fast-twitch fibers enable the sprinter to move the legs more rapidly, although a price is paid in burning up anaerobic energy sources. For short distances, the sprinter's extravagance with energy supplies does not matter.

In recent years, however, it has become apparent that there is a considerable diversity in the structure, biochemistry, and physiology of striated muscle fibers. Most mammalian muscles are made up of different types of muscle fibers. Some of these contract fast and others rapidly. The function of the fast-contracting fiber was perhaps obvious, but it was more difficult to appreciate why muscles should have slow-contracting fibers.

It seems likely, however, that these slow-contracting fibers may be more efficient or more effective in certain functions. In general slow-twitch muscles are more economical than fast-twitch muscles in developing sustained (isometric) tension. Therefore, it would be expected that slow-twitch fibers be involved in maintaining posture and in movements that involve sustained tension.

When more rapid movements are required, it is necessary to use fast-contracting fibers because the slow-contracting fibers are not mechanically effective at higher shortening velocities. They become inefficient once their optimal rate of shortening has been exceeded.

Accordingly, it is not surprising to find that many muscles contain more than one type of fiber. In other words, muscles may possess a two- or three-geared system. This enables the muscles to contract efficiently over a wide range of shortening velocities by progressively recruiting different fiber populations. Although it would appear that shot-putters and high jumpers would have predominantly fast-twitch muscles, they are usually characterized by a more or less even distribution of fiber types. Investigations into slow- and fast-twitch fibers continue. One thing that seems certain is that proper training can improve the function of both types of muscle fiber.[13]

Factors Affecting Contraction

Within all muscles, regardless of type, three major factors are associated with contraction. The first involves the chemical reaction that utilizes adenosine triphosphate (ATP), and the second relates to the force and the velocity of the muscular contraction.[14, 15] The third factor is elasticity, which is the muscle's capacity to recover energy absorbed in the tissue. This elastic quality is one of the main characteristics differentiating the super-athlete from the average participant.

There is a relationship between the force with which a muscle can contract and its velocity.[16, 17] A muscle shortens more rapidly when it is working against lighter weights. This means that there is a damping element in the muscle, which could be compared with a shock absorber. Since this phenomenon was first discovered, it has been suggested that there is something like a mechanical absorber actually present in the muscle. Although research continues, it is currently thought that this damping effect is the property of the force-generating mechanism itself or, more specifically, of the interaction of the actin and myosin protein elements of muscle.[18]

Tendons also have a certain amount of inherent elasticity that contributes further to muscle action. They can act like coil springs, compressing or stretching under force, then snapping back to their original length. Thus, muscles function not only as work performers but also as a suspension system for the body to provide a "smoother ride."[19] For example, a ballet dancer moves with a smoothness no machine can match and a coordination and organization that no computer-driven robot can produce.

Thus, the body is controlled and coordinated by the many mechanisms existing within the cells and under the guidance of the nervous system. Yet with all its complexities and sophistication the human body must still conform to the laws of mechanics described in equation form in the 17th century by Sir Isaac Newton.

LAWS OF MOTION

Mechanical science started with the scholars of ancient Greece, who attempted an understanding of the universe. One of the earliest phenomena that made the Greeks curious was motion. The interaction between a human and the environment is possible only through motion. The first Greek who attempted to quantify the principle of motion was Aristotle. He maintained that each element on Earth had its own characteristics and therefore behaved uniquely according to those features.

The Aristotelian views of motion were accepted for a long time but were later disproved. One of the fallacies of the Aristotelian view was the absence of gravitational effects. According to the ancient approach, if a tennis ball were thrown into the air the air itself would make movement possible, and in the absence of air there would be no movement. It was further believed that different masses would not have the same forces, which of course was later disproved.

The Italian scientist Galileo found experimentally that the Aristotelian view was invalid. Galileo formulated the bases of movement of free-falling bodies. By rolling different masses of balls across an inclined board, he found that balls of different weights rolled down the same inclined plane at the same rate. When the plane was tipped more steeply the balls rolled more rapidly, but all of the balls increased their rates similarly and moved the same distances in the same time.

This means that freely falling bodies move through equal distances in equal times regardless of weight. The explanation of the experiment with falling masses lies in an understanding of acceleration. As discovered by Galileo, the distance traversed by a body rolling down an inclined plane grows progressively greater in successive equal time intervals. This means that the rate of speed is changing. The change in the rate of speed, or more correctly the velocity, is acceleration. For the falling masses, in each second the velocity of the mass increases by the same amount for this particular time interval. On Earth, a body falls at a constant acceleration of 32 feet per second per second.

It was this understanding of acceleration that facilitated Sir Isaac Newton to formulate the *laws of motion*. These laws directly relate to acceleration according to the Newtonian law, which is that the acceleration produced by a particular force acting on a body is directly proportional to the magnitude of the force and inversely proportional to the mass of the body.

The importance of discussing acceleration and forces lies in the fact that movement must begin with force. It is impossible to begin movement without applying force, whether it is an external force, such as gravity, or an internal force, such as muscular contractions. For example, the force applied to a hockey puck on the ice creates an acceleration and moves the puck faster and faster as long as the force is applied. How long that force is applied is therefore important.

In mechanics the product of force and time is called *impulse*. For a given mass, a given impulse results in a particular velocity. The heavier the object, the greater is the impulse needed to achieve the same velocity. It is obvious, therefore, that velocity and mass are related, and in fact the product of mass and velocity is referred to as *momentum*.

The *law of momentum* is extremely important in contact sports in which different masses collide at different velocities. For instance, the principles of this law allow a smaller football player with greater velocity to block a heavier slower player.

In the case of the hockey puck, the puck that possesses a certain mass and is speeding across the ice at a given velocity has momentum equal to its mass times its velocity. If the puck happened to collide with another puck of equal mass moving at the same velocity but traveling in the opposite direction the two pucks would come to an abrupt stop. In other words, the momentum of one puck would be canceled by that of the other. This concept is the *principle of conservation of momentum* and creates much of the enjoyment and challenge of billiards with its interplay of solid balls striking each other at different velocities.

So far only linear movements, with all actions occurring in the same plane, have been considered. In the human body, however, the parts move in rotational fashion primarily because of the anatomic relationship and structure of the bones and joints. Without this rotational motion human actions would resemble those depicted by ancient Egyptian art forms, which portrayed only two dimensions.

Rotational motion can be visualized easily in terms of a wheel with a hub in the center and with spokes connecting it to an outer rim. The hub remains stationary while the parts move about it. Rotational movement requires an understanding of *torque*. A force producing rotational movement is called a torque or *moment of force*. The amount of torque depends on the force and the distance from the center of the rotational object. The product of force and distance is equal to the torque.[20]

The principle of momentum applied to linear movement also applies to rotational motions, and the conservation of angular momentum is one of the most important principles in athletics. Angular momentum is a function of the mass and the rotational acceleration as well as the square of the distance from the center of rotation.

Angular momentum can be expressed in terms of two other important parameters of rotation—*angular velocity* and *moment of inertia*. Angular velocity is represented by the body's rotational speed and direction. For example, if a diver performs a forward double somersault in one second, the magnitude of his average angular velocity is two revolutions per second.

The moment of inertia of a body about an axis represents the body's tendency to resist changes in angular velocity about that axis. It is obvious that massive and extended bodies have a larger moment of inertia than do lighter and smaller ones. In fact, the contribution of each particle or segment in a body to the total moment of inertia about an axis is equal to the mass of the segment times the square of its distance from the axis of rotation. For example, a typical male diver performing a dive that requires his body to be straight with his arms at his sides has a moment of inertia of 14 kg times meters squared about his somersaulting axis. However, in the same dive the moment of inertia about his twisting axis is only 1 kg times meters squared.

Angular momentum is the product of the angular velocity and the moment of inertia about a specific axis. In the example of the diver the angular momentum is the sum of angular velocities around the two axes and the moment of inertia around these axes.

ATHLETIC APPLICATIONS

The shot-put provides a practical application of these concepts. For many years coaches have debated shot-put techniques and argued whether the rotational method is superior to the linear style. In terms of mechanics the rotational technique allows the development of more angular momentum and angular speed. Since the release velocity of the shot is the most important critical factor in achieving maximal distance, the rotational technique provides greater mechanical advantages.

It is this interplay of mechanics and biological systems, including the essential central programming, that biomechanics seeks to quantify. While the basic tenets of mechanics cannot be violated, the variations in competitors's sizes, shapes, strengths, and levels of skill necessitate quantification in order to optimize performance. The combination of biomechanics and computer science enables the scientists, coaches, and athletes to study motions.

Cinematographic analysis provides the simplest form of quantification.[21] This method relies on film from high-speed cameras to record the motion from at least two views simultaneously. The desired joint centers can be traced from each of the camera views, and their recordings can be stored in a computer and processed. Information secured includes displacements, velocities, and accelerations in each of the three planes—x-, y-, and z—as well as the resultants.

Thus, biomechanical analysis provides specific quantification about the individual's actions with subsequent opportunities for improvement. In addition, alternatives can be calculated on the computer until the best strategy for a particular athlete is determined. Only then does the individual actually begin performance modifications.[22]

For example, in the 1976 Olympic games in Montreal it was possible, assuming the ability to generate an equal amount of force, to predict the height that a jumper could attain if he or she changed from the roll style to the flop technique. It was determined from the biomechanical analyses performed that the flop allows a more efficient use of forces for athletes who do not possess extremely powerful legs.

It is important to remember that because of both gross and subtle variations in the neuromuscular system of each human the biomechanical actions of individuals are as unique as fingerprints or a signature. In fact, whether the athlete actually is aware of this or not, he or she is actually trying to establish a pattern of motion that is every bit as precise and reproducible as that person's signature.

As described previously, each individual has a very specific pattern for signing the name. Because this is such a common event, little thought is given to the uniqueness and inherent neurologic requirements involved. For years forgers have attempted to duplicate the appearance of another individual's name. Yet they are ultimately unsuccessful, since they cannot duplicate the neural "program." If a bank or credit institution were to have each of its new customers sign his or her signature into the computer by using special equipment to record the force patterns, it would be impossible for anyone else to duplicate the person's signature. The information in the computer would contain not only the shapes of the letters but the amount of force the individual applied to each loop, line, and curve. With this system, for example, a customer in a store need only sign the receipt on a small force plate or use a pen with a built-in force transducer linked directly to the computer bank. The patterns of force could be compared instantly, and if they were different the discrepancy would be known immediately.

Detection of variations or inconsistencies in human movement has always been one of the most difficult problems facing coaches, trainers, and athletes. If the detection of error is inaccurate or nonspecific, the quality of correction is poor. Failure to recognize the causes of error stems from an inadequate understanding of the forces or from the inability to quantify the actions, or from both. Increasingly, technology is providing newer and better devices for such quantification. The principal factor that must be included regardless of the degree of sophistication of measurement is that the entire body must be incorporated in the analysis even if only the hand is thought to be important. Forces are produced by the whole body with the various links in the system generating patterns of acceleration and deceleration. It is this total integrated involvement that determines whether a boxer knocks out an opponent or a golfer hits a 200-yard drive.

It is inappropriate to analyze only the arm in either of these two examples if the question is how to optimize performance. To perform correctly, it is important to sum the forces exerted on the various joints. This principle is called the *summation of joint forces*. For example, in swinging a golf club the amount of force exerted by the club on the ball depends on how much of the forces summed by the body actually reaches the club.

Additionally, if there is any loss of force owing to poorly timed segments the golf club head will not move at the optimal velocity at the moment of impact. This fact illustrates another important biomechanical principle, which is the *continuity of joint forces*. The coordination of the forces of the leg and trunk segments significantly affects the force impacting the ball. The motion must begin in the first—in this case the larger—segments of the leg and continue through the link system of the trunk and arms. There must be no pause in the flow of motion from the legs to the trunk, to the arms, and finally to the club. A violation of this principle not only results in a smaller force at impact, but also the bad timing generates what the golfer would describe as a "bad feel."

Because club speed is determined by the force applied and the length of time of this force application, the best combination of force application should be determined. In other words, it must be determined which is more effective, a large force in a short time or a small force in a longer time. There is an optimal combination for each activity. The size of the force multiplied by its time of application is called impulse, and it is actually this force-time combination that produces the golf club velocity. The same is true for any ballistic movement such as throwing a football, a shot, or a javelin or as in long jumping. Although compromises in the size of force and duration of application often have to be made in order to achieve the optimal relationship, one such combination to be avoided is a small force applied for a short time.

The size of the force an athlete can produce is determined by the ability to comply with the principles of summation and continuity of joint forces. In the absence of measuring devices, assessing whether the time of force application is as great as possible presents yet another problem. In general, if each joint has gone through a complete range of motion it can be assumed that the maximal time available has been used. However, not only must the range of motion of the joint be complete, but the joint must straighten rapidly and the combined joint motion must be continuous. The concept of the importance of the combined effect of force and duration of application in producing speed changes is called the *principle of impulse*. Violation of this principle causes further errors in performance.

Direction of force application is another important principle. It is not only the direction of the application of force from the body to the golf club that is critical; this force also must be correctly transferred from the club head to the ball. In an optimal situation the force is exactly 90 degrees to the club, and the club head hits the ball exactly at its center.

A final principle is the *summation of body segment speeds*. Especially in throwing, kicking, and striking events, it is important to obtain as great a hand, foot, racket head, or club head speed as possible at the instant of impact or release. The speed of the last segment in the chain, such as the hand, the club, or the javelin, is the total produced by adding the individual speeds of all of the preceding segments with the appropriate timing. Disregarding potentially important segments or using them submaximally results in less skilled performance. This concept is similar to the summation of joint forces and is closely related to it.

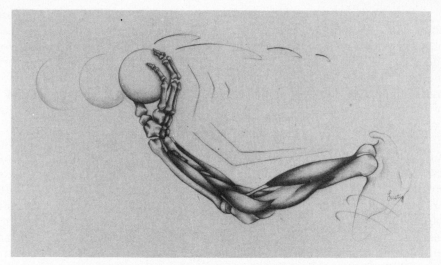

FIGURE 1–1. Anatomic dynamics of the throwing motion.

Javelin Throw, Shot-Put, and Hammer Throw

Examination of three throwing events—javelin throwing, shot-put, and hammer throwing—provides examples of many of these concepts. Perhaps the most important factor to bear in mind is that in trying to optimize or quantify performance the mechanical analysis of movement of an arm must include the entire body. The empirical results presented here reinforce this precept. (See Fig. 1–1.)

Initially, attention focused on the javelin throw. Although the United States (U.S.) may be a land of baseball pitchers and football quarterbacks, smaller countries like Finland and Hungary, which are normally associated with kicking sports, excel in javelin throwing. Biomechanical analyses[23, 24] of a group of U.S. throwers and the six finalists in the 1976 Montreal Olympics were performed in an effort to determine the differences between the more successful Olympic athletes and the U.S. throwers.

Results revealed two opposite styles of throwing that generally employed either (1) runs with a large sideways body twist or (2) straight-ahead runs with limited body rotation. The U.S. athletes employed an approach that kept the sagittal plane of the body perpendicular to the plane of the throw and approached the release with as high an initial running velocity as could be attained. On the other hand, the Olympic athletes showed more rotational torque in their throws. The rotational technique restricted the running velocity prior to release but generated a greater twisting torque of the body immediately prior to release. The rapid and more severe twisting of the trunk by the Olympic throwers produced higher velocities of the throwing hand during release of the javelin and thus longer throws.

A second difference between the six Olympic finalists and the less successful U.S. athletes concerned the hip-shoulder orientation. The U.S. athletes tended to keep their hips in line with their shoulders and ran down the runway with a forward or straight-line motion. This body posture allowed them to run faster and also to decelerate their centers of gravity more efficiently. However, it also served to inhibit both the rotational effect of the trunk twist and the coordination of the lower body-hip system with the upper body.

The Olympic athletes twisted the trunk with the shoulders 90 degrees and the hips 45 degrees out of the plane of the throw. This position prevented maximal speed in the run but allowed significantly greater rotational effects. These throwers demonstrated smooth patterns of acceleration-deceleration beginning with the legs and moving sequentially to the hip, to the shoulder, and then to the arm segments in a twisting or corkscrew fashion. The U.S. throwers, who had not placed their bodies in such an orientation, were not able to utilize their legs or trunk segments as effectively and executed shorter throws.

A second study[25, 26] was conducted to determine the differences in shot-put techniques between the Eastern European throwers, who now dominate this event, and their less successful competitors. Again, comparisons were made between the six finalists in the Montreal Olympic games with some U.S. throwers.

The biomechanical analysis revealed that the most important factor in the shot-put was the velocity of the shot at release. This factor was more important than either the height or the angle of release. Although some attention must also be given to the release angle, the primary goal of the the thrower should be to generate the greatest ball velocity at the point of release. Other factors being approximately equal, the faster the ball is at the release the longer will be the throw. In order to generate this maximal velocity at the release there must be a summation of forces from the various phases of the throw and the various segments.

The movement pattern of the shot-put using the straight-line style can be partitioned into five phases. The first is the starting phase when the athlete accelerates his body and the shot. The rear foot leaves the ground at the end of this phase. The second phase is the glide when the athlete is in the air for a brief amount of time, after which the rear foot again contacts the ground. It is important during this airborne phase for the rear leg to actively and rapidly bring the foot under the body. The third phase is a transitional phase when the rear foot touches the ground at the beginning and the front foot contacts the ground at the end of the phase. In this phase the athlete should minimize the deceleration of the center of gravity and allow transfer of energy to the push-off phase. The fourth phase, the push-off, is the most important. In this phase the front foot touches the ground initially, and the shot leaves the hand at the end of the phase. During the push-off phase the body exerts maximal acceleration of the shot toward the release.

It is this relationship between the transitional and the push-off phases that separates the 50- from the 70-foot throwers. In order to produce maximal velocities at the release it is necessary to achieve specific coordination during all of the previous phases of the throw. Too rapid a start can be as detrimental to producing an optimal final velocity as too slow an initial one. Examination of the acceleration curves of the various throwers revealed that the Olympic finalists exhibited highly symmetric curves, with peak acceleration occurring shortly before release. The shorter throws by the U.S. athletes were found to have maximal acceleration during the beginning phase, followed by a reduction in acceleration during the middle phases, and large acceleration again in the stance phase. In other words, rather than starting with lower acceleration values that increased during each successive phase, reaching a peak at release, these throwers demonstrated an oscillating pattern. They produced large accelerations too early during the throwing motion and were unable to sustain them.

In addition, the Olympic throwers maintained their centers of gravity at approximately the same height throughout the glide, transition, and into the beginning of the push-off phase. The U.S. throwers elevated the center of gravity continuously during all phases of the throw. This deficiency caused them to "open up" before the push-off phase and therefore to lose power in this most important portion of the throw.

Another important factor in successful shot-put performance is that the gliding phase should require as little time as possible. In this phase the athlete cannot accelerate his body, since he is in the air and has nothing to push against. The best throwers minimized the time of the gliding phase and shifted immediately into the transitional phase, which was also of relatively short duration. Conversely, the U.S. throwers remained in the air too long during the glide phase and therefore lost horizontal velocity.

Examination of the velocity of the horizontal component of the center of gravity clearly revealed that the gold and silver medal winners produced higher velocities and subsequently more rapid deceleration of the center of gravity. This stopping action of the heavier body segments transferred momentum to the throwing arm and the shot to cause them to move faster.

The third throwing event for consideration is the hammer throw. As before, comparisons were made between the six finalists in the Olympic games of 1976 and the best U.S. throwers.[27] The U.S. athletes produced shorter throws, which resulted from relatively low velocities during the turns and low linear velocities of the hammer during the delivery. In contrast, the three medal winners demonstrated initially lower speeds but continually increased their speeds throughout the turns to reach maximal acceleration at release.

A second important factor was the ground contact time. The best athletes utilized a two-footed or double support phase. The longer both feet are on the ground, the longer the force can be applied to accelerate the turning body. In addition, the foot placement was adjusted so that the right foot was planted slightly behind the left foot during each turn, which effectively enhanced the ability to extend the double support phase and imparted early and continued acceleration to the hammer. The U.S. throwers were in the air for longer periods, during which they were unable to exert as much force or to generate or sustain adequate shot acceleration.

A third critical component concerned the athlete's center of gravity. A continuous movement of the center of gravity in the direction of the throw was found to be an extremely significant factor in the longest performances. If the body-hammer system moved forward early in the throwing sequence, it ultimately reached a higher horizontal velocity, which resulted in greater transference of momentum to the hammer during the deceleration phase immediately prior to release. However, it was found that maintenance of a positive horizontal center of gravity displacement throughout the turn was of even greater importance. A positive displacement means that the contact foot is between the body's center of gravity and the hammer. In this relative position the athlete can effectively push with the foot to accelerate the hammer. With a negative displacement, the body's center of gravity is between the foot and the hammer. In this position the athlete cannot push against the foot and therefore is unable to pull on the hammer handle to accelerate it.

In addition, the gold medalist demonstrated a low vertical component of his center of gravity. This was the result of deep leg flexion and a forward trunk lean. In this posture the legs were in an advantageous position for horizontal thrust across the throwing circle. The forward lean also caused a reduction in the vertical component of the trunk segment. Owing to a shortened resistance arm a given amount of torque exerted by the lower back and hip muscle on the trunk resulted in a relatively high horizontal force against the hammer handle and thus helped to produce the longest throw.

To assist in conceptualizing the advantage of a proper body center of gravity displacement, the reader may imagine trying to open a closed door that has become stuck. Pulling on the handle of a hammer to accelerate it is similar to pulling on the doorknob to try to open the door. If the person leans forward with the feet behind, he cannot pull back on the doorknob because he has nothing to pull against. In order to have something to pull against, the feet must be placed between the body and the doorknob so that the person can push against the feet in order to pull on the doorknob. If the legs are kept straight as the person leans back he can pull only his body weight. If the legs are bent first the person can push with the leg muscles as he tries to straighten them, producing a force greater than his body weight. Another important consideration is that a person can apply the most force to the doorknob by pulling straight out, rather than at an angle. This means that the body must be lowered so that the arms are parallel to the ground. In other words, greater biomechanical efficiency can enhance opening doors as well as throwing the hammer.

In summary, the human body and the various implements that are used must follow basic scientific precepts. The internal physiologic conditions for optimal health and well-being are no less important than the programming of the central nervous system for skill development. Considerable attention must be given to the mechanical components associated with performance if techniques are to be enhanced or athletic performances maximized. When examining the last element in the system—such as the hand or arm—consideration must be given to the entire interrelated system.

REFERENCES

1. Thorstensson, A. G., Grimby, G., and Karlson, J.: Force-velocity relations and fiber composition in human knee extensor muscles. J Appl Physiol 40:12, 1976.
2. Thorstensson, A., Sjodin, B., and Karlson, J.: Enzyme activities and muscle strength after sprint training in man. Acta Physiol Scand 94:313, 1975.
3. Rosentsweig, J., and Ilinson, M. M.: Comparison of isometric, isotonic, and isokinetic exercises by electromyography. Arch Phys Med Rehabil 53:249, 1972.
4. Arbib, M. A.: The Metaphorical Brain. New York., Wiley-Interscience, 1972.
5. Edgerton, V. R.: Neuromuscular adaptation to power and endurance work. Can J Appl Sport Sci 1:49, 1976.
6. Rodgers, K. L., and Berger, R. A.: Motor-unit involvement and tension during maximum voluntary concentric, eccentric and isometric contractions of the elbow flexors. Med Sci Sports Exercise 6:253, 1979.
7. Barnes, W. S.: The relationship of motor-unit activation to isokinetic muscular contraction at different contractile velocities. Phys Ther 60:1152, 1980.
8. Clark, D., and Henry, F.: Neuromuscular specificity and increased speed from strength development. Res Q 32:315, 1961.
9. Hellebrandt, F., and Houtz, S.: Mechanism of muscle training in man: Experimental demonstration of overload principle. Physiol Ther Rev 36:371, 1956.
10. Wilkie, D.: Muscle. New York., St. Martin's Press, 1968.
11. Perrine, J. J., and Edgerton, V. R.: Muscle force-velocity and power-velocity relationships under isokinetic loading. Med Sci Sports Exercise 10:159, 1978.
12. Wilmore, J. H., Parr, R. B., and Girandola, R. N., et al.: Physiological alterations consequent to circuit weight training. Med Sci Sports Exercise 10:79, 1978.
13. Barnard, R. J., Edgerton, V. R., and Peter, J. B.: Effect of exercise on skeletal muscle. Biochemical and histological properties. J Appl Physiol 28:762, 1970.
14. Clark, D.: Adaptation in strength and muscular endurance. In Wilmore, J. H. (ed.). Exercise and Sport Science Reviews. New York, Academic Press, 1973.
15. Gettman, L. R., Culter, L. A., and Strathman, T.: Physiologic changes after 20 weeks of isotonic vs. isokinetic circuit training. J Sports Med Phys Fitness 1980.
16. Larson, L., Grimby, G., and Karlsson, J.: Muscle strength and speed of movement in relation to age and muscle morphology. J Appl Physiol 46:451, 1979.
17. Moffroid, M. R., and Whipple, R.: Specificity of speed of exercise. Phys Ther 50:1692, 1970.
18. Wilkie, D.: The relation between force and velocity in human muscle. J Physiol 110:249, 1950.
19. Perrine, J. J.: Isokinetic exercise and the mechanical energy potential of muscles, J Health Phys Ed Recreat 39:40, 1968.
20. Scudder, G. N.: Torque curves produced at the knee isometric and isokinetic exercise. Arch Phys Med Rehabil 61:68, 1980.
21. Ariel, G. B.: Computerized biomechanical analysis of human performance. Mechanics Sport 4:267, 1973.
22. Pekka, L., and Komi, P. V.: Segmental contribution to forces in vertical jump. Eur J Appl Physiol 34:181, 1978.
23. Ariel, G. B.: Computerized biomechanical analysis of throwers at the 1975 Olympic javelin camp. Track Field Q Rev 76:45, 1976.
24. Ariel, G. B.: Biomechanical analysis of the javelin throw. Track Field Q Rev 80:9, 1980.
25. Ariel, G. B.: Computerized biomechanical analysis of track and field athletics utilized by the Olympic training camp for throwing events. Track Field Q Rev 72:99, 1972.
26. Ariel, G. B.: Biomechanical analysis of shotputting. Track Field Q Rev 79:27, 1980.
27. Ariel, G. B.: Biomechanical analysis of the hammer throw. Track Field Q Rev 80:41, 1980.

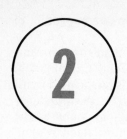

THE PITCHING
MECHANISM

WILLIAM D. McLEOD, Ph.D.

INTRODUCTION

The pitching motion can produce significant injuries to the throwing arm.[1–7] It has been difficult to determine the exact mechanism within the pitching act that produces the various injuries to the throwing athlete's arm. However, with the development of newer diagnostic techniques such as shoulder arthroscopy[8–11] common patterns of injury are becoming more evident. Because the pitching act is a dynamic process involving multiple muscle groups and interaction of tendons, muscles, and bones, it has been quite difficult to study the pitching mechanism. However, attempts have been made to measure the energies and forces developed during the pitching act to identify the segments of this motion that stress the arm the most and that could possibly cause injury.[12]

The joints of the upper extremity that are most prone to injury during the throwing act are the elbow and the shoulder. The common patterns of force overload to the throwing athlete's elbow include tension overload of the medial aspect and compression overload of the lateral aspect of the elbow.[6] Common injuries to the medial aspect of the elbow include overuse musculotendinous stress syndromes and even avulsion fractures of the medial epicondyle.[13] Laterally compression forces can cause significant damage to the capitellum and even to the radial head.[2] A third common pattern that is often seen is caused by extension forces about the elbow. The repetitive forces of throwing can cause limited extension of the elbow joint as a result of prominences and osteophytes of the olecranon process.[7, 12]

Commonly seen pathology about the throwing shoulder includes partial tears of the rotator cuff, tearing of the anterior and superior areas of the glenoid labrum,[14] and tearing of the biceps tendon-labrum complex. The advent of arthroscopy of the shoulder has brought attention to these new patterns of tearing of the glenoid labrum that have traditionally been described as occurring in association with instability of the shoulder[15] or as degenerative lesions in the older population.[13]

This chapter describes the pitching mechanism and evaluates the various aspects of the throwing act as they relate to injuries sustained by the elbow and shoulder.

THE PITCHING MECHANISM

The pitching mechanism can be divided into five phases:

1. Wind-up
2. Cocking
3. Acceleration
4. Release and deceleration
5. Follow-through

1. Wind-up

The wind-up phase is a relatively slow motion phase that prepares the pitcher for the correct body posture and balance to lead into the cocking phase. It starts with both feet planted on the ground and the shoulder shifted away from the direction of the pitch. During the wind-up the opposite leg becomes cocked generally quite high, and the ball is just removed from the glove. The acceleration and deceleration forces during this phase are quite minimal, since this is primarily a balance and preparatory phase (Fig. 2–1).

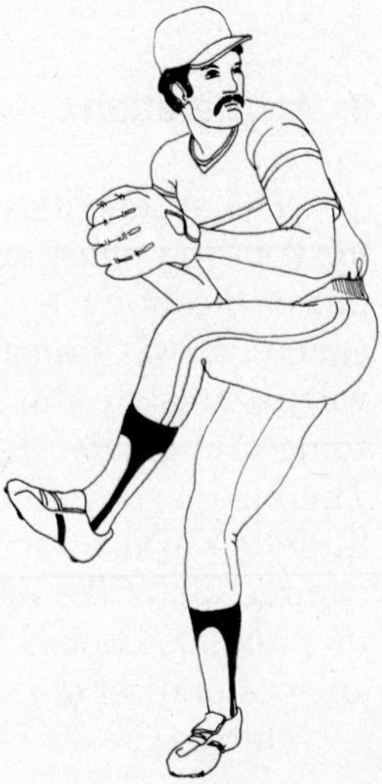

FIGURE 2–1. Wind-up.

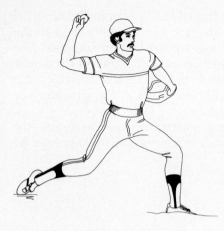

FIGURE 2–2. Cocking.

2. Cocking

This phase is aptly named, because it is a phase that applies maximal tension to all the muscles that will be used in accelerating the ball during the subsequent acceleration phase. The contralateral leg is kicked forward and planted directly in front of the body, the pelvis is internally rotated, and the chest is thrust forward. The shoulder is abducted 90 degrees and the humerus is externally rotated approximately 160 degrees. The anterior capsule of the shoulder is taut, and traction stress is placed on the anterior capsule and the internal rotators of the shoulder. The elbow is flexed approximately 90 degrees and is dynamically cocked by both the flexors and the extensors of the elbow. The ball is not effectively moved forward at all during this phase. The shoulder and chest advance forward to develop extrinsic loading to the pitching arm through a smooth well controlled process (Fig. 2–2).

3. Acceleration

The acceleration phase begins with deceleration of the forward movement of the chest and shoulder and ends just prior to ball release. In this phase the body is brought forward with the arm following behind. The energy that is transferred whips the arm forward and creates tremendous valgus stress to the elbow joint. The ball must be accelerated from zero to somewhat greater than 80 miles per hour in approximately 80 milliseconds. The energy developed by the body moving forward is transferred to the throwing arm to accelerate the humerus. This energy is enhanced by the contraction of the internal rotators as the humerus is internally rotated from its previous cocked position of 160 degrees of external rotation and effects an acceleration of the ball to delivery speed.

During the acceleration phase some deceleration forces are used to stop

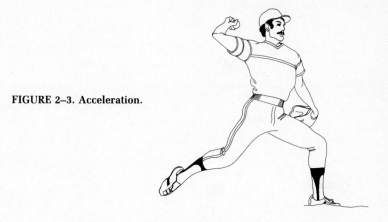

FIGURE 2–3. Acceleration.

the horizontal adduction movement of the humerus as the elbow is brought closer to the pitcher's side. These forces are applied by the three posterior rotator cuff muscles (supraspinatus, infraspinatus, and teres minor). This specific action is generally well controlled but can impose very strong forces of short duration.

During acceleration of the forearm an extension force is placed on the elbow joint. This tendency to extension is resisted by the elbow flexors, primarily the brachialis and biceps muscles. Just before the end of the acceleration phase the forearm is allowed to extend, and the rate of extension can be quite high. This extension allows a spin to be imposed on the ball as it leaves the fingers (Fig. 2–3).

4. Release and Deceleration

This phase was initially described as simply the release phase. However, owing to the importance of the deceleration forces, it is helpful to combine the release and deceleration phases. In general, the deceleration forces are approximately two times as great as the acceleration forces, which, however, act for a much shorter time.

There is no easily definable instant of ball release. The process of ball release starts with the relaxation of the grip, and in most cases the movement of the hand simply starts to decelerate as it pulls away from the ball. The fingers remain on the ball to impart the desired spin required by a certain pitch. As the ball comes away from the thumb the first two fingers are left on the ball to impart the desired spin. Ball release occurs over an approximate eight- to ten-millisecond interval. At the moment of ball release the ball has been accelerated to its maximum velocity, and the arm motion must now be decelerated to maintain the humeral head in the glenoid cavity. Peak deceleration torques after ball release have been shown to approach 300 inch pounds.

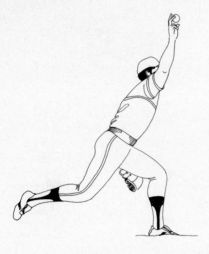

FIGURE 2–4. Release and deceleration.

At the beginning of the deceleration phase the humerus has a relatively high rate of internal rotation and the elbow is rapidly extending. This extension after ball release causes the humeral internal rotation to present itself as a forearm pronation. Thus, great forces are applied to the muscles about the shoulder that are required to decelerate the motion of the arm and to stabilize the humerus in the glenoid cavity during the deceleration phase. In addition, large forces are applied to the muscle groups that cross the elbow joint, primarily the biceps, brachialis, and brachioradialis. These muscle groups decelerate the rapidly moving forearm (Fig. 2–4).

5. Follow-Through

In the follow-through phase the body moves forward with the arm, effectively reducing the distraction forces applied to the shoulder and relieving tension on the rotator cuff muscles. The planted opposite leg is the controlling factor during this phase. This leg control maintains the balance and allows a smooth transition from the violent deceleration forces to recovery (Fig. 2–5).

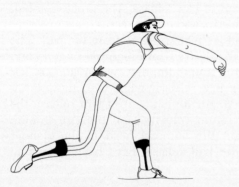

FIGURE 2–5. Follow-through.

EVALUATION OF THE FAST BALL, THE CURVE BALL, AND THE SLIDER

High-speed cinematography and computer analysis[17] were utilized to determine the forces imparted to the throwing arm by pitches such as the fast ball, the curve ball, and the slider.

With regard to the forces imparted to the shoulder, it was found that the fast ball was less traumatic than the curve ball or the slider. The fast ball applied lower peak deceleration forces than either the slider or the curve ball and thus less torque about the shoulder. The curve ball and the slider were generally somewhat slower and were delivered at a reduced level of acceleration because the actual rate of humeral rotation was less for the slider and the curve ball than for the fast ball. Thus, although there was a slower rate of humeral rotation in the curve ball and the slider, the time available to decelerate the shoulder was much less, causing the deceleration torques to be greater for both the curve ball and the slider than for the fast ball. It appeared that the curve ball was the most traumatic and demonstrated the highest combined velocities.

With regard to valgus forces placed on the elbow, the fast ball developed greater torque in the elbow than did either the slider or the curve ball. The rate of elbow extension for the fast ball is relatively smooth and well controlled throughout the full range of motion, as opposed to that during delivery of the curve ball and the slider. The curve ball was shown to have the greatest rate of elbow extension, demonstrating greater shear forces on the elbow joint surface than either of the other two pitches.

DISCUSSION

The pitching mechanism is a highly complex interaction of dynamic forces about the upper extremity that has been quite difficult to study. Attempts are being made, however, to study these forces and to evaluate common injury patterns that are frequently seen in the throwing athlete. Most of the injuries sustained in the throwing athlete's elbow or shoulder appear to occur during the acceleration and deceleration phases, with possibly more injuries occurring in the latter stage.

The shoulder is subjected to tremendous forces as the body rotates forward and the shoulder and arm lag behind, thus causing great momentum to be transferred from the moving body to the throwing arm. When these forces are combined with those of the humerus, which is externally rotated approximately 160 degrees and then rapidly internally rotated, tremendous stress is applied to the throwing athlete's shoulder. Because of these large forces the tendency for the humerus to move anteriorly out of the glenoid cavity must be offset by muscles that provide reverse torque to decelerate this forward movement.

This relationship between acceleration, deceleration, and internal and external rotation of the humerus can be viewed as the "shoulder grinding factor." If the muscles and musculotendinous units about the shoulder are not extremely well conditioned or if there is some lack of coordination or fatigue and tiring of these stabilizing muscles it is possible for the normal apposition and stability of the glenohumeral joint to be upset and for the humeral head to move transiently anteriorly or posteriorly in the glenoid cavity. Even small amounts of abnormal motion brought about by tiring or fatigued muscles can cause damage to intra-articular structures such as the glenoid labrum when the high torsional velocity forces of the humerus are applied as well.

The long head of the biceps tendon may also be responsible for initiating tearing of the glenoid labrum. Of the three muscles available to decelerate the rapidly accelerating elbow (biceps, brachialis, and brachioradialis), the biceps is the only muscle to cross both the elbow and the shoulder joint. The forces imposed by the biceps muscle to decelerate the elbow could be transmitted proximally to its origin near the glenoid labrum and could initiate a traction type of tearing on the anterosuperior aspect of the glenoid labrum during the deceleration phase of throwing. Once this tear is initiated, the hypermobile labrum conceivably could be further torn by the excessive anterior or posterior rolling action of the humeral head in the glenoid cavity during the extremes of motion to which the throwing shoulder is subjected. This type of tearing of the glenoid labrum most likely is not the result of one traumatic episode such as that seen with an anterior dislocation of the shoulder.[15] It is most likely the result of overuse.

While injuries to the shoulder most likely occur during both the acceleration and the deceleration phases, the elbow appears to be in greatest jeopardy during the acceleration phase of throwing. It is during this phase that large valgus forces are applied to the elbow causing medial tension and lateral compression forces. During the high rate of extension the articular surface is compressed and possibly transiently deformed. Because the curve ball has the highest rate of elbow extension theoretically it is the most destructive to the articular surfaces of the radial head and capitellum.[5, 6] These high torques applied to the elbow during the throwing motion are also resisted by the medial surface of the olecranon against the trochlea.[7] Thus, whereas injuries to the medial aspect of the throwing elbow are usually overuse syndromes such as tendinitis and muscle strains, the lateral aspect of the elbow can sustain more serious injuries such as articular cartilage damage to the radial head and capitellum with subsequent degenerative changes within the joint and possibly formation of loose bodies and spurs (see Chapter 23).

SUMMARY

The pitching motion can be divided into five phases: windup, cocking, acceleration, release and deceleration, and follow-through.

Owing to the magnitude of the forces that are applied to the throwing athlete's shoulder and elbow, injuries to both the elbow and the shoulder are frequent. The elbow joint is at risk because of the high acceleration torques and high rate of extension. The elbow is particularly at risk during the delivery of the curve ball because of the especially high rate of extension during this pitch. This extension causes large shearing forces because of the high deformation rate of the articular cartilage and could ultimately cause damage to the lateral articular structures about the elbow. The shoulder joint appears to be at risk because of the combination of acceleration and deceleration forces combined with extremes of external and internal rotational velocities of the humerus. This combination of velocities causes a grinding type of action on the glenohumeral joint. If the stability of the shoulder joint is upset by either fatigue or trauma the intra-articular structures such as the glenoid labrum become vulnerable to injury and could be torn by either the traction of the biceps tendon or by becoming impinged between the humeral head and the glenoid cavity.

Because the throwing mechanism is a complex interaction of multiple musculotendinous units applied in a dynamic fashion over a very short time interval and requiring forces in the range of 300 inch pounds the exact contribution of the individual muscle groups to the various phases of throwing has been quite difficult to ascertain. As more sophisticated methods to evaluate the various forces and injury patterns of the pitching mechanism are developed much more valuable information can be obtained. This information can be applied to the throwing athlete in a practical fashion to lessen his chances of sustaining serious injuries to the shoulder and elbow.

REFERENCES

1. Barnes, O. A., and Tullos, H. S.: An analysis of 100 symptomatic baseball players. Am J Sports Med 6:62, 1978.
2. DeHaven, K. E., and Evarts, C. M.: Throwing injuries of the elbow in athletes. Orthop Clin North Am 4:801, 1973.
3. King, J. W., Brelsford, H. J., and Tullos, H. S.: Analysis of the pitching arm of the professional baseball pitcher. Clin Orthop 67:116, 1979.
4. Neer, C. C., and Welsh, R. P.: The shoulder in sports. Orthop Clin North Am 8:585, 1977.
5. Pappas, A. M.: Elbow problems associated with baseball during childhood and adolescence. Clin Orthop 164:30, 1982.
6. Slocum, D. B.: Classifications of elbow injuries from baseball pitching. Texas Med 64:48, 1968.
7. Wilson, F. D., Andrews, J. R., Blackburn, T. A., and McCluskey, G. M.: Valgus extension overload in the pitching elbow. Am J Sports Med 11:83, 1983.
8. Andrews, J. R., and Carson, W. G.: Arthroscopy of the shoulder. Orthopedics 6:1157, 1983.
9. Andrews, J. R., Carson, W. G., and Ortega: Arthroscopy of the shoulder: Technique and normal anatomy Am J Sports Med 12:1, 1984.
10. Johnson, L. L.: Arthroscopy of the shoulder. In Diagnostic and Surgical Arthroscopy. St. Louis, C V Mosby Company, 1981, pp. 376–398.
11. McGlynn, F. J., and Caspari, R. B.: Arthroscopic findings in the subluxing shoulder. Clin Orthop 183:173, 1984.
12. Jobe, R. W., Tibone, J. E., Perry, J., and Moynes, D.: An EMG analysis of the shoulder in throwing and pitching: A preliminary report. Am J Sports Med 11:3, 1983.
13. DePalma, A. F.: Degenerative lesions of the shoulder joint at various age groups which are compatible with good function. American Association of Orthopedic Surgeons Instructional Course Lectures 7:168, 1950.
14. Pappas, A. M., Goss, T. P., and Kleinman, P. K.: Symptomatic shoulder instability due to lesions of the glenoid labrum. Am J Sports Med 11:279, 1983.
15. Bankart, A. S. B.: The pathology and treatment of recurrent dislocation of the shoulder. J Bone Joint Surg 26:23, 1938.

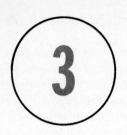

PROPER PITCHING TECHNIQUES

JOHN SAIN / JAMES R. ANDREWS, M.D.

The use of proper body mechanics is the most important way a pitcher can avoid injury caused by repetitive throwing. The purpose of this chapter is to explain proper pitching techniques from the coaching viewpoint. Various types of pitches are described as well as injury patterns and prevention.

Pitching the natural way is probably the major factor in preventing injuries to the throwing arm. If the player fields the ball and takes a step backwards or to the side and then begins a fluid forward overhand motion with a smooth follow-through he is throwing the natural way. The pitcher should throw like an outfielder, handling the ball in a loose and easy manner. When pitching from the mound, the pitcher should first step backwards or to the side to gain control and balance. He should then begin a fluid forward motion and throw the ball overhand toward the plate in a way that feels most comfortable and that is mechanically sound.

The pitcher should avoid hyperextending the planted leg and landing on his heel. This causes a sudden deceleration of the body, which promotes an undue counter force on the throwing arm. Quite frequently this hyperextension of the planted leg is seen in pitchers who are "overthrowing" and trying to get more velocity on their fastball. The maneuver can injure the young and inexperienced pitcher.

The planted foot should always point in the direction in which the ball is to be pitched, that is, toward home plate. This orientation promotes a natural rhythm and prevents "opening up" too soon (with pelvic rotation toward the target), which creates an increased stress, or valgus vector, on the inside of the elbow of the throwing arm. "Staying closed" too long, planting of the foot toward the third-base side of home plate by a right-

30

handed pitcher, can also be detrimental to the natural way of pitching. This flaw in delivery takes away the body's momentum, and the pitch has to be delivered entirely by the arm. The pitcher's motion is a smooth deceleration and acceleration of the center of gravity toward the target. The large muscle groups should position the throwing arm in the most advantageous position to avoid fatigue and thus injury. A fluid follow-through across the body helps to gradually decelerate the tremendous forces generated during the acceleration phase of pitching and is very important in allowing controlled deceleration of the throwing arm.

In pitching the natural way, all pitches, including the fastball and all types of breaking balls, are associated with a natural pronation of the forearm after ball release. Pronation is an internal rotation of the forearm as the arm comes over the top during ball release and across the body with follow-through. The forearm, however, is in relative supination at the release point of a curve ball.

Another important concept is pitching to keep the arm in shape. Recently this idea has been deemphasized. It is common to find pitchers who only pitch prior to the beginning of spring training. They will not throw at all during the off-season. The act of pitching itself is an exercise and should be used to keep the arm in shape. The specific-adaptation-to-imposed-demand (S.A.I.D.) principle, by which the athlete gradually increases the amount of force to which the body is subjected, can be applied here.

During the off-season a pitcher should throw for five days at half speed, including both a long toss (150 feet) and a short toss (60 feet). He should do this for five days and then have two days of complete rest. This schedule keeps the pitching arm in shape. The number of pitches should be counted and should not exceed 60 long toss and 60 short toss pitches.

To keep his arm in shape during the season a pitcher must throw more often than just at his turn in the game's regular rotation. The amount of time spent pitching depends on whether he is in a four- or five-day rotation.

Many different pitching rotation schedules are being used by Major League baseball organizations today. However, the authors have found that a pitching rotation with the pitcher performing in a game every fourth or fifth day is the most effective. At present the authors prefer the four-day pitching rotation with a pitcher pitching on a given day and then having three days of rest before his next game. Over the duration of the Major League season this rotation enables the better pitchers on a club to perform in six or eight more games per season.

The following rotation is one that coach Sain has used during 14 years of coaching in the Major Leagues, 11 years of pitching in the Major Leagues, and 6 years of pitching in the Minor Leagues. The four-day pitching rotation (three days of rest between workouts) is as follows:

1. The pitcher performs on the first day, usually pitching for seven, eight, or nine innings.

2. The pitcher rests the arm on the following day, with the exception of some light overall exercise such as running or gentle throwing.

3. On the second day after pitching the arm is rested once more. However, running and a slight increase in the gentle throwing is suggested. The pitcher should be involved in a toss program at 40 feet and 50 per cent speed.

4. The third day after pitching consists of running again and more throwing in an attempt to remove all stiffness and soreness. The pitcher should throw for 15 minutes off the mound.

The goal of having pitchers throw between games is to maintain mobility and range of motion, and to avoid stiffness. If no exercise is performed between starts it usually takes at least five or six days for the pitcher to regain motion. A pitcher's goal between starts should be to reestablish a pain-free full range of motion and muscle stamina.

During the season a pitcher pitches approximately 120 pitches per game. At this rate he averages about 15 pitches per inning.

ARM POSITIONS

With the normal pitching motion the arm is almost always at 90 degrees of abduction. Misconceptions exist that the overhead pitch allows the arm to be abducted more than 90 degrees at the shoulder level. High-speed cinematography has shown that the various types of arm positions all carry the shoulder at 90 degrees of abduction. The pitcher's body position determines whether the pitch will be over the top or a side-arm delivery.

In pitching over the top the elbow is bent or flexed, with the three-quarter delivery the elbow is flexed less, and in the side-arm position the elbow is flexed even less. The submarine pitch is a different position and can almost be considered an underhand type of pitch.

TYPES OF PITCHES

The spin applied by the fingers of the throwing hand determines the type of pitch.

In throwing a *fastball* the hand and thumb point to home plate at ball release. The index and middle fingers apply the power and the movement to the ball. A fastball can be thrown by using a two- or four-seam grip. With the four-seam grip the ball is gripped across the seams, and with the two-seam grip the fingers are placed along the seams. This creates more movement on the ball. Back spin is directed up and back toward the pitcher and away from the batter and makes the fastball appear to rise. This pitch may look as if it rises to a batter because as he levels off to hit it, he lowers his body height by "squaring" his stance at ball impact.

Gravity, always a factor in pitching, naturally causes the baseball to drop. However, a good pitcher throwing a fastball at 90 miles per hour or faster can throw it so hard and so fast that gravity's effect is lessened. Speeds in this category certainly give the batter the impression that the ball rises.

Breaking pitches are thrown by turning the hand just slightly either inward or outward. This type of pitch is controlled by a very slight variation in pressure of one finger or the other, not by breaking the wrist, as is commonly thought. Most breaking pitches have one thing in common, that they break downward. They can either break down and in or down and out from a right-handed batter.

Of all breaking pitches the *slider* is probably the most popular and most often used in baseball. The slider actually came into its own in the late 1950s or early 1960s and has had a tremendous impact on baseball. It is partially responsible for doing away with the .400 batting average in the Major Leagues. It is thrown in the same manner as the fastball, but with the slider the index finger comes off the ball just slightly at the release point. Some pitchers throw it by slightly turning the hand a quarter turn away from the batter (as in turning a door knob) to create rotation on the ball. Using a seam grip, as the ball is released the index finger comes off the ball just as in pointing a finger at someone. This maneuver creates uneven pressure on the seam, which comes from the middle finger and causes the ball to "break" slightly down and in. In most cases the ball actually breaks 1 foot horizontally and 3 to 4 inches downward. This pitch looks just like a fastball to the batter but has less speed than the normal fastball. Therefore, it has the advantage of being an off-speed pitch that breaks while looking like a fastball.

The *curve ball* was developed as the original breaking pitch. In the past the wide curve was very popular. At both the elite amateur level and the professional level a tight curve is by far the predominant type of curve ball thrown today. In the past the wide curve has been blamed as a cause of injury to the Little Leaguer's elbow. The pitch was usually improperly taught. This pitch is notorious for generating vector velocity forces about the elbow and causing injury. Very seldom is a wide curve ever taught by knowledgeable coaches today.

The technique for throwing a curve ball is fairly simple. The hand is flexed at the wrist and turned inward with the palm facing the pitcher's body. There is a misconception that a curve ball is thrown by breaking the wrist, that is, by turning the wrist over with external rotation or supination of the forearm. The middle finger is the controlling finger, and the index finger is the guide finger for throwing a curve ball. The motion is always over the top and downward, with pronation and internal rotation of the forearm and fluid deceleration across the body.

A *sinker ball* is the mirror image of a slider but is more difficult to throw. The hand turns outward from the plate or away from the pitcher's body. Pressure is put on the index finger rather than the middle finger, as is done in throwing a slider. Seam concentration, therefore, is reversed, and the ball is given a counterclockwise rotation when it is thrown by a right-handed pitcher. It looks like a fastball to the batter but sinks and dives suddenly. The sinker, when thrown by a right-handed pitcher, breaks down and in toward a right-handed batter.

A *change-up* is a pitch in which the body and arm mechanics look like those used in throwing a fastball. This pitch is designed to take the finger power off the ball and to leave the arm power on. The ball then slips out of the hand prematurely, which gives it less forward momentum. This pitch is very effective at keeping a hitter off balance, since the delivery looks just like that of a fastball. However, the difference in speed may be as great as 10 miles per hour. A change-up is usually gripped with the ball back in the hand against the palm or thrown with three fingers on the ball to slow it down and allow it to slip out of the control of the fingers and palm.

Many pitches fall into the category of "junk" balls. Two examples are the *knuckle ball* and the *fork ball*. A *knuckle ball* is thrown by gripping the baseball with two to four knuckles. This grip takes all the spin off the ball, which causes it to float toward the plate. A knuckle ball moves in an unpredictable way both horizontally and vertically.

A *fork ball* is thrown by placing the ball between the index and middle fingers, with pressure being applied to the ball from these two fingers. This pitch appears to come straight to the batter but drops straight down as it approaches the plate.

INJURY PATTERNS

Most injuries to the throwing arm occur because of overextension. This can mean overextension from a physiological standpoint or from an anatomic standpoint, as in actual overextension of the shoulder or the elbow joint.

Certain throwing patterns correlate directly with shoulder injuries. The fastball creates 600 inch-pounds of forward momentum at ball release. Deceleration of this momentum occurs during the deceleration or follow-through phase of the pitching act. Certainly, 600 inch-pounds of momentum is a considerable force to be absorbed by the shoulder and in particular by the rotator cuff. For this reason the authors suspect that the rotator cuff itself fails under the stresses of the release and deceleration phase of the pitching act, since this is where peak forces occur. By repeatedly throwing a 90 mile per hour fastball a young pitcher eventually should injure his rotator cuff unless he can learn how to throw this pitch correctly.

Breaking balls appear to create more stress to the elbow than does a fastball. Throwing a slider too hard and too often can certainly create a predictable injury pattern in the elbow. The curve ball, especially a wide curve, can create tremendous forces and has been responsible for a majority of the injuries to the skeletally immature athlete's elbow. When a pitcher throws a curve ball improperly, as by breaking or turning the wrist over with eversion or supination, even greater forces are generated across the elbow. Throwing a tight curve with the proper technique decreases the possibility of injury.

Hyperextension of the elbow in the true sense of the word is also responsible for elbow injuries. When there is a lack of deceleration of the elbow at ball release this creates a "valgus extension overload" injury to the elbow. A pitcher can prevent this by learning to "shorten the elbow," that is, to increase elbow flexion strength, or by learning to control deceleration at the release of the ball.

INJURY PREVENTION

Proper body mechanics are the key to injury prevention. Taking stress off the arm and distributing these forces throughout the body are the goals of proper body mechanics. The planted foot should always be pointed toward the plate during pitching. This allows fluid body motion with the natural deceleration process of the pitching act. Injuries can also be prevented by teaching a pitcher how not to overextend his elbow. He must understand what "shorten the arm" means, that is, the fluid control of the deceleration forces across the elbow. Taking a step backwards or to the side to begin the throwing act and throwing the natural way are important as well. Injuries can be caused by changes in throwing technique in young pitchers. It is very important in the prevention of throwing injuries for coaches to take what a player naturally has and to refine it and not to try to make drastic changes in the technique and body form that a young pitcher has developed through the years.

Pitchers of high school age or younger should throw only one or two types of pitches. A Little Leaguer should attempt to perfect one good type of pitch. Generally, this should be a fastball, since it takes less expertise on both the coach's and the young pitcher's part to perfect. A young pitcher should develop his skills in the following order: (1) velocity, (2) consistent mechanics (control), (3) changeup, sinker, and cross seam pitches, and (4) breaking pitches. Off-season training is also a key to the prevention of injury to the throwing arm. It is important for pitchers to realize that they must pitch to stay in shape and use the S.A.I.D. principle. During the off-season the throwing athlete should throw at half or three-quarter speed at short intervals. If he is to pitch 25 to 30 minutes each day it would be better to break up the total pitching time into 8-minute intervals with 4 minutes being devoted to the long toss and 4 minutes to the short toss. He should rest for 20 to 30 minutes and then pitch for another 8-minute interval. Interval pitching prevents the fatigue that can cause injuries to the throwing arm.

An off-season weight-lifting program is also very important. Many specific weight-lifting programs have been described. These off-season weight-lifting programs are built around light weights to promote endurance, particularly in the rotator cuff. Muscle imbalance is to be avoided and should be considered in any off-season weight-lifting program. The anterior shoulder muscles are generally stronger than the posterior shoulder muscles, and the weight-lifting program should emphasize the posterior shoulder musculature. Emphasis should be placed on flexibility as well as strength in a complete program.

An in-season weight-lifting program is equally important. During the season a pitching arm actually weakens as a result of the stresses applied to it during the daily act of pitching a baseball. An in-season weight-lifting program using light weights along with a flexibility program is mandatory.

The warm-up is a major aspect of injury prevention. It has been said, "Warm-up to pitch, don't pitch to warm-up." After an initial period of stretching the pitcher should follow a prescribed sequence. The pitcher should begin with a total body warm-up followed by general body stretching. For example, the sequence could be ankles, hamstrings and quadriceps, hip extensors and flexors, pelvic rotation, spine, neck, shoulder, and elbow. The pitcher should begin to throw while using a short stride, continue this for two to three minutes, and then begin to stretch. It is particularly important not to hyperextend the planted leg in the initial warm-up.

Most injuries occur during spring training or during the early part of the season because many players do not report to spring training with their bodies or their arms in shape. The throwing athlete should report to early season training already in proper physical condition; otherwise he may immediately begin to overextend himself physically because of the presence of the coach, the manager, or the owner on the field. In the attempt to impress someone with his ability his tendency to overextend the arm can cause an injury.

Physical fitness must always be emphasized as a way to prevent injuries. A general fitness program should be followed during the baseball season as well as the off-season. A baseball player should run sprints as well as distance each day to promote anaerobic as well as aerobic fitness.

With all that is known today about the throwing arm young pitchers still ruin their arms by only throwing a fastball and never learning to throw an off-speed pitch. The elbow and the shoulder both need rest from the vector velocity forces generated when throwing a 90 mile per hour fastball. A pitcher must learn to throw an off-speed pitch. A young "fireball" who throws nothing else will inevitably ruin his throwing arm.

Recognizing the tired pitcher is important in preventing injuries. Communication between the pitcher, the coach, and the trainer is crucial during the rigors of a season. A good indicator to follow is the number of pitches that have been thrown. For example, if a pitcher has thrown 110 pitches in six innings, the coach or trainer should watch for fatigue that would make him prone to injury. Ball control is also an indication of fatigue. If a pitcher has thrown too many high pitches, given up too many hits, or walked too many batters, he may be getting tired. He should also be watched for a change in tempo or pitching rhythm. Fatigue is probably the primary factor in rotator cuff injuries. Above all, a pitcher must be honest with himself and communicate with his coach when he is becoming tired.

Undue pain in the throwing arm or elbow during pitching should always be evaluated. The pitcher should differentiate between sharp joint pain and aching pain from muscle fatigue caused by exercise. As the pitcher begins to have increased pain that is unnatural to him, an evolving injury should be suspected. Particular attention should be paid to pain that persists through the hitting portion of an inning when the pitcher is at rest.

Improper pitching mechanics that can cause injury can often be detected by high-speed–shutter video recordings or high-speed cinematography. These observations can be studied by the coach, the player, the trainer, and the physician. All of these individuals can play a part in promoting proper body mechanics, which is the primary means of preventing injury.

Acknowledgments

The authors thank the persons listed below for their technical assistance and contributions to this chapter.

George Medich, M.D., is an orthopedic resident at the University of Pittsburgh. He is a former Major League pitcher.

Jeff Heathcock is a pitcher in the Houston Astros organization. He began his professional career in 1980 as a first-round draft choice of the Astros. After four years in the farm system, he ended the 1983 season on the Major League team in Houston.

George Cappuzzello began his professional career in 1972. He has pitched for the Detroit Tigers and the Houston Astros and spent the 1983 season in the New York Yankees' organization.

Johnny Sain is considered one of the best pitching coaches in baseball. In 17 seasons as a Major League coach, he guided 10 20-game winners. For six consecutive seasons he has been with the Atlanta Braves Minor League organization as a pitching coach. He began the coaching phase of his career in 1959 and joined the Braves' organization in 1976.

Sain began his professional career in 1936 and starred for the Boston Braves and the New York Yankees. He ended his active career as a member of the Kansas City Athletics in 1955. He was chosen National League Pitcher-of-the-Year in 1948 and pitched in three World Series games as a member of the New York Yankees.

Sain is both a great teacher of the mechanics of pitching and a remarkable student of human nature. In his view the ultimate burden of improvement rests with the pitcher and not with the coach.

THE CURVE BALL AND
THE ELBOW

CHARLES P. GREENE, PH.D.

Since arm injuries occur after a prolonged period of constant throwing and not usually as a result of one sudden isolated effort, it is imperative that an athlete possess the best possible throwing technique in order to eliminate or delay the onset of arm injury. Repetitious throwing with a fundamentally unsound delivery can hasten the occurrence of a serious tear or rupture. Sound pitching mechanics are therefore vital to prevention.

The fundamentals of the delivery must be mastered long before any sophisticated or "trick" deliveries are attempted. This is particularly true of the curve ball and its effect on the elbow joint.

Contrary to the accepted theory that the arm is supinated when throwing a curve, it now can be seen through careful analysis of slow-motion photography that the forearm actually pronates right after the ball has been released. It has long been thought that the athlete releases the ball out in front with the ball rolling off the middle and index fingers. However, further review of the film consistently shows the ball being released about 15 degrees forward of perpendicular and not out in front as traditionally has been accepted. The visualization or most pitchers' perception of how a curve ball is thrown is contrary to what actually occurs. The continual attempts to supinate the curve ball can cause the elbow to work against its natural inclination and cause constant irritation to that joint area. The ulnar nerve on the inner side of the elbow can be injured by improper throwing technique and overuse. The ligaments and muscles on the inner side of the elbow may also be strained by the attempt to supinate at a high velocity.

Since pronation is the natural action of the arm when throwing a curve ball or any other pitch, it is recommended that pitchers not work against this action but rather utilize it and go with it.

To properly throw a curve or breaking ball emphasis should be placed on positioning the middle and index fingers on the top right side of the ball during release. It is thought that by putting pressure on the right side of the ball and *not* attempting to supinate as the ball is being released, the athlete exerts less pressure on the elbow joint. In addition, it has been the author's experience that a much more effective breaking ball results. By experimenting with this right side theory a pitcher can find the proper pressure point for him and pitch accordingly. It is also considered that the more to the right side the pressure is exerted the bigger and slower is the break and conversely that the more to the top of the ball the pressure is exerted the smaller and faster is the break.

If thrown properly the curve ball should not be any more dangerous to the elbow joint than any other pitch. It is in working against the normal action of the arm (pronation) that the susceptibility to injury is increased. The important thing is to help the pitcher understand the true mechanics of the pitching delivery and to guide him to adapt his curve ball technique to those mechanics.

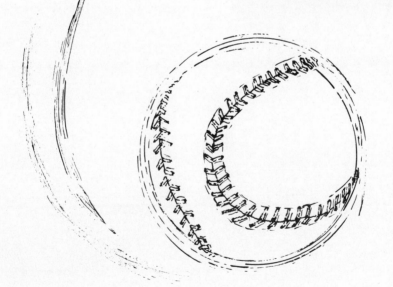

PART
TWO

THE
SHOULDER
IN THE
THROWING
ATHLETE

FUNCTIONAL ANATOMY OF THE SHOULDER*

JACK C. HUGHSTON, M.D.

THE SHOULDER GIRDLE

The shoulder girdle consists of three bony structures, the *clavicle*, the *scapula*, and the *humerus*. They make up four joints, the *sternoclavicular*, the *acromioclavicular*, the *scapulothoracic*, and the *glenohumeral joints*, which work together functionally as a single joint (Fig. 5–1). The total unit is almost completely dependent on the synergism of musculotendinous units for functional stability. Fifteen muscles are involved with motion of the scapula. Nine muscles provide glenohumeral motion. Six muscles support the scapula on the thorax.

The synergism of these muscles and joints allows maximal rotation of the shoulder with minimal rotational stress on the proximal fixation point, the sternoclavicular joint. The clavicle, being an unstable bony structure itself, articulates with the body by its attachment to the sternum. The clavicle is primarily stabilized dynamically by the trapezius and deltoid and the subclavius muscles. The clavicle is thereby the key supporting element, acting as a "yardarm" to hold the scapula at the proper degree of abduction and external rotation on the thorax in order to allow maximal function of the glenohumeral joint.

Some of the joints must be considered separately in order to demonstrate the amount of motion present in each under varied circumstances.

---

*This work was supported in part by the Hughston Sports Medicine Foundation, Inc., 6262 Hamilton Road, Columbus, Georgia 31995.

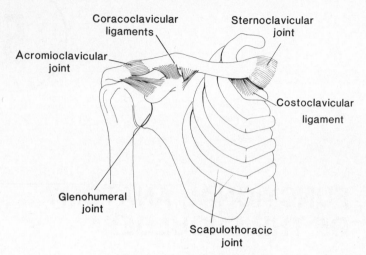

FIGURE 5–1. The shoulder girdle.

Thus, if the scapula were attached to the thorax, and abduction of the humerus from the body at the glenohumeral joint were attempted with the humerus held internally rotated, abduction would be possible to only 60 degrees before the greater tuberosity became compressed against the underside of the acromion. Such compression would produce impingement and prevent further abduction (Fig. 5–2). With the scapula fixed and the humerus externally rotated at the time of abduction, motion at the glenohumeral junction would allow 120 degrees of abduction (Fig. 5–3). Obviously, it is impossible to attach the scapula to the thorax, and these assumptions are made merely to illustrate that the humerus does externally rotate at the glenohumeral joint as abduction occurs.

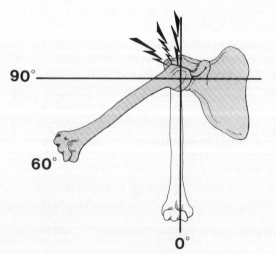

90°

60°

0°

FIGURE 5–2. Abduction at the glenohumeral joint with the humerus internally rotated is possible to only 60 degrees before impingement of the greater tuberosity leads to compression against the underside of the acromion and prevents further abduction.

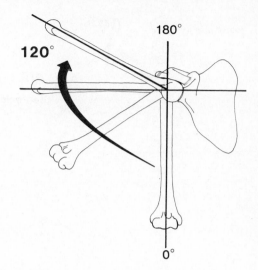

FIGURE 5–3. If external rotation of the humerus occurs simultaneously with abduction at the shoulder joint but without scapular motion, abduction is possible to 120 degrees. However, this illustration is meant only to demonstrate the glenohumeral motion, since normally the scapula rotates with abduction.

The Scapula

If the scapula is allowed to rotate on the thorax, the usual amount of rotation is 30 degrees at the scapulothoracic joint and 60 degrees at the glenohumeral joint in order to achieve 90 degrees of abduction. When the arm is abducted to 180 degrees, as it is in the pitching motion, the scapula rotates 60 degrees, and the glenohumeral joint rotates 120 degrees (Fig. 5–4).

Proper function of the scapulothoracic and glenohumeral joints is completely dependent on the clavicle, its length, and its normal motion at both the sternoclavicular and acromioclavicular joints.

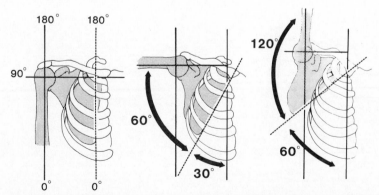

FIGURE 5–4. Normal abduction of the shoulder takes place with the humerus externally rotating at the glenohumeral joint and with the scapula rotating on the thorax. The ratio of glenohumeral to scapulothoracic motion is 2:1.

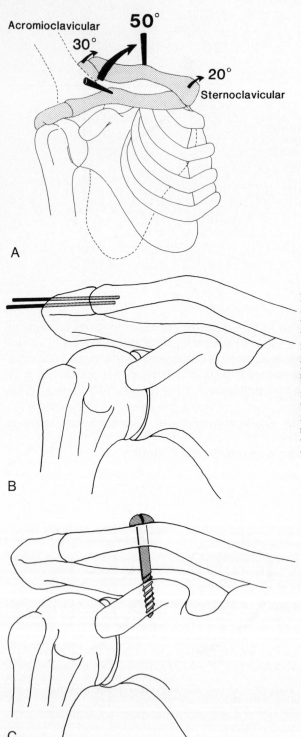

A

B

C

FIGURE 5–5. *A.* When shoulder abduction reaches 180 degrees, the outward rotation of the clavicle is 30 degrees at the acromioclavicular joint and 20 degrees at the sternoclavicular joint. *B.* Fixation of the clavicle by transfixion pins at the sternoclavicular joint prevents rotation and thereby prevents normal abduction motion. *C.* The same clavicular rotation is prevented by a screw from the clavicle to the coracoid process.

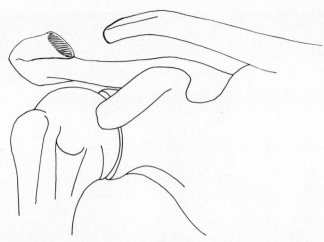

FIGURE 5–6. Excision of the distal end of the clavicle, as is sometimes performed for acromioclavicular arthritis, removes the bony stability of the entire shoulder girdle.

The Clavicle

The clavicle allows abduction of the glenohumeral joint by virtue of its S-shape and rotates on itself 50 degrees to allow 180 degrees of abduction of the shoulder, which is necessary in the pitching motion (Fig. 5–5A). When the acromioclavicular joint is fixed with a pin rotation in the acromioclavicular and sternoclavicular joints cannot occur, and abduction of the glenohumeral joint is compromised (Fig. 5–5B). If the clavicle is fixed to the coracoid process by a rigid screw, such as with the Bosworth type of fixation of the clavicle for immobilizing an acromioclavicular dislocation, rotation of the clavicle is eliminiated (Fig. 5–5C). If an excision of the distal end of the clavicle is carried out in the treatment of an acromioclavicular dislocation or for arthritic deterioration of the joint, the clavicular distance is shortened and the scapula rotates internally on the thorax and may become fixed in this position by scar tissue between the distal end of the clavicle and the scapula (Fig. 5–6). This anterior subluxation of the scapulothoracic joint causes alteration of the humeral rotators, especially the pectoralis major and the latissimus dorsi muscles, which work from the thorax rather than from the scapula (Fig. 5–7A,B,C).

THE ROTATOR CUFF

The function of the rotator cuff is to stabilize the glenohumeral joint and at the same time to aid in the abduction and rotation of the joint. The rotator cuff muscles are the fine tuners of the glenohumeral joint and the shoulder girdle, whereas the latissimus dorsi, deltoid, and pectoralis major muscles are the powerful rotators and abductors. Therefore, loss of stabili-

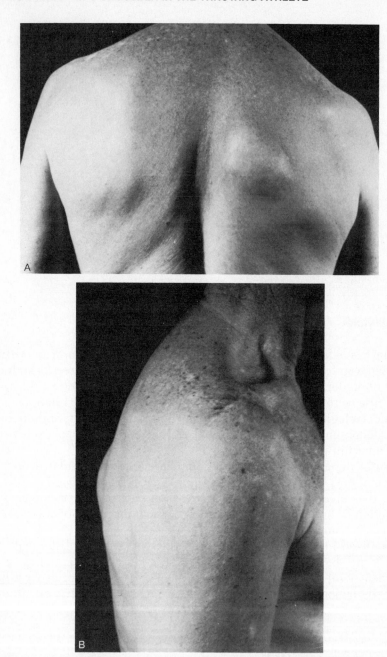

FIGURE 5–7. Excision of the distal end of the clavicle removes the bony stability of the shoulder girdle and allows forward subluxation of the scapulothoracic joint. This patient had excision of the distal end of the clavicle with resultant forward subluxation of the scapulothoracic joint and depression of the scapula on the involved right side, as seen in the posteroanterior *(A)* and lateral *(B)* views. Thus, abduction of the shoulder produces an abnormal scapulothoracic motion and abnormal glenohumeral motion with loss of strength and function *(C)*.

Illustration continued on opposite page

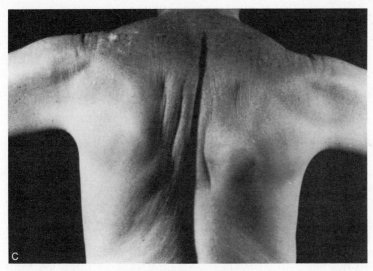

FIGURE 5–7. *Continued.*

zation of the glenohumeral joint by the rotator cuff produces disability. The rotator cuff deteriorates primarily owing to disuse and traction ischemia and secondarily owing to compression on the acromion and the coracoclavicular ligament. In the athlete in particular, it is necessary to recognize deterioration of the rotator cuff in its early stages so that it may be corrected in order to restore good function. Obviously, it is impossible to restore good function once the rotator cuff has ruptured completely and shortened. On the other hand, acute tears of the rotator cuff can occur with violent forces in the absence of any deterioration and acute repair of these can result in a normally functioning shoulder. Recognition of this condition is difficult, and an arthrogram is necessary for diagnosis. The acute complete tear is rarely painful and rarely involves any limitation of active motion of the shoulder on clinical examination. There is relative weakness and mild soreness. The history and the physical examination are extremely important for young athletes who incur this acute type of rupture. This disorder should be immediately recognized and repaired.

The Long Head of the Biceps

The long head of the biceps is frequently the site of painful tenosynovitis necessitating an injection or a surgical tenodesis to the humeral head to alleviate the pain. It is the author's experience that tendinitis of the biceps tendon is most often a secondary disorder. It is important to search for the causes of these symptoms. The long head of the biceps is a dynamic suspensory ligament of the glenohumeral joint. When there is a malfunction additional strain is placed on the tendon of the long head of the biceps causing pain and localized tenderness. Loss of the long head of the biceps by rupture or by surgical tenodesis transfers the entire suspensory load of fixation of the humeral head in the glenoid cavity to the rotator cuff muscles. In the throwing arm such a loss can produce inferior subluxation of the shoulder with resultant malfunction. Therefore in cases of biceps tenosynovitis the primary causative factor producing the strain must be recognized and corrected through either rehabilitation or appropriate surgical means.

The Glenohumeral Joint

The glenohumeral joint is quite shallow, and its depth is slightly increased by the presence of the glenoid labrum (the meniscus of the shoulder joint). If there is tearing of the glenoid labrum, which is not an infrequent disorder of the pitching and throwing shoulder, the mechanics of the glenohumeral joint are altered, so that they often produce pain and popping but not necessarily a subluxation of the glenohumeral joint. Further injury to the bony structure of the glenoid is most often associated with sufficient lack of support for the humeral head so that recurrent subluxation or dislocation does begin to occur with forceful motions of the shoulder.

The Glenoid Labrum

Until the last five to six years, the glenoid labrum had not received much attention or blame for malfunction of the glenohumeral joint, except in association with glenohumeral dislocations. Over the past few years the author has had several patients with tears of the glenoid labrum with no associated dislocation or subluxation of the glenohumeral joint. At first the approach used was surgical excision of the tear, which is a procedure similar to removing the meniscus of the knee. More recently, the arthroscope has been used for removal of torn tissue with less resultant surgical trauma. Although the glenoid labrum is a cartilaginous element producing a deepening of the glenoid socket for the humeral head, only a few patients have been seen in whom subluxation of the shoulder occurred after the removal of the torn labrum. As with treatment of any disorder of the shoulder girdle, gradually increasing degrees of rehabilitation to complete function are necessary and time-consuming even after arthroscopic removal of the glenoid labrum.

SUMMARY

The shoulder girdle has very little static or ligamentous stability. Its stability is dynamic and requires almost perfect synergism of all of the muscles. Structural defects to any of the bony or musculotendinous units involved prevent perfect function.

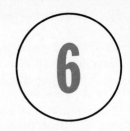

PHYSICAL EXAMINATION OF THE SHOULDER IN THROWING ATHLETES

JAMES R. ANDREWS, M.D. / SCOTT GILLOGLY, M.D.

The physical demands placed on the throwing shoulder are quite different from those of the nonthrowing shoulder. The extreme stresses placed on the dynamic stabilizing structures of the shoulder joint by rapid and forceful contractions of the external muscles during the throwing motion lead to adaptive changes. It is these same rapid acceleration and deceleration forces that often predispose the throwing shoulder to injury. It is essential for the physician examining the shoulder in throwing athletes to have an appreciation of the baseline physical characteristics, which may differ in the throwing and nonthrowing shoulders, and a basic understanding of the mechanics of the throwing motion.

PHYSICAL CHARACTERISTICS OF THE THROWING SHOULDER

The most readily apparent characteristic on examination is the amount of hypertrophy evident in the shoulder girdle muscles beyond that normally associated with dominant handedness. This hypertrophy can at times make it difficult to palpate specific underlying structures unless certain maneuvers are undertaken during the actual examination. The hypertrophy also

51

accentuates recognition of any muscle wasting that may be present with chronic injury or nerve damage.

Throwing athletes typically show a marked increase in external rotation of the throwing shoulder and relative loss of internal rotation when compared with the nonthrowing side. It is important to correctly interpret this physical finding and not to diagnose an abnormal internal rotation contracture. In fact, should the throwing shoulder not show this combination of increased external rotation, this is more likely an indication of pathology.

Throwing shoulders usually exhibit hyperextensibility. This may be an adaptive change in the throwing shoulder or may reflect overall joint hypermobility. This common feature in a competitive throwing athlete undoubtedly contributes to subluxation or dislocation injuries and associated lesions.

BASIC MECHANICS OF THROWING

The throwing motion is a highly complex and integrated motor function that places maximal stress on the structures of the shoulder. In the throwing athlete these extreme stresses occur just under the maximal tolerance of the tissues. When the tolerance of the tissues is exceeded, injury occurs.

While the repetitive task of the throwing motion has led to gradual adaptive changes and hypertrophy of the tissues about the shoulder, even minor alterations in throwing mechanics can lead to disruption of the fine balance between maximal stress and maximal tolerance. By having an understanding of basic throwing mechanics, the physician can not only diagnose and guide rehabilitation of the injured throwing shoulder but also aid in prevention of recurrence of injury.

The throwing motion can be divided into five phases: wind-up, cocking, acceleration, release and deceleration, and follow-through.

During wind-up the thrower is relatively relaxed and coils the arm and body to shorten the muscles and relax the accelerators. This allows the unleashing of maximal energy during the later phases of throwing. It is important to have this position correctly aligned to provide maximal thrust while maintaining balance. The cocking phase completes the loading of the arm and does not involve forward motion of the ball. The contralateral leg steps forward, rotating in the line of the throw just prior to planting the feet. This causes the hips to open up, building a large moment of rotation to be transferred to the shoulder. At this point the arm is in extreme external rotation, and the anterior muscles and fibrous structures are extrinsically loaded.

Next the acceleration phase starts, with the humerus accelerating and pulling the forearm and hand to cause slight further external forward rotation of the forearm and hand. About halfway through the acceleration phase, the humerus starts to decelerate, transferring the momentum into internal rotation of the forearm. The loaded internal rotators contract just as the hand has passed slightly in front of the head.

Following ball release, deceleration occurs. This is the most violent phase in throwing. The anterior fibrous tissues and muscles are suddenly relaxed. The posterior muscles jarringly contract as the force is dissipated in energy transfer to the shoulder structures during follow-through.

HISTORY

As with any examination, the patient's history is the first step. The usual questions of duration and location of pain and aggravating factors need to be addressed. The nature of the pain can give important clues to the diagnosis: a dull aching pain, often felt at night, is characteristic of a rotator cuff tear; a stabbing or burning pain is more typical of bursitis or tendinitis.

The location of the pain can be diagnostic. For example, the acromioclavicular joint is close to the surface and can easily be localized. Pain that is generalized usually comes from a deeper structure, such as the rotator cuff, or is referred from a distant source. Radiation of pain, paresthesias, or numbness can indicate compressive neuropathies such as thoracic outlet syndrome or entrapments of specific nerves such as the suprascapular nerve on the scapula or axillary nerve in the quadrilateral space.

History of prior injuries also should be assessed, since previous subluxations or dislocations may have produced a Hill-Sachs lesion or Bankart lesion that has become symptomatic. Previous inflammatory conditions can recur after a period of quiescence, particularly following an off-season break from training. Patients may complain of feeling or hearing noises such as a pop with certain motions, possibly indicating a glenoid labrum tear. Crepitus or grinding can occur with degenerative disease in the acromioclavicular joint or from chronic bursitis. A pop or snap could also indicate a subluxating biceps tendon.

The patient should be questioned as to the phase in the throwing motion during which symptoms occur. If possible, the patient should demonstrate the aggravating position. Other factors such as change in the throwing style or specific technique or grip changes should be correlated to the onset or type of symptoms.

PHYSICAL EXAMINATION AND DIAGNOSIS

The physician should establish a consistent routine for performing physical examination of the throwing shoulder. This not only insures completeness but allows the examiner to simplify the diagnostic formulation by logically relating the functional anatomy of throwing to the physical findings on examination. The normal anatomic characteristics of the throwing shoulder should be kept in mind, and the uninjured shoulder should always be included in the examination.

Initial examination begins with inspection of the various contours of the shoulder. This can usually be started while the examiner is conversing with the patient, taking a history, observing the patient undressing, and moving to the examination table. Obvious asymmetry, atrophy, hypertrophy, erythema, and swelling can be recognized. The patient's overall functional status can also be evaluated during this period by observing the degree of discomfort caused by the simple maneuvers of undressing.

The active portion of the examination is begun from the posterior aspect of the throwing shoulder with the patient in the sitting position. Rotation is first checked with the arm at 90 degrees of abduction, with both external and internal rotation noted in this position. When this rotation is compared with that of the contralateral side, the excessive external rotation and loss of internal rotation is readily apparent. Overhead abduction is then checked by having the patient raise his arms directly overhead (Fig. 6–1). It is important to watch the scapula during abduction to see whether it rides out laterally. Next the sternoclavicular joint is examined with the arm in full abduction, and the normal 50-degree rotation of the clavicle is noted.

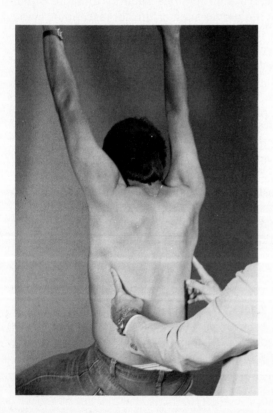

FIGURE 6–1. Method of demonstrating overhead abduction.

The sternoclavicular joint is commonly overlooked and can be a source of pain and crepitus in the throwing shoulder. The clavicle is palpated distally for tenderness extending to the acromioclavicular joint. The acromioclavicular joint is also palpated for dislocation, pain, and crepitus in various degrees of abduction and flexion. Dislocation of this joint can occur in the anterior or posterior direction as well as in the superior direction.

The next test is for strength of the supraspinatus muscle by having the shoulder in 90 degrees of abduction and 30 degrees of forward flexion and full internal rotation (Fig. 6–2). The patient maintains this position as the examiner exerts downward force. Weakness or pain can indicate superior rotator cuff pathology or neuropathy of the supraspinatus nerve.

The impingement test is carried out with the patient sitting and abducting his arm fully overhead. Impingement against the coracoacromial arch can be detected by manually depressing the scapula as the patient abducts the arm (Fig. 6–3).

Anterior stability can be examined with the patient in the sitting position. The throwing arm is held by the examiner at 90 degrees of elbow flexion. The shoulder is slowly rotated externally (Fig. 6–4). Apprehension or pain felt by the patient as this maneuver is increased implies subluxation or prior dislocation. Diffuse pain alone during the apprehension test can indicate a rotator cuff tear rather than glenohumeral subluxation. While the apprehension test is being performed, the anterior glenoid rim should be palpated. Tenderness can be found in instances of anterior subluxation. The examiner should always be prepared to reduce a dislocation if this occurs during the testing maneuver.

The patient stands while the posterior musculature is examined for

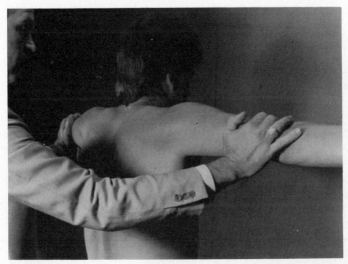

FIGURE 6–2. Testing for strength of the supraspinatus and deltoid muscles.

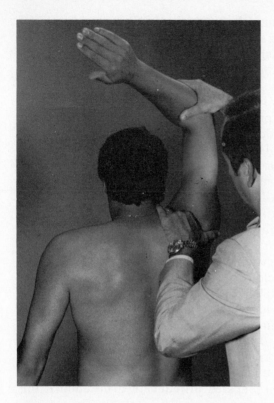

FIGURE 6–3. Testing for impingement against the coracoacromial
arch.

hypertrophy of the teres minor, a common finding in the throwing shoulder
(Fig. 6–5). The posterior musculature can be accentuated by having the
patient place his hands on his hips and tighten his muscles. The posterior
muscles are palpated to detect tenderness. Internal rotation can be measured

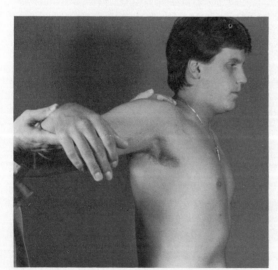

FIGURE 6–4. Testing for anterior
stability.

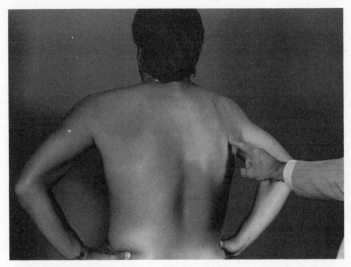

FIGURE 6–5. Examining the posterior muscles to detect hypertrophy of the teres minor muscle.

for both shoulders by recording the spinous process that the patient can touch with his thumb (Fig. 6–6). This measurement points out the relative lack of internal rotation on the throwing side. The patient then pushes against the wall to check for winging of the scapula, indicative of weakness in the serratus anterior muscle or injury to the long thoracic nerve, or both (Fig. 6–7). With the arms in the overhead position the rotation of the scapula in relation to the thoracic wall should be noted. It should be remembered that scapulothoracic motion is an important component of the throwing motion at the shoulder. Inferior glenohumeral stability can be tested in the

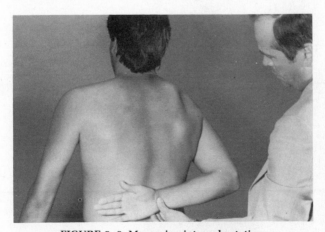

FIGURE 6–6. Measuring internal rotation.

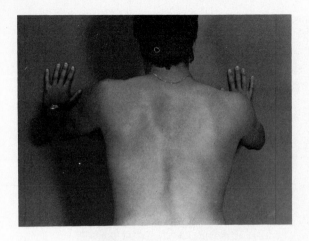

FIGURE 6–7. Checking for winging of the scapula, a sign of weakness in the serratus anterior muscle or injury to the long thoracic nerve, or both.

standing position by pulling straight down on the arm while palpating in the axilla.

The next step is to have the patient lie supine and to again observe the rotation on both sides with the arm abducted 90 degrees (Fig. 6–8). The increased external rotation of the throwing shoulder and relative loss of internal rotation should be noted. Rotation should also be recorded with the arms in the full overhead position. Horizontal adduction across the body is checked, as well as tightness in the motion necessary for follow-through at the end of the deceleration phase of throwing (Fig. 6–9).

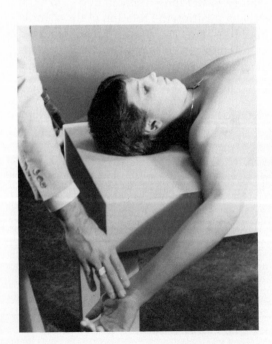

FIGURE 6–8. Observing external rotation of both shoulders with the arms abducted 90 degrees.

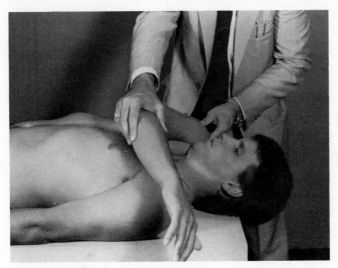

FIGURE 6–9. Measuring horizontal adduction across the body.

Tightness within the glenohumeral joint itself can be checked by holding the scapula posteriorly fixed with one hand while putting the arm through attempted full abduction overhead.

The patient is positioned supine to reexamine the shoulder for signs of anterior subluxation. With the patient's shoulder at 90 degrees of abduction and the elbow flexed 90 degrees, the examiner places one hand on the glenohumeral joint with the fingers posteriorly on the humeral head and the thumb anteriorly, with the other hand supporting the arm. The examiner applies an anteriorly directed stress to the humeral head to lever it anteriorly (Fig. 6–10). This maneuver is repeated at various degrees of increasing abduction up to the full overhead position while the examiner feels for anterior subluxation.

Posterior instability is assessed next. Frequently, throwing athletes demonstrate considerable posterior laxity, a normal finding for the throwing shoulder. The throwing arm is flexed forward and abducted while the examiner's hand provides a posteriorly directed stress with the thumb on the humeral head. The examiner can feel the posterior subluxation with his fingers placed posteriorly (Figs. 6–11 and 6–12). The posterior subluxation is reduced as the arm is brought back to an abducted position.

The prevalence of glenoid labrum tears in the throwing shoulder has recently been recognized. Therefore, it is important that this potentially correctable lesion be diagnosed clinically. The authors use the "clunk test" to make the clinical diagnosis of an anterior labrum tear (Fig. 6–13). This test is performed with the patient in the supine position. The examiner's hand is placed posteriorly on the humeral head, and the opposite hand holds the humeral condyles at the elbow to provide a rotating motion. The

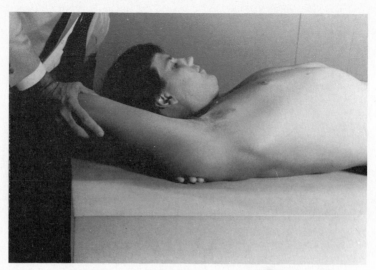

FIGURE 6–10. Testing for anterior subluxation.

patient's arm is brought into full overhead abduction, and the examiner's hand on the humeral head provides an anterior force while the opposite hand rotates the humerus. A "clunk" or grinding can be felt in the shoulder as the humerus hits or snaps on the labral tear to indicate a positive "clunk test."

Impingement of the greater tuberosity or rotator cuff against the acromion process or coracoacromial ligament can occur in throwing shoulders.

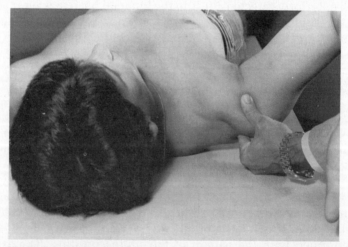

FIGURE 6–11. Assessing posterior instability. The examiner's hand provides posteriorly directed force using pressure of the thumb on the humeral head.

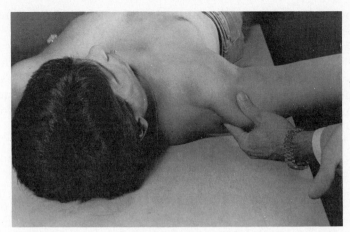

FIGURE 6–12. Posterior subluxation can be reduced when the arm is brought back to an abducted position.

This can lead to primary attrition tears of the rotator cuff and produce inflammation and edema in the subacromial bursa and biceps tendon. To elicit impingement, the arm is abducted with the shoulder in slight forward flexion. The scapula is fixed by firmly holding the top of the shoulder. Impingement also can be checked by internal rotation of the forward flexed arm with the scapula held in a fixed position. These tests can be done with the patient sitting or supine. In a large athlete the supine position is better.

It should be emphasized that contrary to what is found in the general

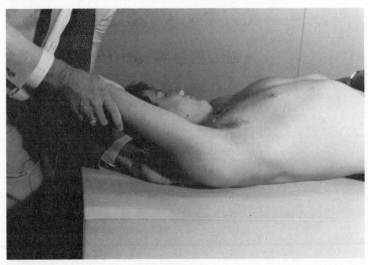

FIGURE 6–13. Method of performing the "clunk test" to diagnose anterior labral tear.

patient population, high-performance throwing athletes quite frequently develop tears in the rotator cuff that begin on the deep rather than the superficial portion of the rotator cuff. Presumably this is caused by extreme tension on the undersurface of the cuff during the throwing motion and the rapid deceleration of the shoulder. Hence, findings on examination for these types of lesions do not necessarily mimic the typical findings in nonthrowing athletes, and the examiner must observe closely for subtle clues.

The biceps tendon area can be palpated while the patient is in the supine position. With the shoulder at 90 degrees of abduction and neutral rotation, the bicondylar axis of the elbow is grasped by the examiner with elbow in one hand while the other hand palpates the anterior shoulder (Fig. 6–14). The elbow is then internally rotated 15 degrees to point the biceps tendon and bicipital groove directly toward the ceiling and to make it easily palpable. Palpation of the biceps tendon can be facilitated by lowering the arm off the table toward the floor, to bowstring the tendon and make it more prominent. Next the humerus is internally and externally rotated while the biceps tendon and groove are palpated. This motion allows the examiner to feel any snap or pop if the tendon is subluxating out of the bicipital groove. Pain elicited along the biceps tendon or the groove suggests bicipital tendinitis or injury to the biceps tendon-labrum complex.

The anatomic landmarks are again identified anteriorly. The anterior acromion and coracoid processes act as reference points to guide further palpation of the anterior muscles in search for tenderness (Fig. 6–15). The anterior deltoid muscle can be palpated. The arm is internally rotated and

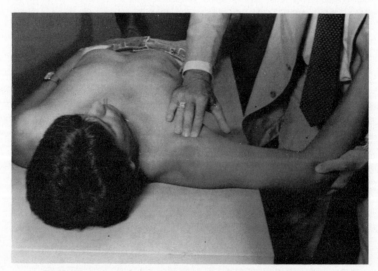

FIGURE 6–14. Palpating the long head of the biceps tendon.

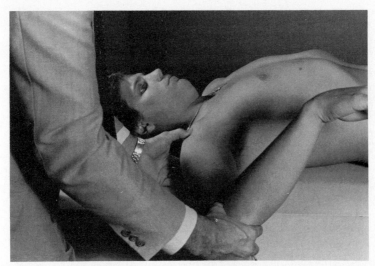

FIGURE 6–15. Palpating the anterior muscles to look for isolated tenderness.

adducted across the patient's chest to allow palpation of the supraspinatus tendon area just anterior to the acromion process. The infraspinatus tendon muscle can also be palpated more posteriorly, as can the teres minor. Rotator cuff tears in throwing athletes more commonly involve the supraspinatus or infraspinatus tendons, or a combination of both, rather than the teres minor.

The final position of the patient for examining the throwing shoulder is lying in the prone position. The throwing arm is allowed to fully relax and is lowered over the side of the examining table with the elbow extended and pointing directly toward the floor. This brings the posterior deltoid muscle forward and allows further palpation of the posterior rotator cuff muscles (Fig. 6–16). The quadrilateral space can also be palpated inferior to the teres minor muscle near its insertion, anterior to the long head of the triceps, and posterior to the humerus. This area very rarely can be the site of compression on the axillary nerve and posterior humeral circumflex artery as they exit the quadrilateral space.

With the patient in the prone position the posterior capsule can be palpated just above the teres minor muscle at the glenohumeral joint. The posterior capsule can be a source of chronic inflammation owing to stretching or even avulsion from its scapular attachment. This injury can cause localized calcification of the posterior capsule that can be diagnosed using radiographs.

True internal and external rotation of the glenohumeral joint can be confirmed once again while the patient is lying in the prone position. The examiner holds the scapula fixed and internally and externally rotates the humerus to the extremes of motion while the shoulder is held at 90 degrees

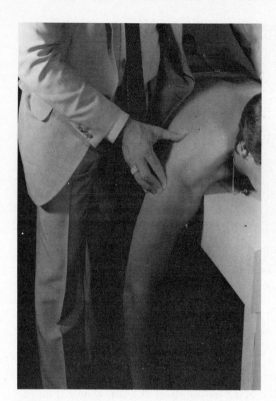

FIGURE 6–16. Palpating the posterior cuff muscles: the teres minor and infraspinatus.

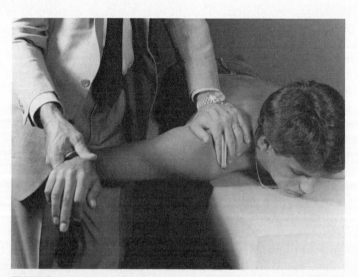

FIGURE 6–17. Measuring true internal and external rotation of the glenohumeral joint in the prone position.

of horizontal abduction (Fig. 6–17). This maneuver can lead to diagnosis of contractures of the glenohumeral joint.

ADDITIONAL DIAGNOSTIC PROCEDURES

Radiographic examination should include an anteroposterior view in internal and external rotation and a transaxillary lateral view and occasionally the West Point view. Other diagnostic studies that can be performed are double contrast shoulder arthrography or arthrotomography. Diagnostic arthroscopy provides an outstanding method of evaluating shoulder pathology in throwing athletes, since it allows examination under anesthesia.

Shoulder evaluation should routinely include a full neurologic assessment and examination of related areas such as the cervical spine and elbow that can cause shoulder symptoms.

SHOULDER ARTHROTOMOGRAPHY IN THE EVALUATION OF THE INJURED THROWING ARM

JOHN ALBRIGHT, M.D. / GEORGES EL KHOURY, M.D.

INTRODUCTION

A detailed history, skillful physical examination, and proper interpretation of appropriate baseline radiographic studies are usually sufficient to establish the correct diagnosis and proper treatment for most shoulder disorders. On the other hand, persistent pain, particularly in the shoulder of the pitcher, quarterback, javelin thrower, gymnast, or swimmer, presents a challenging problem in both diagnosis and management. The purpose of this article is to describe arthrotomography and its role in the evaluation of the throwing athlete's shoulder. Knowledge in this field, indications, and limitations will be updated, especially with respect to an earlier report on this subject.[1]

In athletes with persistent symptoms subluxation should be considered as a possible underlying cause. Until proved otherwise, a subluxating shoulder should be considered to be the result of a tear of the anterior glenoid labrum and/or an excessive degree of capsular laxity.[2] However, the diagnosis of subluxation is often very difficult to establish, since the complaints are usually vague and varied. On examination it is difficult to sort out symptoms caused by subluxation and those from other causes.

Arthroscopy has improved the diagnostic accuracy in disorders of the shoulder joint. However, this technique is invasive and requires general anesthesia and a significant recovery period. With the development of arthroscopy the need still existed for a simple outpatient diagnostic technique not requiring general anesthesia. The authors therefore devised the technique of arthrotomography, which is a radiographic technique combining the standard method of double contrast arthrography with the unique clarity of multidirectional tomography.

THE TECHNIQUE

Although the radiographic technique has been described in detail elsewhere,[3] it is reviewed here. Routine anteroposterior and axillary views are obtained prior to performing arthrotomography. The patient is then placed in a supine position under the fluoroscope. The shoulder is prepared and draped to create a sterile field. The skin is anesthetized with lidocaine 1 per cent. Four ml of 60 per cent Renografin and 10 ml of room air are injected from an anterior direction into the shoulder joint under fluoroscopic control through a 22-gauge spinal needle. After confirmation that the double contrast material is within the joint, the needle is withdrawn. The patient is asked to sit up and to move the shoulder about gently. A routine anteroposterior film can be obtained to rule out rotator cuff tear or to look for excessive intra-capsular volume.

For the tomographic procedure exact positioning is required: the patient's arm is extended superiorly, and the axilla is forced flush to the table top so that the glenoid surface and the scapular wing are oriented perpendicularly to the plane of the film. Thin-section multidirectional tomography is then performed at 3-mm intervals. With this technique consistently fine detail can be obtained for a diagnostic examination that outlines the glenohumeral joint in cross section, including the entire labrum, the chondral surface, the bony architecture, and the capsule. This positioning also allows identification of the clavicle and the anterior portions of the rib cage to assist the interpreter in the orientation of the film. Small numbers on the film indicate the depths of focus that correlate with the inferior portion of the labrum.

INTERPRETATIONS

Normal Anatomy

The labrum is a hoop of pliable fibrous tissue attached to the peripheral edge of the saucer-like glenoid cavity. In cross section the labrum is triangular, with its thin edge pointing outward. It has a base-to-apex height

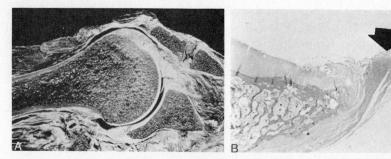

FIGURE 7–1. Normal anatomy. *(A)* Cross section of the glenohumeral joint showing the contiguous articular surfaces of the glenoid cavity and labrum. *(B)* Microscopic section of the glenoid-labrum junction. Note the smooth transition from the hyaline articular cartilage of the glenoid cavity to the fibrous tissue at the tip of the labrum *(arrow)*. (Reprinted, with permission, from McGlynn, F. J., EI-Khoury, G., and Albright, J. P., "Arthrotomography of the glenoid labrum in shoulder instability." *Journal of Bone and Joint Surgery* 64A:515, 1982.)

of about 0.5 cm. Both the glenoid and the labrum are joined to articulate with the oversized humeral head at the lateral border of the scapula. The fibrocartilaginous zone at the base of the labrum has a smooth transition from the fibrous tissue of the outer rim to the hyaline cartilage lining of the slightly concave glenoid cavity (Figure 7–1). The glenohumeral joint is the most mobile joint in the body, and the small fulcrum provided by the glenoid fossa is never in contact with more than one quarter of the articular surface of the humeral head.[4] The glenoid labrum makes this small bony saucer somewhat wider and deeper. Its function appears to be to provide a restraint to abnormal translational "slipping" of the oversized humeral head during use of the shoulder.

The glenoid labrum is often compared to the knee meniscus because they are similar in color, consistency, and triangular shape. However, the structure and function of the labrum are quite dissimilar to those of the meniscus. First, the labrum is a redundant portion of capsule that consists mostly of fibrous tissue with many elastic fibers.[5, 6] Secondly, its base attaches directly to and is contiguous with the glenoid articular surface. Third, rather than being interposed between incongruent bony surfaces, the free labral edge extends beyond the limits of the glenoid cavity. Finally, the labrum does not function as a shock absorber in the same manner as does the knee meniscus.

In the arthrotomogram of the normal glenohumeral joint the anterior and posterior lips of the labrum appear in all sections as sharp lucent triangles that are continuous with the lucent articular cartilage covering to the glenoid cavity. The labrum extends beyond the bony edge of the glenoid cavity. In most views the anterior labrum has the configuration of an elongated triangle[1] with an acute angle at the apex of the free edge. The free edge of the posterior labrum is normally more rounded but often is symmetric with its anterior counterpart. The peripheral surface of the posterior labrum is usually more completely outlined by contrast media than is the anterior labrum, owing to filling of the posterior capsular recess.

Pathologic Findings

Contrast material violates the free triangular edge of the glenoid structure on more than one consecutive exposure when there is pathology of the glenoid rim and labrum. The authors classify the pathologic findings in three grades radiographically according to the type and location of pathology: (I) a well-defined defect in the body of the labrum; (II) complete absence of the labrum but a normal contour of the glenoid rim; and (III) a defect involving the bony structure of the glenoid cavity itself.

Degenerative changes in the joint cause subtle thinning or irregularity of the normally even and smooth articular surfaces. Bony indentations seen on polytomographic views can be caused by Hill-Sachs lesions that are large enough to also be seen on plain films. Excessively distended joint capsules have been noted in patients with recurrent multidirectional instability. Rupture of the capsule and rotator cuff in the area of the supraspinatus tendon attachment allows contrast material to flow into the subdeltoid bursa. Degeneration of the rotator cuff may be detected by thinning of the capsule in this area, but this is a very subtle finding.

Grade I Labral Defects. In the authors' experience the most common tears of the labrum occur through the attachment of the base of the labrum to the anterior bony glenoid rim (Fig. 7–2). Recently such tears have also been seen in the posterior aspect of the joint. Occasionally injury to the fibrous substance of the labrum is detected, including distinct midbody tears, as well as irregularities, attenuation, or blunting of the lucent triangle. This latter situation may represent disruption and even displacement of the outer rim fragment. Such displacement leads to comparison of labrum tears

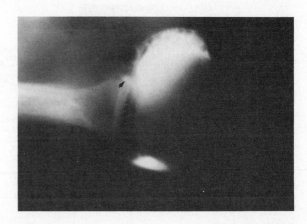

FIGURE 7–2. Grade I labral defect. Contrast material obscures the base of the normally lucent triangle *(arrow)*.

of knee menisci; both phonomena are associated with catching, popping, and locking symptoms.

Grade II Labral Defects. Complete segmental absence of the labrum, without damage to the glenoid rim, has been seen in many patients with long-term histories of recurrent dislocations (Fig. 7–3). At the time of surgery the authors have documented absence of the glenoid rim and frequently have observed capsular redundancy. Although no fracture fragment can be identified, a periosteal reaction may be seen at the site of capsular attachment. This reactive tissue also may be identified on plain axillary views. Occasionally a concomitant indentation of the posterior humeral head (Hill-Sachs lesion) has been noted.

Grade III Labral Defects. Shoulders in which a bony lesion extends through the substance of the glenoid rim are included in this category. This lesion was first described by Bankart in 1923.[7] There may be a fracture fragment (Fig. 7–4) as well as blunting of the usually sharp edge of the glenoid (Fig. 7–5). A Hill-Sachs lesion may also be present. Both Bankart and Hill-Sachs lesions are often seen in the unstable joint after multiple dislocations. Although the pathology may remain undetected until the time of the arthrotomogram, routine anteroposterior and axillary views often establish the diagnosis in this category.

INDICATIONS

Multidirectional tomography of the shoulder with double contrast material is the most useful technique for evaluating the cross-sectional profile of the glenoid labrum, the articular surfaces of the joint, as well as the bony architecture of the glenoid fossa and the head of the humerus. Plain "scout film" radiographs taken before as well as after injection of double contrast material are also useful in assessing the integrity of the

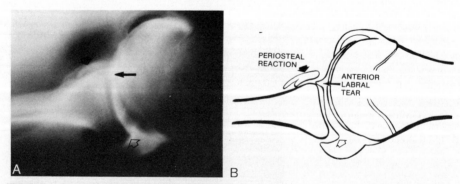

FIGURE 7–3. Grade II labral defect. The posterior labrum is intact *(outlined arrow)*. The anterior labrum is absent, but bony integrity is intact *(thin solid arrow)*. Note the periosteal reaction at the attachment of the capsule *(arrowhead)*.

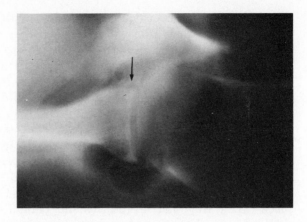

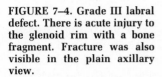

FIGURE 7–4. Grade III labral defect. There is acute injury to the glenoid rim with a bone fragment. Fracture was also visible in the plain axillary view.

capsule and rotator cuff, the volume of the synovial cavity, and the status of the biceps tendon in its groove.

Arthrotomography can be useful in situations in which the patient has shoulder pain, weakness, or instability but the diagnosis cannot be made using less expensive means.

As reported earlier,[1] the majority of patients who had this procedure performed at the University of Iowa were either athletes or active individuals who required vigorous shoulder use. With few exceptions all patients had one or more of the following findings: (1) a history of recurrent dislocations; (2) a positive apprehension test result for anterior or posterior dislocation; (3) the ability to voluntarily dislocate the shoulder; (4) evidence of excessive glenohumeral translation during stress testing; (5) positional differences in isometric arm strength; (6) a history of persistent painful locking, popping, or sudden "giving way" of the shoulder; or (7) a "dead arm" type of weakness emanating from deep within the shoulder, even in the absence of clinical instability.[8]

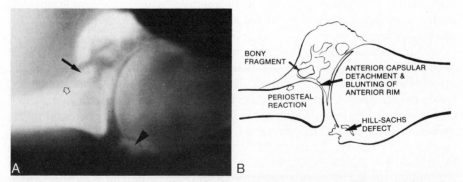

FIGURE 7–5. Grade III labral defect. The patient had chronic shoulder instability after multiple dislocations. Erosion of the glenoid rim, a Hill-Sachs lesion of the humeral head, a detached fragment of the glenoid rim, and a periosteal reaction are apparent.

When the subtle instability associated with subluxation is suspected, the stress and strength tests mentioned earlier have proved very helpful. For the *translational stress test* the patient lies supine with the involved shoulder closest to the examiner. The humerus is then abducted to 90 degrees and flexed or extended to the position in which symptoms usually occur. One of the examiner's hands is placed deep in the patient's axilla over the glenohumeral joint line or at least over the most proximal portion of the humeral head that is palpable. The other hand is placed on the humeral head on the side directly opposite the first. With the patient's muscles relaxed, attempts are then made to translate the humeral head on the glenoid in all directions. Subluxation is defined as excessive translational motion to the point at which the joint is recognized as being "out of place" in a way that reproduces the patient's symptoms. The type of subluxation is determined by the direction in which the humeral head was forced out of the glenoid cavity.

The second test for subtle shoulder joint instability involves the demonstration of positional differences in shoulder girdle strength by the patient. For the *positional strength test* the patient again lies supine on the examination table with the examiner standing at the patient's side, just caudal to the level of the shoulders. Then with the patient's arm in the overhead position and his hand held directly above his head, the examiner grasps the middle to distal forearm in order to provide resistance from a mechanically advantageous position. After being informed of the nature of the test, the patient is then instructed to push forward against the examiner's resisting hand with a maximal effort while stabilizing himself with his opposite hand. This strength test is then repeated several times with the arm moved progressively forward, through a neutral plane of adduction, to positions in which angles of 135, 90, and 45 degrees are created with the frontal plane of the body.

For the sake of comparison, a semiquantitative assessment of the force generated and the symptoms produced is noted for each position of the arm. While strength is expected to be relative to position, any sudden or dramatic differences throughout the arc of motion should be compared with the opposite side.

A remarkable loss in strength becomes obvious when the patient is asked to generate a maximal straight-arm isometric flexion force with the arm held in a position in which the suspected portion of the labrum is being called upon to provide a fulcrum against the shear forces generated across the glenohumeral joint: more specifically, the position cranial to the glenohumeral joint. The diagnosis of instability is made with greater assurance if the weakness found on examination is associated with the symptoms of subluxation and if that sensation reproduces the patient's symptoms during throwing, serving in tennis, using the Nautilus upper extremity machine, and in other activities.

Positional differences in strength of patients with posterior glenohumeral subluxation are best tested for in the push-up position with the arm abducted 90 degrees and the elbow flexed. The patient is then asked to push directly forward against the examiner's hand from a variety of positions of shoulder flexion-extension in which the elbow lies posterior, even, and anterior to the glenohumeral joint when the force is being generated. Apparent positional weakness should be obvious in comparison with the opposite arm. The weakness and sensations of subluxation should also correlate with the patient's history of difficulty during attempted bench presses, push-ups, basketball chest passes, warding off opposing blockers in football, and so forth.

These two tests, when used as part of the routine shoulder examination, are useful for differentiating excess physiologic laxity in athletes involved in repetitive throwing from pathologic conditions.

Routine radiographs are taken prior to arthrotomography to detect pathology. These include axillary as well as anteroposterior radiographs with the humerus rotated about 70 degrees internally and externally. Computed tomographic scans of both shoulders are obtained whenever there is a question concerning the angle of the glenoid surface or the extent of a bony defect.

Examination under anesthesia and diagnostic arthroscopy are not part of the routine screening procedure. They are used mainly (1) when the diagnosis remains unclear after arthrotomography, and (2) when the surgical treatment of the suspected defect of the labrum is to be attempted through the arthroscope.

LIMITATIONS AND CONTRAINDICATIONS

Sensitivity to iodine or any other component of the injection material and the presence of an active skin infection are both contraindications to this procedure. The authors have had no adverse reactions to shoulder arthrotomography. A history of previous surgery makes it more difficult to inject the contrast materials into the joint. However, this may not present a major technical difficulty after some expertise has been developed. Although the situation has not yet been encountered, there may be cases in which the pathology is located in the superior glenoid near the attachment of the biceps tendon. A change in the position of the patient on the table may make it easier to demonstrate the pathology in this instance.

RESULTS AND DISCUSSION

In 1982 the authors reported their initial results after reviewing 38 arthrotomograms from the first 37 patients[1] who had either subluxation

(28), pain without subluxation (7), or voluntary instability (2). Twenty-five of the 28 patients with painful subluxation demonstrated obvious pathology on arthrogram, while none of the other 9 patients did. For the 21 patients who underwent a surgical procedure there was a 95 per cent correlation between the results of the radiograpic studies and the operative findings.

The authors have now performed 110 procedures. This additional experience has not changed indications for the procedure or the accuracy of arthrotomography in making a diagnosis in disorders of the shoulder joint. Although the formal review of the updated results has not yet been completed, several comments about the continuing experience with this procedure are appropriate.

The stress and strength tests developed to screen for instability in the awake patient have continued to be reliable predictors that pathology of the labrum is to be found with arthrotomography. This is in conflict with the results recently reported by Kleinman et al.,[9] who found that over one half of the patients with tears of the labrum had no clinical evidence of instability. This difference may be explained by a variation in the method and the sensitivity of the physical examinations used.

In findings similar to those of Pappas and coworkers,[1] the authors did find a small number of cases of functional instability in which Grade I tears with filling defects in the labral body were documented at arthroscopy. These cases were longitudinal tears of either the incomplete "bucket-handle" or free-end type. The patients had stable shoulders at examination but complaints of intermittent pain and weakness, popping, or locking. The authors' limited experience supports the observation that when the mobile labrum fragment is displaced, blunting and irregularity of the remaining attached portion are often the only visible evidence of pathology.

The authors have been encountering of an increasing number of posterior labral defect over the past several years. Of the original 37 patients, there were only one with a posterior and 24 with anterior defects of the labrum. However, more recent experience is more consistent with that of Boyd, with approximately 10 to 15 per cent of positive studies demonstrating posterior pathology.[10] The possibility that a posterior defect exists can have a great bearing on the course of treatment. The authors had one patient who had both anterior and posterior labral tears in the same shoulder.

Symptomatic shoulder subluxation appears to be much more common than previously had been thought and is often associated with pathology of the glenoid labrum.[1, 2, 11–22] The role that minor glenohumeral instabilities and impingement may play in these conditions is gradually becoming more clear as knowledge of this joint increases. Kleinman et al. reported that the greatest utility for shoulder arthrotomography may be for patients with pain but without clinical evidence of instability.[8]

The authors' experience is similar to that of others[2, 9] that patients with negative arthrographic results usually respond well to nonoperative treatment. On the contrary, patients with pathology of the labrum are unlikely to obtain relief of symptoms without surgical intervention.

SUMMARY

Arthrotomography of the shoulder is a simple and accurate tool that can be used in the diagnosis of shoulder disorders. It is a minimally invasive screening method for detecting intra-articular pathology. The authors believe it is the best radiograpic technique for demonstrating abnormalities of the glenoid labrum. The most common indications for the procedure are to confirm the diagnosis when subluxation is suspected or to diagnose the shoulder with pain or weakness, or both.

REFERENCES

1. McGlynn, F. J., El-Khoury, G., and Albright, J. P.: Arthrotomography of the glenoid labrum in shoulder instability. J Bone Joint Surg 64A:506, 1982.
2. Pappas, A. M., Goss, T. P., and Kleinman, P. K.: Symptomatic shoulder instability due to lesions of the glenoid labrum. Am J Sports Med 11:279, 1983.
3. El-Khoury, G. Y., Albright, J. P., and Abu Yousef, M. M., Montgomery, W. J., and Tuck, S. L.: Arthrotomography of the glenoid labrum. Radiology 131:333, 1979.
4. Bost, F. C., and Inman, V. T.: The pathological changes in recurrent dislocation of the shoulder. A report of Bankart's operative procedure. J Bone Joint Surg 24A:595, 1942.
5. Gardner, E.: The prenatal development of the human shoulder joint. Surg Clin North Am 43:1465, 1963.
6. Moseley, H. F., and Overgaard, B.: The anterior capsular mechanism in recurrent anterior dislocation of the shoulder. Morphological and clinical studies. J Bone Joint Surg 44B:913, 1962.
7. Bankart, A. S. B.: The pathology and treatment of recurrent dislocation of the shoulder joint. Br J Surg 26:23, 1938.
8. Rowe, C. R., and Zarins, B.: Recurrent transient subluxation of the shoulder. J Bone Joint Surg 63:163, 1981.
9. Kleinman, P. K., Kanzarin, P. K., Goss, T. P., and Pappas, A. M.: Axillary arthrotomography of glenoid labrum. Am J Roentgenol 142:993, 1984.
10. Boyd, H. B., and Sisk, T. D.: Recurrent posterior dislocation of the shoulder. J Bone Joint Surg 54A:799, 1972.
11. Blazing, M. E., and Satzman, J. S.: Recurrent anterior subluxation of the shoulder in athletics—a distinct entity. J Bone Joint Surg 51A:1037, 1969.
12. Booth, R. E., Jr., and Marvel, J. P., Jr.: Differential diagnosis of shoulder pain. Orthop Clin North Am 6:353, 1975.
13. Bateman, J. E.: The Shoulder and Neck. 2nd ed. Philadelphia, W. B. Saunders Company, 1978.
14. DePalma, A. F.: Surgery of the Shoulder. 2nd ed. Philadelphia, J. B. Lippincott Company, 1973.
15. LeClerc, J.: Chronic subluxation of the shoulder. In Proceedings of the Dewar Orthopaedic Club. J Bone Joint Surg 51B:778, 1969.
16. Morton, K. S.: The unstable shoulder: Recurring subluxation. J Bone Joint Surg 59B:508, 1977.
17. Neer, C. S., II, and Foster, C. R.: Inferior capsular shift for involuntary inferior and multidirectional instability of the shoulder. A preliminary report. J Bone Joint Surg 62A:879, 1980.
18. Protzman, R. R.: Anterior instability of the shoulder. J Bone Joint Surg 62A:909, 1980.
19. Rockwood, C. A., Jr.: Subluxation of the shoulder: The classification, diagnosis, and treatment. Orthop Trans 4:306, 1979.
20. Rowe, C. R., Pierce, D. S., and Clark, J. G.: Voluntary dislocation of the shoulder. A preliminary report on a clinical, electromyographic, and psychiatric study of twenty-six patients. J Bone Joint Surg 55A:445, 1973.
21. Rowe, C. R., Patel, D., and Southmayd, W. W.: The Bankart procedure. A long term end-results study. J Bone Joint Surg 60A:1, 1978.
22. Rutledge, B. J.: In O'Donoghue, D. H. (ed.): Treatment of Injuries to Athletes. Philadelphia, W. B. Saunders Company, 1976, p. 211.

ARTHROSCOPY OF THE SHOULDER: TECHNIQUE

BERTRAM ZARINS, M.D.

Shoulder arthroscopy is the direct visualization of the interior of the glenohumeral joint through a small-diameter telescope. This new method allows the precise diagnosis of most intra-articular causes of shoulder dysfunction. Shoulder arthroscopy has improved the accuracy of diagnosis and treatment of athletic injuries to the shoulder and has caused modifications in many time-honored concepts of shoulder pathophysiology. This chapter describes a standard technique of shoulder arthroscopy and stresses details of the operative setup and selection of portal locations.

GENERAL PRINCIPLES

Arthroscopy is performed under sterile conditions in the operating room. The patient is positioned lying on the side with the arm held abducted by skin traction. The arthroscope is introduced through a posterior portal. The procedure can be carried out under local or general anesthesia. A standard 4- or 5-millimeter 30-degree oblique arthroscope is used. The joint is kept distended with saline or Ringer's lactated solution. Intermittent inflow and outflow to maintain clear visualization are accomplished through the arthroscope sheath. Accessory instruments for arthroscopic surgery or inflow can be introduced through an anterior or second posterior portal.

PROCEDURE

Patient Positioning

After satisfactory induction of general anesthesia with endotracheal intubation, the patient is positioned in the lateral decubitus position with the shoulder to be examined by arthroscopy directed upward (Fig. 8–1). The upper knee in this position is flexed, and a pillow is placed between the two knees. The pelvis is stabilized with 4-inch–wide adhesive tape going across the iliac crest and secured to the operating table. Skin traction straps are applied to the forearm and held in place with elastic bandages. The straps are connected by a rope to a 10-pound weight via a pulley. The pulley is attached to a pole that is held to the operating table in a stirrup holder clamp. The clamp is in place on the side of the table toward the anterior aspect of the patient at approximately the level of the knees. The pole is elevated to a height of approximately 4 feet above the table. This keeps the arm in a position of approximately 45 degrees of abduction and 30 degrees of forward flexion. Attaching the pulley and weight to the operating table adds a safety factor to prevent excessive traction on the arm if the table is suddenly lowered.

Draping

Routine skin preparation is carried out. Sterile drapes, including a waterproof sheet, are placed around the shoulder. A towel covers the forearm and is wrapped with a circular gauze bandage. This bandage is covered lengthwise with an adhesive sterile drape.

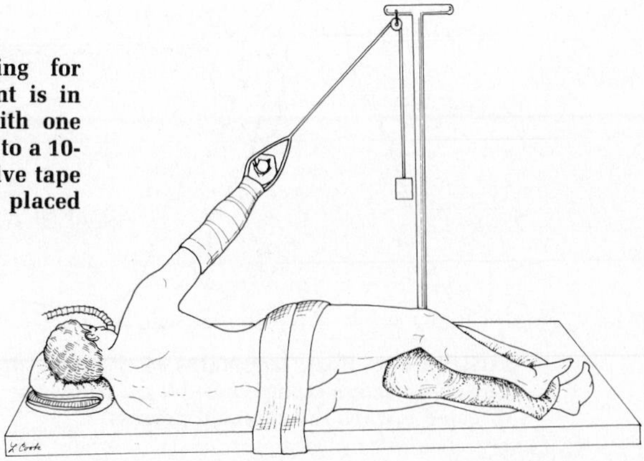

FIGURE 8–1. Patient positioning for shoulder arthroscopy. The patient is in the lateral decubitus position with one arm suspended with skin traction to a 10-pound weight by a pulley. Adhesive tape stabilizes the pelvis; a pillow is placed between the knees.

Introducing the Arthroscope

The acromion, the acromial angle, and the posterior border of the acromial process should be palpated. A soft spot is located approximtely 1 to 2 cm below the acromial angle on the posterior aspect of the shoulder. This area is infiltrated with 5 ml of bupivacaine 0.5 per cent with epinephrine 1:200,000. A 20-gauge spinal needle is passed into the posterior site by aiming slightly below the acromial process toward the tip of the coracoid. A finger of the physician's free hand is placed on the tip of the coracoid process to serve as a landmark. The shoulder joint is distended with 50 cc of saline or Ringer's lactated solution. Backflow of the fluid confirms correct placement of the needle in the joint. A 5-mm skin incision is made. The arthroscope sheath with a sharp obturator is passed in the same direction as the spinal needle entering the posterior aspect of the glenohumeral joint. The instrument is directed slightly below the acromion process and aimed toward the coracoid process (Fig. 8–2). A pop into the shoulder joint and outflow of fluid confirm correct placement in the superior aspect of the glenohumeral joint. The arthroscope is inserted, and the inflow and suction tubing are connected directly to the sheath.

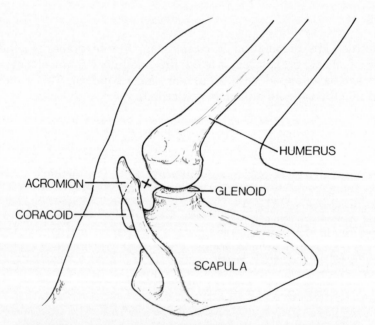

FIGURE 8–2. Bony landmarks of the right shoulder, posterior view. The arthroscope is introduced 2 cm below the acromial angle (x) and directed toward the coracoid process.

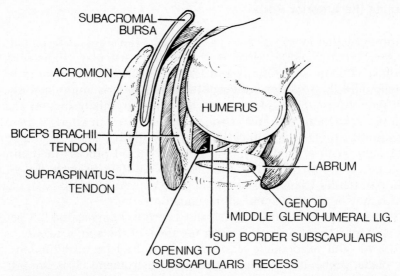

FIGURE 8–3. Anatomic landmarks, right shoulder, as seen by arthroscopy through the posterior portal. The arthroscope can also be introduced into the subacromial bursa to view the rotator cuff from above. LIG. = ligament; SUP. = superior.

Systematic Visualization

The long head of the biceps brachii tendon inserting into the postero-superior aspect of the glenoid cavity is consistently the most useful intra-articular landmark with which to begin visualization (Fig. 8–3). After identification of the biceps tendon the arthroscope is rotated to look toward the proximal aspect of the joint. This area is the supraspinatus tendon that inserts into the humerus. The supraspinatus tendon is followed medially to the superior glenoid recess. Visualization is continued along the posterior glenoid recess to the inferior glenoid recess. In this way the inferior portion of the glenohumeral joint is reached. Next the glenoid labrum is traced starting from its inferior aspect along the posterior rim of the glenoid recess to return to the superior aspect (to the origin of the biceps tendon). Proceeding distally along the anterior aspects of the joint leads to a vertical structure, the superior border of the subscapularis (incorrectly called middle glenohumeral ligament on occasion). Just proximal to the subscapularis tendon, close to the glenoid, is the opening into the subscapularis bursa. With the assistant applying manual traction on the patient's arm to distract the glenohumeral joint, visualization should proceed along the anterior glenoid labrum. The physician should look for the middle and inferior glenohumeral ligaments. The articular cartilage of the glenoid cavity should be inspected along with the attachment of the labrum to the glenoid. The articular surface of the humeral head is viewed by rotating the humerus to increase the area that is seen.

Selecting the Anterior Portal

Intra-articular landmarks are used to select the site for placement of an accessory anterior portal (Fig. 8–4). An intra-articular triangle can be identified as bounded by the biceps tendon superiorly, the glenoid labrum medially, and the superior border of the subscapularis anterolaterally. The tip of the arthroscope is advanced to the center of this triangular space to touch the synovium. The area is transilluminated in an effort to detect the light shining through the skin of the anterior shoulder. The coracoid process is palpated. With a position lateral to the coracoid process maintained, a spinal needle is introduced, aiming toward the light to enter the joint in the intra-articular triangle. The telescope is withdrawn slightly to visually confirm the correct placement of the spinal needle.

When the proper location has been selected, bupivacaine 0.5 per cent with epinephrine is infiltrated along the track of the spinal needle as it is withdrawn. This exact angle of entry must be used for introduction of the knife blade, probe, arthroscope, or surgical instruments. It is important to stay lateral to the coracoid process with this portal to avoid neurovascular structures.

Second Posterior Portal

If a second posterior portal is required, it is positioned 2 to 3 cm distal to the first, at the same distance from the glenoid cavity. The arthroscope that is already in the joint is used as an external guide for proper angle and

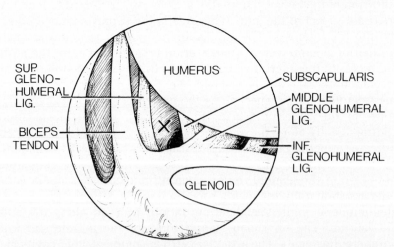

FIGURE 8–4. Intra-articular landmarks used to select the location of an anterior portal (x). The biceps tendon (superior) and the subscapularis tendon (inferior) are the most consistent and easy to locate. LIG. = ligament; INF. = inferior.

position of the second posterior portal. To avoid injury to the axillary nerve this portal should not be positioned more distally than the limit of the articular cartilage on the humeral head.

Technique Under Local Anesthesia

Patient positioning and basic technique are the same as when using general anesthesia. A mixture of equal volumes of lidocaine 0.5 per cent with epinephrine 1:200,000 mixed with bupivacaine 0.5 per cent should be used. The extra-articular tissues leading to the posterior portal should be infiltrated using this solution. The spinal needle is introduced from the posterior approach, and 50 cc of lidocaine 1/8 per cent solution is instilled to distend the joint.

Finishing

At the close of the arthroscopic procedure, the joint is thoroughly irrigated, and excess fluid is aspirated. The portals are closed very loosely using simple sutures. A sling can be worn for several days for patient comfort. Pendulum exercises are begun early to maintain passive joint motion.

Arthroscopy of Subacromial Bursa

The arthroscope can be introduced through a posterior approach into the subacromial bursa to view the rotator cuff from the superior aspect. This approach can give good visualization of the supraspinatus tendon to look for rotator cuff tears, tendinitis, and calcification. The portal for entry into the subacromial bursa is located on the posterolateral aspect of the shoulder slightly less than 1 cm below the level of the acromion just lateral to the acromial angle. A posterolateral rather than a straight lateral approach is best.

PRECAUTIONS AND POTENTIAL COMPLICATIONS

Patient Positioning and General Setup

The endotracheal or respirator tubing must not be secured to a tube holder that is fixed to the operating table. The patient is often pulled forward and backward when traction is applied to the arm to distract the joint. This motion can dislodge the endotracheal tube. Careful positioning of the patient on the operating table is necessary to avoid excessive pressure points.

Applying excessive traction to the arm with the patient under anesthesia and muscle relaxation is a potential hazard. Traction must not be applied in positions of elevation above 90 degrees. The rope that attaches to the skin traction straps must not be secured to an immovable object such as a hook on the wall because if the table is inadvertently lowered excessive traction can be applied to the shoulder.

Location of Portals

The location of the axillary nerve should be considered in making a distal posterior portal. For anterior portals, instruments should be kept lateral to the coracoid process to avoid injury to neurovascular structures. If the patient is not completely in the lateral decubitus position, external landmarks are altered. When manual traction is applied to the arm, the lateral decubitus position may be altered during the procedure.

General Problems

The soft tissues around the shoulder joint infiltrate quickly with fluid used to distend the joint. The irrigation fluid leaks out more easily than it does in the knee, and extravasation of fluid into the soft tissues becomes a time-limiting factor.

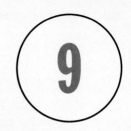

ARTHROSCOPY OF THE SHOULDER: NORMAL ANATOMY

WILLIAM G. CARSON, JR., M.D.

INTRODUCTION

Arthroscopy of the shoulder has been shown to be particularly effective in evaluating the throwing athlete's shoulder.[1-5] To be effective, however, arthroscopic examination of the shoulder must be performed in a systemic and reproducible fashion. In addition, a knowledge of the normal anatomy of the shoulder and variations of normal are necessary for those performing this procedure.

This chapter describes the normal arthroscopic anatomy of the shoulder as seen from the posterior approach. The technique of gaining entrance into the shoulder joint through this approach is discussed in the preceding chapter.

ARTHROSCOPIC ANATOMY

To insure a thorough and reproducible examination of the shoulder, arthroscopy should be performed in a systematic fashion. These structures (Fig. 9–1) should be identified in sequential order: (1) the biceps tendon, (2) the humeral head, (3) the glenoid cavity, (4) the glenoid labrum, (5) the superior, middle, and inferior glenohumeral ligaments, (6) the subscapularis tendon and recess, (7) the rotator cuff, and (8) the superior recess.

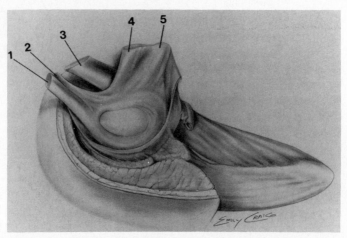

FIGURE 9–1. Arthroscopic anatomy of a right shoulder with the arm abducted 70 degrees: (1) long head of the biceps tendon, (2) superior glenohumeral ligament, (3) subscapularis tendon, (4) middle glenohumeral ligament, and (5) inferior glenohumeral ligament. The authors wish to thank *The American Journal of Sports Medicine* for permission to reprint material which appeared in Vol. 12, No. 1:1–7, Jan/Feb 1984.

Biceps Tendon. The biceps tendon is the first structure to be identified after entrance has been gained into the shoulder. This structure is the key to maintaining proper orientation during the examination. With the patient positioned in the lateral decubitus position, as described in the preceding chapter, the biceps tendon courses through the shoulder joint in a nearly vertical fashion, oriented approximately 10 to 15 degrees away from an imaginary vertical line. The tendon attaches to the supraglenoid tubercle at the posterosuperior aspect of the glenoid cavity and in this area is intimately related to, and continuous with, the glenoid labrum (Fig. 9–2). The normal biceps tendon should appear glistening, smooth, and free of adhesions, fraying, or partial tearing.

Humeral Head and Glenoid Cavity. After inspection of the biceps tendon is complete and proper orientation has been gained, the articular surfaces of the humeral head superiorly and of the glenoid cavity inferiorly are examined. The portion of the articular surface of the humeral head that can be examined from this angle is oriented at 30 degrees of retroversion and includes approximately one third of its circumference. Examination of the entire articular surface is facilitated by rotating the arthroscope superiorly and by rotating the humeral head into internal and external rotation. The glenoid cavity, a pear-shaped fossa approximately one fourth the size of the humeral head, should also be examined; it is important to keep in mind that the long head of the biceps tendon attaches to the posterosuperior aspect of the glenoid rim.

FIGURE 9–2. Arthroscopic anatomy of a right shoulder with the arm abducted 70 degrees as seen through the posterior portal: (1) superior recess, (2) long head of the biceps tendon, (3) subscapularis recess, (4) humeral head, (5) subscapularis tendon, and (6) glenoid labrum. Detachment of the anterior labrum from the glenoid (Bankart lesion) should be noted. The authors wish to thank *The American Journal of Sports Medicine* for permission to reprint material which appeared in Vol. 12, No. 1:1–7, Jan/Feb 1984.

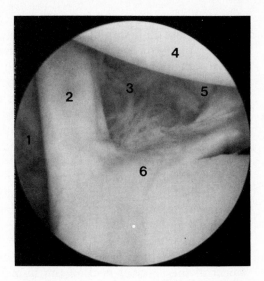

Glenoid Labrum. The glenoid labrum is a wedge-shaped structure that forms the border of the glenoid fossa and deepens this cavity to provide some inherent stability to the glenohumeral joint. The glenoid labrum restricts anterior and posterior humeral head excursion.[6, 7] The glenoid labrum has been described as consisting of cartilage, fibrocartilage, and fibrous tissue and having a surface continuous with the hyaline cartilage of the glenoid cavity; the capsular surface blends with the joint capsule.

The glenoid labrum should appear smooth without fraying, hypermobility, or tearing. Inspection begins at the long head of the biceps tendon's insertion through the superior portion of the labrum into the supraglenoid tubercle. The labrum is then followed anteriorly and inferiorly. Further distraction of the arm with the traction apparatus at this point facilitates visualization of the inferior rim. The posterior rim is examined by slightly retracting the arthroscope and rotating it posteriorly.

Glenohumeral Ligaments. The superior, middle, and inferior glenohumeral ligaments (Fig. 9–1) are thickenings of the anterior portion of the shoulder joint capsule that provide reinforcement to the anterior and inferior portions of the shoulder joint. These are visualized quite readily arthroscopically. Although much variation of these ligaments has been described,[8–12] their contribution to the stability of the shoulder joint has been well documented.[11, 13, 14]

When viewed arthroscopically the glenohumeral ligaments are anteriorly displaced secondary to fluid distension within the shoulder joint. In the normal physiologic state these ligaments lie much closer to the glenoid labrum. Occasionally they can be seen to have distinct labral origins rather than the usual capsular origins.

The superior glenohumeral ligament may be visualized near the insertion of the biceps tendon into the superior aspect of the glenoid cavity. This ligament courses laterally to insert on the anterior aspect of the anatomic neck of the humerus. Anatomic dissections have revealed the superior glenohumeral ligament to be the most consistent of the glenohumeral ligaments.[8] However, arthroscopically the superior glenohumeral ligament often is obscured by the biceps tendon.

The middle glenohumeral ligament extends from just beneath the superior glenohumeral ligament along the anterior border of the glenoid cavity to the junction of the middle and inferior one third of the glenoid rim. This ligament blends with the capsule of the anteroinferior aspect of the shoulder joint and also at times with the posterosuperior aspect of the subscapularis tendon. With the arm abducted 70 degrees the middle glenohumeral ligament is put in somewhat of a stretched position and is visualized quite readily.

The inferior glenohumeral ligament is a triangular ligament that arises from the anteroinferior margin of the labrum and inserts into the inferior aspect of the surgical neck of the humerus. It is located just beneath the middle glenohumeral ligament and is also visualized quite readily arthroscopically with the arm abducted 70 degrees.

With the arm abducted 70 degrees the posterosuperior edge of the subscapularis tendon (Fig. 9–1) is well visualized over the anterior aspect of the shoulder between the superior and middle glenohumeral ligaments. The subscapularis tendon may be obscured by the middle glenohumeral ligament and may appear to blend with this ligament.

The subscapularis recess is the area beneath the subscapularis tendon that is visualized over the anterior aspect of the shoulder joint in the region of the middle glenohumeral ligament (Fig. 9–3). There is much variation in the relationship between the middle glenohumeral ligament, the subscapularis tendon, and the subscapularis recess. Care should be taken not to diagnose a variation in the normal anatomy of the middle glenohumeral

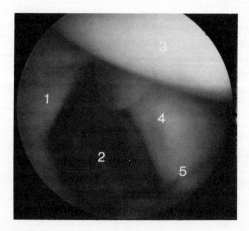

FIGURE 9–3. Area of the subscapularis tendon in a right shoulder as seen through the posterior portal: (1) long head of the biceps tendon, (2) subscapularis recess, (3) humeral head, (4) subscapularis tendon, and (5) middle glenohumeral ligament. The authors wish to thank *The American Journal of Sports Medicine* for permission to reprint material which appeared in Vol. 12, No. 1:1–7, Jan/Feb 1984.

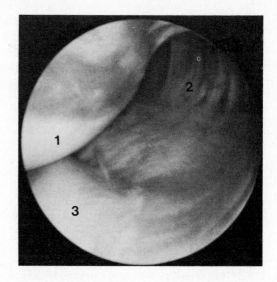

FIGURE 9–4. Arthroscopic view in a right shoulder as seen from the posterior portal. The arthroscope is directed posteriorly and superiorly, facilitating visualization of (1) the humeral head, (2) the posterior rotator cuff, and (3) the posterior portion of the glenoid labrum. The authors wish to thank *The American Journal of Sports Medicine* for permission to reprint material which appeared in Vol. 12, No. 1:1–7, Jan/Feb 1984.

ligament and subscapularis bursa as a traumatic rent in the anterior capsule. DePalma[7, 8] noted that in 41 per cent of his cadaveric dissections there was a superior subscapularis recess above the middle glenohumeral ligament and a second inferior subscapularis recess below it. In 32 per cent of his dissected specimens only one subscapularis recess was present, which was located superior to the middle glenohumeral ligament.

Rotator Cuff. Arthroscopic examination of the rotator cuff begins by once again identifying the biceps tendon and obtaining proper orientation. The supraspinatus tendon portion of the rotator cuff is visualized at a location just superior to the biceps tendon. Visualization is facilitated by rotating the arthroscope superiorly and slightly toward the humeral head. Slight posterior retraction of the arthroscope demonstrates the insertion of the tendinous cuff in the humeral head. The infraspinatus and teres minor tendon portions of the rotator cuff may be visualized by directing the arthroscope posteriorly and superiorly (Fig. 9–4).

Superior Recess. The superior recess is the area that is superior and slightly anterior to the insertion of the long head of the biceps tendon extending into the superior aspect of the glenoid cavity.

CONCLUSION

Shoulder arthroscopy is an effective means of evaluating and diagnosing the patient with chronic shoulder complaints, particularly the throwing athlete. For arthroscopy of the shoulder to be effective, the examination needs to be performed in a systematic fashion, utilizing the long head of the biceps tendon as the orienting landmark. Knowledge of the normal anatomy of the shoulder, as seen arthroscopically, as well as the variations of normal, is essential for the arthroscopic examination to be successful. The technique described in Chapter 8 and the technique of sequentially identifying the anatomic structures of the shoulder as described in this chapter have proved effective in producing a successful arthroscopic examination.

REFERENCES

1. Andrews, J. R., and Carson, W. G.: Arthroscopic surgery in throwing athletes with glenoid labrum tears. Orthop Trans 8:44, 1984.
2. Andrews, J. R., Carson, W. G., and Hughston, J. C.: Operative arthroscopy of the shoulder: A preliminary report. Orthop Trans 5:499, 1983.
3. Andrews, J. R., and Carson, W. G.: Shoulder joint arthroscopy. Orthopedics 6:1157, 1983.
4. Andrews, J. R., Carson, W. G., and Ortega, K.: Arthroscopy of the shoulder. Technique and normal anatomy. Am J Sports Med 12:1, 1984.
5. Carson, W. G., McLeod, W. D., and Andrews, J. R.: An analysis of the long head of the biceps tendon in relation to glenoid labrum tears. Am J Sports Med (accepted for publication).
6. Bankhart, A. S. B.: The pathology and treatment of recurrent dislocation of the shoulder joint. Br J Surg 26:23, 1938.
7. DePalma, A. F.: Surgery of the Shoulder. Philadelphia, J. B. Lippincott Company, 1973.
8. DePalma, A. F., Callery, G., and Bennett, G. A.: Variational anatomy and degenerative lesions of the shoulder joint. In Instructional Course Lectures of the American Academy of Orthopaedic Surgeons. Ann Arbor, Edwards, 6:255, 1949.
9. DePalma, A. F.: Degenerative lesions of the shoulder joint at various age groups which are compatible with good function. In Instructional Course Lectures of the American Academy of Orthopaedic Surgeons. Ann Arbor, Edwards, 7:168, 1950.
10. Flood, V.: Discovery of a new ligament of the shoulder joint. Lancet 672, 1829.
11. Mosely, J. F., and Overgaard: The anterior capsular mechanism in recurrent anterior dislocation of the shoulder. J Bone Joint Surg 44B:913, 1962.
12. Weitbrecht, J.: Syndesmology, or A Description of the Ligaments of the Human Body. Translation by E. B. Kaplan. Philadelphia, W. B. Saunders Company, 1969.
13. Rowe, D. R., and Zarins, B.: Recurrent transient subluxation of the shoulder. J Bone Joint Surg 63A:863, 1981.
14. Turkel, S. J., Panio, M. W., Marshall, J. L., and Girgis, F. G.: Stabilizing mechanism preventing anterior dislocation of the glenohumeral joint. J Bone Joint Surg 63A:1208, 1981.

SUGGESTED READING

1. Caspari, R. B.: Shoulder arthroscopy; a review of the present state of the art. Contemp Orthop 4:523, 1982.
2. Johnson, L. L.: Arthroscopy of the shoulder. Orthop Clin North Am 11:197, 1980.
3. Johnson, L. L.: Diagnostic and Surgical Arthroscopy. St. Louis, C V Mosby Company, 1981, pp. 376–389.
4. Lombardo, S. J.: Arthroscopy of the shoulder. Clin Sport Med 2:309, 1983.

OPERATIVE ARTHROSCOPY OF THE SHOULDER IN THE THROWING ATHLETE

JAMES R. ANDREWS, M.D. / WILLIAM G. CARSON, Jr., M.D.

INTRODUCTION

During the past decade arthroscopy has become firmly established, as both a diagnostic and a surgical modality, especially with regard to the knee joint. Its use for the evaluation of the shoulder joint has been less firmly established; however, several reports concerning its use do exist.[1–7]

Operative arthroscopy of the shoulder offers several advantages over more conventional techniques of shoulder surgery, including a low infection rate, less blood loss, and more rapid return to function. Thus surgical arthroscopy of the shoulder is well suited to the needs of the throwing athlete in that it may return the athlete to his sport more rapidly and requires less rehabilitation than more conventional surgical techniques.

This chapter describes the indications for operative arthroscopy of the shoulder as it relates to the throwing athlete and outlines the technique of this procedure. In addition some of the more frequent pathologic processes seen arthroscopically in the throwing athlete are discussed.

INDICATIONS FOR OPERATIVE ARTHROSCOPY OF THE SHOULDER

Operative arthroscopy of the shoulder is a relatively new advancement in the field of arthroscopy, and thus the indications for its use are still being determined. With regard to the throwing athlete the authors use techniques to perform the following operative arthroscopic procedures about the shoulder: (1) resection or debridement of a torn glenoid labrum, (2) debridement of a partial tear of the rotator cuff, (3) debridement of a partial tear of the long head of the biceps tendon, and (4) removal of loose bodies.

Two other indications for arthroscopy of the shoulder in the throwing athlete are (1) evaluation of shoulder instabilities and (2) evaluation of the chronically painful shoulder that has not responded to nonoperative conservative measures.

PATHOLOGY

During the past three years the authors have seen a large number of throwing athletes in whom tears of the glenoid labrum have been demonstrated on arthroscopic examination of the shoulder.[8–10] Glenoid labrum tears have classically been described as occurring in association with shoulder instability,[11–15] and there has been little mention of glenoid labrum tears occurring as an isolated entity. Injuries of the glenoid labrum occurring as an isolated entity in the throwing athlete's shoulder have been mentioned very little,[16] although glenoid labrum tears have been described as occurring as degenerative lesions in the older population.[17]

In a recent review of 73 throwing athletes who underwent arthroscopic examination of the shoulder, all 73 demonstrated tears of some portion of the glenoid labrum.[9] In this series 80 per cent of the tears were located over the anterosuperior portion of the glenoid labrum near the attachment of the long head of the biceps tendon in the glenoid cavity (Fig. 10–1). Of this same group of throwing athletes 33 patients (45 per cent) had a partial tear of the supraspinatous portion of the rotator cuff and 7 (10 per cent) had a partial tear of the long head of the biceps tendon near its origin in the glenoid labrum. Of this group of 73 throwing athletes 51 were involved in baseball, with 35 of these being pitchers. Other throwing sports included football (quarterback), softball, tennis, volleyball, racquetball, and javelin throwing. Eighty-eight per cent of these athletes achieved satisfactory results following arthroscopic surgery and returned to their sports.[9]

Thus, arthroscopy of the shoulder has demonstrated an exceedingly high yield of positive pathologic findings as noted in this series. This level of pathology in the throwing athlete's shoulder has brought more awareness of the great stresses to which the throwing athlete's shoulder is subjected.

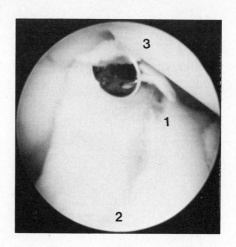

FIGURE 10–1. Arthroscopic view of a torn anterior glenoid labrum in a right shoulder. Note the proximity of the tear of the glenoid labrum to the insertion of the long head of the biceps tendon. *1 = labrum; 2 = biceps brachii tendon; 3 = humeral head.*

OPERATIVE TECHNIQUE

The technique of diagnostic arthroscopy of the shoulder is described in Chapter 8. Operative arthroscopy of the shoulder is performed in a similar fashion with the patient placed in the lateral decubitus position with the affected shoulder up. The arm is placed in the traction apparatus, and the shoulder is abducted approximately 70 degrees and flexed forward 15 degrees. The posterior portal is utilized for the introduction of the arthroscope; this placement is located approximately 3 cm inferior to the posterolateral border of the acromion.

Operative arthroscopy of the shoulder requires additional portals to be placed for operating instruments. These are placed through the anterior portals. The anterior portal is established by bisecting the distance between the coracoid process and the anterolateral edge of the acromion. A spinal needle is placed halfway between these palpable bony landmarks and directed posteriorly toward the center of the joint. Exact placement of the spinal needle is aided by direct intra-articular visualization provided by the arthroscope already in place through the posterior portal. After this placement has been confirmed the needle is removed, and the desired instrument or cannula is inserted. A second anterior portal required for additional inflow of fluid is placed directly adjacent to the first anterior portal, with the desired instrument or probe entering the joint capsule on the opposite side of the biceps tendon from the previously placed anterior instrument (Figs. 10–2A, B).

A 4-mm 30-degree angled arthroscope is utilized for arthroscopic examination. A hand-held video camera is connected to the arthroscope for ease of visualization and for documentation with video recording.

Tears of the glenoid labrum are resected with intra-articular knives or punches and usually a motorized suction instrument. The instruments for re-section of glenoid labrum tears located at the anterior rim are placed through

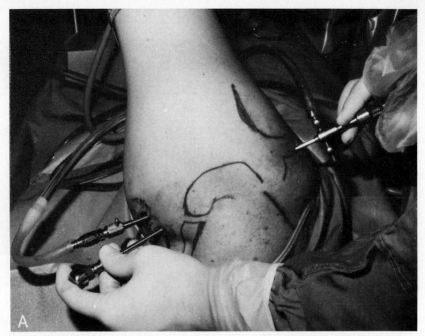

FIGURE 10–2A. The operative arthroscopic system. The arthroscope has been placed through the posterior portal in this right shoulder, and the motorized instrument has been placed through the anterior portal. An additional anterior portal has been placed for the inflow cannula.

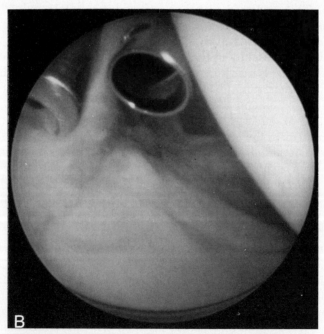

FIGURE 10–2B. Posterior arthroscopic view of operating instruments as they enter the shoulder through the anterior portals. The motorized instrument is located on one side of the biceps tendon, and the inflow cannula is on the opposite side.

the anterior portals. When partial tears of the rotator cuff or the biceps tendon are debrided the motorized suction instruments are usually required and are placed through the anterior portals.

At the completion of the procedure, 30 cc of a local anesthetic is injected into the shoulder, and bulky soft dressings are applied to the anterior and posterior puncture wounds. Immobilization of the shoulder is usually not required.

REHABILITATION FOLLOWING ARTHROSCOPIC SURGERY OF THE SHOULDER

Postoperative rehabilitation is initiated utilizing pendulum exercises as soon as these can be tolerated by the patient. Once the pain has subsided active and active assisted exercises are begun to regain full motion of the shoulder. When full motion has been achieved the patient starts progressive resistive exercises, stressing low weight with numerous repetitions. Of particular importance are the internal and external rotation exercises performed with the shoulder in the overhead position. The patient performs these internal and external rotational exercises at 90-degree abduction, 135-degree abduction, and full abduction. When satisfactory range of motion, strength, and endurance have been achieved and pain is absent the patient gradually returns to the previous athletic activity. Baseball pitchers gradually return to throwing by utilizing a long toss, short toss regimen as described in Chapter 3. Most of the throwing athletes can begin an actual throwing program at six to eight weeks after arthroscopy. The average return to full throwing activity after arthroscopic surgery is usually three to four months following resection of the glenoid labrum tear and four to six months following resection of the glenoid labrum tear when combined with resection of a partial tear of the rotator cuff.[9]

DISCUSSION

Arthroscopy of the shoulder is a new technique in the field of arthroscopy. The arthroscopic technique described has been quite successful in allowing safe and reproducible arthroscopic examination of the shoulder. The most technically demanding aspect of operative shoulder arthroscopy is gaining the initial entrance into the glenohumeral joint. Unlike arthroscopy of the knee, in which the instruments traverse only skin, subcutaneous fat, capsule and a retinaculum, shoulder arthroscopy requires the instruments to pass through thicker layers of fat, muscle, and a thick capsule. Because the glenohumeral joint is located deep relative to these multiple layers proper orientation is essential to avoid damage to nearby neurovascular structures. By adhering to the techniques outlined in this and previous chapters a safe and reproducible diagnostic and surgical arthroscopic procedure can be performed.

Shoulder arthroscopy has provided a unique opportunity to visualize the intra-articular pathology of the throwing athlete's shoulder. Pathologic processes such as glenoid labrum tears or partial tears of the rotator cuff or biceps tendon are much more frequent than previously was thought. Why the incidence of glenoid labrum tears appears to be so high in the throwing athlete is still unknown. These tears possibly can be initiated by a traction phenomenon by the long head of the biceps tendon; possibly the hypermobile torn glenoid labrum may be further torn by becoming impinged between the humeral head and the glenoid cavity during the extremes of motion to which the throwing shoulder is subjected.

Operative shoulder arthroscopy also has provided a unique opportunity to treat certain pathologic processes about the shoulder and to return the throwing athlete to his sport with relatively little morbidity and a rapid rehabilitation phase.

As more sophisticated arthroscopic instrumentation is developed and the technique of shoulder arthroscopy, both diagnostic and operative, is refined, arthroscopy of the shoulder will gain in usefulness. In addition, the multiple pathologic processes that are seen in the throwing athlete's shoulder can be better described and their causes better understood.

REFERENCES

1. Andrews, J. R., and Carson, W. G.: Shoulder joint arthroscopy. Orthopedics 6:1157, 1983.
2. Andrews, J. R., Carson, W. G., and Ortega, K.: Arthroscopy of the shoulder: Technique and normal anatomy. Am J Sports Med 12:1, 1984.
3. Caspari, R. B.: Shoulder arthroscopy: A review of the present state of the Art. Contemp Orthop 4:523, 1982.
4. Johnson, L. L.: Arthroscopy of the shoulder. Orthop Clin North Am 11:197, 1980.
5. Johnson, L. L.: Diagnostic and Surgical Arthroscopy. St. Louis, C V Mosby Company, 1981, pp. 376–389.
6. Lombardo, S. J.: Arthroscopy of the shoulder. Clin Sports Med 2:309, 1983.
7. Wiley, A. M., and Older, M. B.: Shoulder arthroscopy. Investigation with a fibro-optic instrument. Sports Med 8:31, 1980.
8. Andrews, J. R., Carson, W. G., and Hughston, J. C.: Operative arthroscopy of the shoulder: A preliminary report. Orthop Trans 5:499, 1983.
9. Andrews, J. R., and Carson, W. G.: The arthroscopic treatment of glenoid labrum tears in the throwing athlete. Orthop Trans 8:44, 1984.
10. Pappas, A. M., Goss, T. P., and Kleinman, P. K.: Symptomatic shoulder instability due to lesions of the glenoid labrum. Am J Sports Med 11:279, 1983.
11. Bankhart, A. S. B.: The pathology and treatment of recurrent dislocation of the shoulder joint. Br J Surg 26:23, 1938.
12. Blazina, M. E., and Satzman, J. S.: Recurrent anterior subluxation of the shoulder in athletes: A distinct entity. J Bone Joint Surg 51A:1037, 1969.
13. Protzman, R. R.: Anterior instability of the shoulder. J Bone Joint Surg 62A:909, 1980.
14. Rowe, C. R., Patel, D., and Southmayd, W. W.: The Bankhart procedure. A long term end results study. J Bone Joint Surg 60A:1, 1978.
15. Rowe, D. R., and Zarins, B.: Recurrent transient subluxation of the shoulder. J Bone Joint Surg 63A:863, 1981.
16. Bateman, J. E.: Athletic injuries about the shoulder in throwing and body contact sports. Clin Orthop 23:75, 1962.
17. DePalma, A. F., Callery, G., and Bennett, G. A.: Variational anatomy and degenerative lesions of the shoulder joint. In Instructional Course Lectures of the American Academy of Orthopaedic Surgeons. St. Louis, C V Mosby Company, 6:255, 1949.

THROWING INJURIES
TO THE SHOULDER

FRANK C. McCUE, III, M.D. / JOE H. GIECK, Ed.D., ATC, RPT /
JAMES O. WEST, Ed.D.

THE THROWING MOTION

The action of throwing is an extremely complex motion that involves parts of the entire body to varying degrees in a coordinated manner. The mechanism of delivery varies greatly, depending on the sport and the weight of the object to be propelled. The heavier the object and the greater the distance thrown, the greater is the power that is needed in propulsion and the more parts of the body that are required. These can range from the entire body in throwing of the hammer and shot put to only the hand, arm, and shoulder in the act of simply tossing the ball into the air while serving in tennis.

The act of throwing consists of five steps: (1) initial stance, (2) wind-up, (3) cocking phase, (4) acceleration of the arm, and (5) follow-through phase.

The shoulder acts as a base to support the arm that is holding the ball. This behaves in a similar fashion as the handle of a whip, with the arm acting as a lash having a weighted tip on the end. Coordination in the pivoting motion of the lower extremities that includes ipsilateral and contralateral leg motion is essential to optimal delivery.

The athlete is exposed to unique forces on his body in various sports. This varies from the preteenager in Little League baseball or football to the elderly bowler or tennis player. Each sport presents its own particular problems, varying in degree and location, depending on the stress and strain generated.

The majority of injuries occurring in throwing sports involve the soft tissue structures. Injuries to the musculotendinous unit, ligaments, and joints usually occur when these tissues are overstretched. Injury can also involve the contracting unit of the muscle; this usually occurs near the midpoint of contraction and involves the muscle fibers. The nature of the injury is affected by many factors. These include myostatic contracture of the joints and muscles, age and maturity of the patient, weight and type of object to be propelled, the nature of propulsion, weakness, fatigue, or incoordination of the motion, chronic degenerative changes, and prior injury.

Biomechanics are very important in the analysis of the throwing act and in understanding the method in which leverage is applied in throwing. Successful throwing involves the following elements:

1. Exertion of forces in the proper direction.
2. Exertion of forces in the proper time.
3. Exertion of forces in the proper sequence.
4. Exertion of forces over the greatest practical range.
5. Maintenance of ground contact until release.

Baseball throwing imparts a great deal of repetitive stress to the upper extremity. A program for prevention of injuries can be designed specifically for baseball pitchers but altered and adjusted for any sport involving throwing. The initial steps in preventing injury begin with the preseason and off-season training programs. These programs should also be followed during the season with pregame preparation, daily care, and postgame treatment in individual cases. The off-season is utilized to allow previous injuries to heal, since even the most minor injury can develop into a chronic disability. Most injuries heal by scarring with fibrous tissue. Therefore, the injured part may never completely return to a normal condition, particularly in the case in which repetitive motion occurs. It is important to keep the thrower under constant surveillance to prevent improper delivery, which could cause permanent disability. This continual monitoring includes observation not only of the upper extremity but of all parts of the body. The act of delivery includes arm motion, footwork, leg action, hip and trunk rotation, as well as action of the opposite arm. Injuries of any type that break up this coordinated movement can cause abnormal strain to an area. Repeated throwing further compounds the injury and delays healing.

Baseball pitching consists of many variations, ranging from the overhand delivery to the three-quarter delivery, the side-arm delivery, and even the underhand or "submarine" type. In other sports there is a great variation in delivery as well. The thrower begins with the wind-up, then reaches back to the limits of external rotation, abduction, and extension of the shoulder. This motion is followed by the whipping forward of the arm into internal rotation and adduction of the shoulder and extension of the elbow.

This is the motion in which extreme valgus strain is placed on the elbow. The motion progresses to follow-through, at which time the pitcher seems to be attempting to actually throw the shoulder at the batter to obtain maximal speed. Different types of delivery produce varying stresses with the overhand delivery exerting maximal stress on the shoulder, wrist, and back and the side-arm delivery producing stress primarily to the elbow and back.

There are a variety of causes of overuse injury to the shoulder. Factors that are important include the athlete's state of physical conditioning, flexibility, and strength. Proper pregame warm-up can help prevent some injuries. The type of delivery, the force of delivery, and variations of stance are other factors. The age of the athlete and the presence of degenerative changes play a role. Throwing weather conditions such as cold or extremely hot weather can cause undue fatigue and result in injury. The presence of other factors such as obesity, infection, illness of any type, or mental tension add to the problem. Collision injuries sustained while sliding into base can damage the shoulder that is used to throw. Physical immaturity of the individual, such as in Little League, predisposes to different types of injuries from repetitive throwing. Abnormal delivery or change of delivery to compensate for a musculoskeletal injury can place abnormal stress on the throwing shoulder.

COMMON THROWING INJURIES TO THE SHOULDER

Injuries to the shoulder may be classified into groups ranging from the acute, consisting largely of soft tissue injuries, through subacute to chronic. In the latter type, acute flare-ups or recurrences can occur periodically.

Few injuries occur in initial stance and the early part of the wind-up. However, as the shoulder goes into the late wind-up and cocking phases, the anterior structures are placed under stretch prior to muscle contraction in the acceleration phase. The excess stress that can occur with stretching and muscle contraction can cause microtears at tissue insertions, with a resultant inflammatory response.

A discussion of acute throwing injuries of the shoulder can be simplified by grouping them according to anatomic region. Anterior injury usually occurs from stretching when the pitcher attempts to gain power by increasing external rotation of the shoulder. Posterior shoulder injury occurs when elongation of posterior structures occurs in follow-through. Acute injuries also occur when muscle power is impaired as a result of weakness, fatigue, incoordination, and improper position in the muscle length-tension curve. A discussion of shoulder injuries according to anatomic region follows:

The Anterior Structures

The major anatomic structures in the anterior section of the shoulder that are most commonly injured in the throwing motion are:

1. The capsule
3. Pectoralis major muscle
4. Latissimus dorsi muscles
5. Teres major muscles
6. Subscapularis muscle
7. Long head of biceps brachii muscle

The pectoralis major muscle is placed under stress during the cocking phase. The site of injury is usually at the insertion into the humerus posterior to the bicipital groove. Injury is most often seen in baseball and javelin throwers.

The fibers of the anterior deltoid and pectoralis major muscles and other internal rotators can be injured in the early acceleration phase. When the subscapularis muscle is injured, symptoms include localized pain and tenderness over its insertion at the lesser tuberosity.

Acute muscle or tendon ruptures occur but are rare. The latissimus dorsi, which is prone to internal rotation myostatic contracture, and the pectoralis major are the muscles most apt to tear.

Bicipital tenosynovitis is a relatively common cause of anterior shoulder pain. In this condition tenderness can be elicited along the long head of the biceps tendon. This injury is especially seen in overhead throwing and in tennis, when the tendon tends to ride over the lesser tuberosity during external rotation-abduction.

Anatomic variations of the bicipital groove occur. The small, tight-roofed, sharp-walled canal is more apt to cause irritative changes in the tendon, while the canal with a small, lax, transverse humeral ligament, with a shallow obliquely angled wall is more apt to result in tendon subluxation.

The biceps tendon usually subluxates medially because of the angle that is formed as the tendon passes from the bicipital groove to the glenoid cavity. Subluxation occurs when the shoulder goes from internal rotation to external rotation and back again. This is more commonly seen in football quarterbacks because of the heavy object to be thrown and the need for additional pushing action. It is also prevalent in underhand throwing, as in softball, because of the forceful supinator strain, plus arm and forearm flexion. A proximal rupture of the long head of the biceps tendon can occur, most often in the middle-aged athlete.

The Rotator Cuff and Environs

The anatomic structures in the functional unit of the rotator cuff include:

1. Rotator cuff muscles:
   a. Supraspinatus
   b. Infraspinatus
   c. Teres minor
   d. Subscapularis
2. Long head of biceps brachii tendon
3. Acromion process
4. Coracoacromial ligament
5. Acromioclavicular joint

Complete tears of the rotator cuff are uncommon in the young athlete. The injury is diagnosed by clinical loss of rotator cuff function and a positive arthrographic result. Small tears and partial tears are more common but difficult to diagnose accurately even by arthroscopy.

Chronic rotator cuff problems, subacromial bursitis, and subsequent impingement syndromes are more common in the middle-aged athlete and veteran pitcher. These injuries occur in the mid-portion or acceleration phase of the throwing act. The impingement syndrome can be produced by repetitive sliding of the supraspinatus tendon, the biceps tendon, or the greater tuberosity of the humerus against the coracoacromial arch. Microtrauma from repetitive throwing can lead to inflammation that causes swelling. This increases the volume of the musculotendinous unit in an already tight space, increasing the risk of further injury.

The acromion process, coracoacromial ligament, and coracoid form the arch under which the humeral head and rotator cuff glide during the throwing act. For younger individuals, particularly swimmers, excision of the coracoacromial ligament alone has frequently been helpful in relieving impingement. This same procedure has not been successful in many adults with impingement syndrome.

The acromioclavicular joint can be involved in injuries during throwing. Excision of the distal end of the clavicle when degenerative changes are present is occasionally helpful in relieving the symptoms. In chronic cases, spurring at the acromioclavicular joint can cause subacromial impingement.

The Posterior Structures

Structures in the posterior aspect of the throwing shoulder that can be injured are:

1. Posterior capsule
2. Long head of triceps muscle
3. Teres minor muscle

Repeated stretching of the posterior structures during follow-through can cause inflammatory changes at the attachment of the rotator cuff. Chronic injury can also be found at the origin of the long head of the triceps on the posterior-inferior glenoid cavity. Teres minor muscle strain results from a similar mechanism but with pain radiating along the axillary border of the scapula as well as overlying muscle. Ossification at the attachment of the tendon can occur with progression to spur formation. This can lead to impingement and possible fracture of the spur. By this same process, loose bodies can be extruded into the glenohumeral joint.

The Glenohumeral Articulation

The major injuries that involve the glenohumeral joint are:

1. Dislocation
   a. Anterior
   b. Posterior
   c. Multidirectional
2. Subluxation
   a. Anterior
   b. Posterior
   c. Multidirectional
3. Glenoid labrum tears
4. Humeral head degenerative changes
5. Glenoid cavity spurring
6. Loose bodies
7. Epiphyseal injuries

Shoulder subluxation can occur during the cocking phase from repetitive stress but is more commonly caused by trauma. In loose-jointed individuals, multidirectional laxity is difficult to diagnose. When severe multidirectional laxity is present, treatment is difficult even by surgical means.

Posterior subluxation of the shoulder can occur during follow-through as the humerus is brought down into adduction and internal rotation.

Degenerative changes in the glenoid labrum have been described by Andrews; arthroscopic debridement has been reported to be successful. However, these cases have not been followed long enough to determine whether the satisfactory postsurgical results hold up with time.

The humeral head can undergo traumatic osteoarthritic changes. Ridging can be caused by the repetitive external rotation motions forcing repeated compression of the humeral head against the glenoid cavity. This groove is more inferior in the humeral head than that seen in the Hill-Sachs lesion of recurrent anterior dislocation.

Glenoid cavity spurring and loose bodies either from fracture of the arthritic spurs or osteochondral fragments from the articular surface can be seen in veteran throwers.

In children with open epiphyseal plates, stress can cause injury to the growth cartilage itself or to the adjacent bone. Osteochondrosis of the proximal humeral epiphysis has been described. This condition responds well to rest and rarely causes long-term disability.

Rare Causes of Posterior Shoulder Pain

The following clinical conditions are infrequent but can cause problems for the throwing athlete:

1. Suprascapular nerve compression
2. Quadrilateral space compression
3. Myositis ossificans
4. Latissimus dorsi muscle contracture

Subscapular nerve compression can cause localized discomfort in the posterior shoulder and atrophy of the supraspinatus and infraspinatus muscles.

The *quadrilateral space compression syndrome* is an uncommon condition that is caused by compression of the posterior humeral circumflex artery and axillary nerve or one of its major branches in the quadrilateral space. The pain of this syndrome is poorly localized to the anterior aspect of the shoulder. The paresthesias have a nondermatomal distribution in the arm, forearm, and hand. Forward flexion or abduction, or both, and external rotation of the humerus aggravate the symptoms. Discrete point tenderness is usually found posteriorly in the quadrilateral space. The diagnosis can be confirmed by a subclavian arteriogram. The diagnostic arteriographic finding is occlusion of the posterior humeral circumflex artery with the arm in abduction and external rotation. Surgical decompression should be considered if the patient has sufficient symptoms to warrant surgery and no relief after a long course of conservative care. The authors have seen patients in whom the arteriogram is negative for thoracic outlet syndrome who have a compressed posterior humeral circumflex artery when the humerus is positioned in abduction and external rotation.

Myositis ossificans can be seen about the shoulder. It is caused by trauma, usually to the vascular area in the posterior shoulder. *Contracture of the latissimus dorsi* results in limitation of external rotation and may be painful in the posterior shoulder area.

Vascular Shoulder Problems

The axillary artery is divided into three portions. The first lies proximal, the second deep, and the third distal to the pectoralis minor muscle. During the cocking phase of throwing, the arm is brought into abduction, extension, and external rotation or the so-called *hyperabduction position*. In this shoulder position, the second portion of the axillary artery can be occluded by the pressure of the overlying pectoralis minor muscle. If transient occlusion occurs with each pitch, and if sufficient local injury occurs to produce intimal damage, thrombosis can ensue. The arm fatigues, and axillary tenderness, absent pulses, cyanosis, and decreased skin temperature can be observed. The treatment is surgical. Sympathectomy has been temporarily successful in certain individuals.

So-called *effort thrombosis* of the subclavian vein has occurred in throwers, but the exact causes are still unknown. One currently held concept is that the syndrome results from mechanical obstruction, with or without concomitant venous thrombosis of the subclavian vein at one or more points as the vein passes out of the thoracic inlet. This condition usually occurs on the dominant arm in a young active male. It is characterized by acute onset of diffuse swelling and distension of the superficial veins accompanied by cyanosis. The patient feels a sensation of heaviness associated with the increase in size of the arm and elevated venous pressure. The onset is often sudden and may disappear when the arm is held in the neutral position. The compression occurs most commonly between the clavicle anteriorly and the first rib posteriorly. Other factors such as the fibrotic anterior scalene muscle, abnormal fibrous bands, the costoclavicular ligament, or an extremely tight pectoralis minor muscle also possibly can cause compression.

Fractures

Osteochondral fractures of the humeral head can be caused by direct contact of the humeral head against the glenoid cavity. An example is the posterior humeral head compression fracture seen in anterior dislocation, called a *Hill-Sachs lesion*. The anterior rim of the glenoid cavity can also fracture in this type of injury.

Stress fractures can occur in the first rib and usually involve the nondominant side. The fracture occurs at the thinnest portion of the rib, in the subclavian groove between the attachment of the scalenus anticus and scalenus medius muscles. The serratus anterior muscle also attaches at this level. Similar fractures in the lower three floating ribs have been described as well. Repetitive vigorous contraction of the external oblique muscles, interdigitating with the latissimus dorsi, serratus posterior, serratus inferior, and internal oblique muscles at the tips of the 10th, 11th, and 12th ribs can cause stress fractures of these ribs.

Stress fractures can develop at the epiphyseal or apophyseal growth plates. These can disrupt not only bone integrity but also affect future bone growth to varying degrees. While this situation is most common in the medial humeral epicondyle at the elbow, other areas, including the proximal humeral epiphysis, may be involved.

INJURY IN OTHER THROWING MOTIONS

The throwing of a football differs from the throwing of a baseball in that there is a short wind-up, less forward action, and a weaker follow-through. Football throwing uses a larger heavier object and greater pushing action.

Throwing of a javelin requires a similar mechanism as in baseball, but the majority of stress is to the elbow.

In putting the shot, a strong pushing motion of the heavy object to be propelled and its forceful follow-through put tremendous stress on the muscles anchoring the shoulder girdle.

The hurling of the discus or hammer substitutes centrifugal force for linear force, with different terminal movements at the release. These forces seldom cause serious problems, but with improper release can cause traction-type injuries.

The underhanded throwing mechanism required in bowling, softball, and curling is mostly a flexion action with a shorter excursion and less force that is applied on the biceps muscle and anterior shoulder capsule.

The racquet sports cause different types of stresses to the shoulder than in baseball throwing. The shoulder serves chiefly as a fulcrum for the forearm, since a great deal of force is taken by the elbow and forearm. In tennis, especially on higher competitive levels, significant stress is imparted on the shoulder.

DIAGNOSIS

An accurate history along with the physical examination usually lead to the correct diagnosis. Radiographs, including multiple views (such as axillary views), are needed. Arthrography has proved very helpful, especially in cases of rotator cuff injuries. Cineradiography has been of value in cases of suspected instability. Radiograms of the bursa, image intensifiers, fluoroscopy, electromyograms, laminograms, and other tests are rarely useful. The use of both diagnostic and operative arthroscopy is becoming more common.

Manual muscle testing and stretching the musculotendinous unit aid in the diagnosis of strain.

PREVENTION

Year-Round Training Program

A year-round training program helps to prevent injuries, increases the effectiveness of the athlete, and prevents recurrence of pre-existing problems. Some suggestions that can be tailored to fit the individual include:

1. Treat the initial injury properly to minimize scar formation.
2. Prevent weight gain by dietary discipline.
3. Adhere to a program of running, at least three days a week, during the early part of the off-season and daily when the season nears.
4. Study the previous year's films to understand faulty throwing habits.
5. Participate in other sports such as golfing and handball to improve coordination, self-control, precision, and reflexes.
6. Adhere to an exercise program tailored to fit specific needs, including stretching and muscle strengthening exercises. Perform daily stretching exercises, including hanging from a horizontal bar.
7. Check for any systemic diseases, postural imbalance, or abnormalities of the back, feet, and legs in preseason physical examination.
8. Swing a weighted bat, walk with weighted shoes, and throw a weighted ball.

Early Season Practice

The players should be checked carefully to assess general physical condition. Particular note should be taken of weight, speed, and endurance. The conditioning program should involve running to build strength and endurance of the legs.

Pitchers must not be allowed to throw the ball hard at the start of the practice season. The fast ball can cause early season problems. Hard breaking curves should not be thrown during the first week. Pitchers may be allowed to spin curves on the first day but not to throw the ball to break hard.

Gradual increase in the force of throwing must be carried out. General conditioning, proper balance, and the correct delivery are important and should be carefully observed and corrected if any deficiency is found.

In the early practice season the number of innings pitched should be limited, beginning with each pitcher throwing two to three innings (depending on the number of pitches thrown) and gradually adding an inning each game or period of time until the individual can go the full route. The amount of time necessary for each individual to rest following a game varies, but typically is three to four days.

During the period between pitching, general conditioning exercises should be carried out, especially running. Individual muscle strengthening and stretching exercises are also performed. Other modalities and physical therapy can be used.

Pregame Injury Prevention

The following are some suggestions that can be carried out prior to the game and tailored to fit the individual's needs:

1. Moist heat is applied for 20 minutes. This can be followed by an ice rub or cold wet towel rub.

2. Upper extremity stretching exercises are performed. Not only does stretching loosen up the arm, making it more flexible for optimal delivery, but stretching may save as many as 20 pitches from the pitcher's pregame warm-up. The authors' pregame routine is divided into 12 parts.

POSITION

A. SIDE-LYING
   1. Massage of the shoulder with an analgesic
   2. Scapular press
   3. Abduction
   4. Rotation, external-internal
   5. Extension
B. BACK-LYING
   1. Extension-adduction
   2. Rotation, external-internal
   3. Horizontal flexion
   4. Abduction
   5. Forearm range-of-motion exercises
   6. Wrist and finger range-of-motion exercises
   7. Shaking of the extremities
C. HANG-STRETCH
   1. This is an exercise to use after stretching with the horizontal bar. The pitcher's full body weight is suspended from one arm reaching to the horizontal bar. In this position the pitcher's body revolves slowly for 30 to 60 seconds, stretching the shoulder and arm muscles to distract and loosen the joint structures.
   2. Calisthenics should be used prior to progressive warm-up.
   3. The pitcher must keep warm until ready to pitch, regardless of climatic conditions.

Pregame Warm-Up. It is extremely important to warm-up in order to obtain the optimal degree of preparation of the throwing arm. Each sport may require a different type of warm-up to meet its specific needs. It has been noted that external rotation of the shoulder increases with a concomitant decrease in internal rotation during warm-up. This is a consistent finding in the veteran pitcher.

1. Limbering exercises should be used without throwing.

2. The player should work up a sweat by use of calisthenics before going into the pitching box.

3. Warm-up should begin at a distance shorter than from the pitcher's box to home plate.

4. The distance should be increased gradually as the arm limbers up.

5. Warm-ups should begin with slow pitches, with gradually increasing speed as the arm loosens up.

6. Curve balls should not be thrown until the arm has warmed up.

7. The pitcher must always throw at the mitt as a target.

8. The pitcher must never throw to bases as in pick-offs unless the arm is thoroughly warmed up.

9. The arm should be kept under wraps at all times when not pitching.

10. On cold or windy days additional massage may be necessary—beginning with the fingertips, moving gradually into the wrist, the elbow and the shoulder—and should include the neck and back. An analgesic rub is also helpful in maintaining warmth in the throwing arm.

A specific pregame warm-up routine may consist of a total of 15 to 20 minutes spent pitching (1) 30 straight balls of medium velocity, (2) 10 curve balls, (3) 10 sliders, (4) 10 fast balls at increased velocity, and (5) alternate with sets, 5 pitches of varying types, for a total of approximately 80 pitches; finally, there should be a five-minute rest prior to the start of the game.

Postgame Care

Strenuous use of the arm during throwing causes an increase in vascularity of the soft tissues and edema. In severe cases this can be treated by compression (intermittent compression machine), oral enzymes, and gentle massage, beginning distally, in an attempt to express the edema fluid from the extremity.

The authors have found the ice bath regimen to be helpful in certain cases. This consists of immersion of the arm in the ice bath for 5 seconds, then removal for 5 seconds, with the process repeated for 10 seconds, then 15, until the athlete is able to keep the arm in the bath for 15 to 20 minutes. Only the areas of irritation need to be immersed in the ice bath.

Once the pitcher is in good physical condition and in a regular pitching rotation (pitching every four or five days), the following regimen is used (naturally, this varies with some pitchers):

1. The same limbering-up exercise as in pregame warm-up should be used every day except two days prior to pitching.

2. The pitcher should throw either during batting practices or on the side every day, except two days prior to pitching. At least 70 pitches should be thrown after warm-up.

3. General exercise, as mentioned in the training program, should be

used with at least 30 minutes of running each day, except the day before pitching. The pitcher should be sure to run long distance as well as short sprints.

4. The day before pitching the pitcher should not throw, run, or exercise.

After an injury or a period of inactivity, the following can be used to allow gradual return to normal throwing:

1. Throw long, easy lobs from deep outfield for 30 minutes on two consecutive days followed by resting the arm for one day.
2. Throw from midoutfield on five to six bounces for 30 minutes on two consecutive days followed by resting the arm for one day.
3. Throw from short outfield along a straight trajectory on one bounce for 30 minutes on two days followed by rest for one day.
4. Return to the mound or other position for usual activities.

TREATMENT

Conservative therapy of the throwing arm includes the use of the following:

1. Rest
2. Physical therapy modalities
3. Heat and cold
4. Exercises
5. Technique
6. Medications
   a. Analgesics
   b. Enzymes
   c. Anti-inflammatories
   d. Steroids
   e. Muscle relaxants
7. Reassurance

Rest. Rest is essential for soft tissue healing. This is especially true of the acute injury but also in flare-ups of chronic cases.

The exact period of rest varies widely with the type, severity, and location of the injury, as well as the needs of the patient.

Physical Therapy Modalities and Heat and Cold. Thermotherapy and cryotherapy are important adjuncts in the treatment of the throwing arm. They can be employed alternately or separately. Both are antispasmodic and analgesic. Heat is usually applied initially to stimulate circulation and facilitate warm-up. Ice is usually utilized after an exercise session to reduce swelling and inflammation. Prevention of swelling is important. One of the main values of these modalities is that they relieve pain and allow the athlete to begin exercise.

Exercise and Technique. Exercise, even minimal tension isometrics, should begin as soon as possible, since between 1 and 3 per cent of the athlete's strength is lost with each day's rest after injury. Therefore, early exercise, performed in a pain-free range of motion, reduces the athlete's recovery time. The program should include flexibility, strength, and endurance exercises throughout shoulder forward flexion, backward extension, horizontal flexion, horizontal extension, abduction, adduction, internal rotation, and external rotation; elbow flexion, extension, supination, and pronation; and wrist flexion, extension, abduction, and adduction. The movements should be exercised individually and collectively, with the athlete progressing from isometric to isotonic or isokinetic exercise, or both.

With exercise and the return of strength, flexibility, and endurance, the athlete begins his normal throwing routine. At this stage technique and coordination are essential. The athlete who changes his throwing form because of an injury often invites repeat injury or associated injury to other structures. At this point the coach or trainer who is familiar with the athlete's throwing style is the most important individual in the athlete's treatment. The athlete is not allowed to throw until he can do so in a virtually pain-free manner using normal form. His exercise session is halted when he begins substitution or deviation from this form.

Cardiovascular conditioning must be maintained throughout the athlete's treatment period. The exercise bicycle is an excellent cardiovascular conditioning device for the individual who cannot run. A minimal program of 30 minutes a day, maintaining the pulse rate above 120 beats per minute, is mandatory.

Medications. Medications do not prevent injury. They are used as aids in curing, regulating, and comforting the patient.

Analgesics are used to relieve pain. These are divided into those used for mild pain, the prime example being salicylates, and those used for severe pain, such as morphine. Salicylates are occasionally helpful when administered 20 to 30 minutes prior to a game in cases of mild inflammation.

Injectable enzymes combined with lidocaine and a steroid can be used to break up localized hematomas but are not commonly used for throwing injuries. Oral enzymes are of questionable value.

Nonsteroidal anti-inflammatory medications have been widely used in athletic treatment. They are useful in chronic inflammatory conditions and also in acute injuries. These drugs should be used for short periods of time.

The authors use a graduated schedule of phenylbutazone or a derivative thereof in dosages of 200 mg four times a day for two days, then 200 mg three times a day for two days, and finally 100 mg three times a day for three days.

Similar nonsteroidal anti-inflammatory drugs that may be useful are Indocin, Motrin, Tolectin, and Naprosyn.

Oral administration of corticosteroids is used infrequently if at all. In selected cases injections of a steroid are useful around a tendon or into a joint but not repeatedly. For example, a series of not more than three injections two weeks apart may be used in the acromioclavicular joint for a sprain.

Muscle relaxants such as methocarbamol or carisoprodol and tranquilizers may be used orally to relieve muscle spasm and occasionally intravenously for severe acute spasm. Many muscle relaxants, especially the tranquilizers, give some sedation and may aid in this fashion.

Reassurance. The average athlete is strongly motivated to resume athletic activity on recovery, but a small percentage lack sufficient motivation. Each person has a different reaction to injury, and the reaction may vary for some reason during the period of recovery.

Many factors, such as release from an unpleasant obligation, fear of pain, disability, repeat injury, and loss of social status, may be psychologic factors in delay in recovery. They may also be used to salvage pride and rationalize decreasing performance in the aging athlete.

This phase of treatment is extremely important. The best treatment is prevention. If this aspect is ignored, complete recovery may never occur.

General Treatment Principles

Mild injuries are treated with a relatively short period of rest, medication, and modalities aimed at rapid return to function with minimal reconditioning required.

Moderate injuries need a more prolonged period of rest, medication, and therapy with an individualized rehabilitation and exercise program prior to return to activity.

Severe injuries often need surgical reconstruction with subsequent prolonged rest and more extensive rehabilitation and exercise.

CONCLUSION

The upper extremity plays a critical role in most sports. The sites that sustain the most trauma are the shoulder, elbow, and upper back. The action of throwing is a very complex motion coordinated to involve the body as a whole.

The mechanism of delivery varies greatly depending on the sport and the weight of the object to be propelled. Each sport presents its own individual problems, varying in degree and location. The majority of injuries involve the soft tissue structures.

The musculotendinous unit is the main source of power. Injuries can occur by overstretching the elastic fibers (extrinsic loading) or by contraction of the muscle, usually near its midpoint (intrinsic loading).

The nature of the injury is modified by many factors, including myostatic contracture of the joints and muscles, the age of the patient, the weight and type of object to be propelled, the nature of propulsion, the presence of weakness, fatigue, or incoordination of motion, the degree of chronic degenerative changes, the presence of previous injury, and repetitive microtrauma.

The most common injuries have been discussed, along with treatment. Because of the paramount importance of the throwing arm in sports, it is imperative that a generalized year-round training program, preseason and early season conditioning programs, careful pregame care and warm-up, and diligent postgame care be used to help prevent disabilities and increase the efficiency of the athlete.

SUGGESTED READING

1. Adams, J. E.: Bone injuries in the very young athlete. Clin Orthop 58:129, 1968.
2. _____: Injury to the throwing arm: A study of traumatic changes in the elbow joints of boy baseball players. Calif Med 102:127, 1965.
3. _____: Little League shoulder. Calif Med 105:22, 1966.
4. Adams, J. T., DeWeese, J. A., and Mahoney, E. B., et al.: Intermittent subclavian vein obstruction without thrombosis. Surgery, 63:147, 1958.
5. Andrews, J. R., et al.: Musculotendinous injuries of shoulder and elbow in athletes. The 1975 Schering Symposium on Musculotendinous Injuries; The Journal of National Athletic Trainers Association II:68, 1976.
6. Bateman, J. E.: The Shoulder and Neck. St. Louis, C V Mosby Company, 1972.
7. Brogden, B. S., and Crow, M. D.: Little Leaguer's elbow. Am J Roentgenol 83:671, 1966.
8. Cahill, B. R., and Palmer, R. E.: Quadrilateral space syndrome. J Hand Surg 8:65, 1983.
9. Charrette, E. J. P.: Symptomatic non-thrombotic subclavian vein obstruction. Vasc Surg 7:220, 1973.
10. Ellman, H.: Unusual affections of the pre-adolescent elbow. J Bone Joint Surg 49A:203, 1967.
11. Fauls, D.: The Arm Stretch. The Journal of the National Athletic Trainers Association 3, 1960.
12. Gaylis, H.: Radical approach to venous thrombectomy. Surg Gynecol Obstet 138:864, 1974.
13. Gitlin, G.: Concerning the gangliform enlargement (pseudoganglion) on the nerve to the teres minor muscle. J Anat 91:466, 1957.
14. Hughes, E. S. R.: Venous obstruction in the upper extremity (Paget-Schroetter's syndrome). International Abstracts of Surgery 88:89, 1949.
15. Lord, J. W., Jr., and Rosati, L. M.: Thoracic-outlet syndromes. Clin Symp 23, 1971.
16. Lowenstein, P. S.: Thrombosis of the axillary vein—an anatomic study. JAMA 82:854, 1924.
17. McCleery, R. S., Kesterson, J. E., and Kirtley, J. A., et al.: Subclavius and anterior scalene muscle compression as a cause of intermittent obstruction of the subclavian vein. Ann Surg 133:593, 1951.
18. McLaughlin, C. W., and Popma, A. M.: Intermittent obstruction of the subclavian vein. JAMA 113:1960, 1939.
19. Neij: Nord Med 20:1956, 1943.
20. Ochsner, A., and DeBakey, M.: Surgery 5:491, 1939.
21. Paget, J.: Clinical Lectures and Essays. London, Longmans, Green & Company, 1875.
22. Rabinowitz, R., and Goldfarb, D.: Surgical treatment of axillosubclavian venous thrombosis: A case report. Surgery 70:803, 1971.
23. Roos, D. B.: Transaxillary approach for first rib resection to relieve thoracic outlet syndrome. Ann Surg 163:354, 1966.
24. Sampson, J. J., Saunders, J. D., and Capp, C. S.: Am Heart J 19:292, 1940.
25. Schroetter von L.: Erkrankungen der Gefasse. Nothnagel Handbuch der Pathologie und Therapie. Wein: Holder 1884.

26. Seldinger, S. I.: Catheter replacement of the needle in percutaneous arteriography. A new technique. Acta Radiol 39:368, 1953.
27. Slocum, D. B.: The mechanics of some common injuries to the shoulder in sports. Am J Sports 98:394, 1959.
28. Tullos, H. S., Wendell, D. E., Woods, G. W., Wukasch, D. C., Cooley, D. A., and King, J. W.: Unusual Lesions of the Pitching Arm. Houston, Division of Orthopedic Surgery, Baylor College of Medicine; The Surgery Section, Texas Heart Institution; and Texas Medical Center. Clin Orthop 88:169, 1972.
29. Tullos, H. S., and King, J. W.: Throwing mechanism in sports. Orthop Clin North Am 4:709, 1973.
30. Urschel, H. C., Paulson, D. L., and McNamara, J. J.: Thoracic outlet syndrome. Ann Thorac Surg 6:1, 1968.
31. Waris, W.: Elbow injuries in javelin throwers. Acta Chir Scand 93:563, 1946.
32. William, R. J.: Edinburgh Medical Journal 20:105, 1918.
33. Wright, I. S.: Am Heart J 29:1, 1945.
34. Wright, R. S., and Lipscomb, A. B.: Acute occlusion of the subclavian vein in an athlete: Diagnosis, etiology and surgical management. Journal Sports Med II:343, 1974.

THE TREATMENT OF COMMON THROWING INJURIES TO THE SHOULDER

ROBERT K. KERLAN, M.D.

The purpose of this chapter is to present the author's method of evaluating and treating common shoulder injuries caused by throwing.

EXAMINATION

Examination of the throwing shoulder begins by obtaining a detailed history with emphasis on anatomy and the mechanism of injury. This requires a thorough working knowledge of the anatomic structures as they are utilized in each part of the throwing motion. It is often helpful to ask a patient, "When was the last time your arms felt normal?" and then to have the patient explain in his own words the first time the pain was noticed. Often the stressful part of the motion can be correlated with a specific part of the anatomy of the shoulder. It may be helpful to have the patient identify the location of the pain within one of four quadrants: anterior, lateral, posterior, or superior. Only after a detailed history has been obtained should physical examination be begun. The physical examination is divided into five components: inspection, palpation, motion, strength, and stability. A combination of the history and physical examination provides a preliminary group of diagnoses that must be differentiated.

One common area of pain in the throwing shoulder is that related to the anterior quadrant. The patient indicates that pain starts just prior to ball release and associates this pain with the anterior quadrant. One common entity that has such a clinical picture is that of *bicipital tendinitis.* Once this diagnosis is entertained it must be proved by a combination of knowledge of the anatomy of the shoulder and by injections. The author prefers to place the patient in a position to verify the suspected pathology by physical examination and by putting the suspected area of pathology in a place that is easily palpated. Once the inflamed area has been located, a therapeutic test with a mixture of lidocaine and steroid administered with a 25-gauge ⅝-inch needle is often useful. The steroid is added because it can provide significant anti-inflammatory action and treat at the same time that a diagnosis is confirmed. In addition, often this therapy allows the athlete to return to throwing while a long-term treatment regimen is still under consideration.

For injection of the biceps tendon in the bicipital groove the patient is placed in a supine position with the arm over the table and the elbow bent,

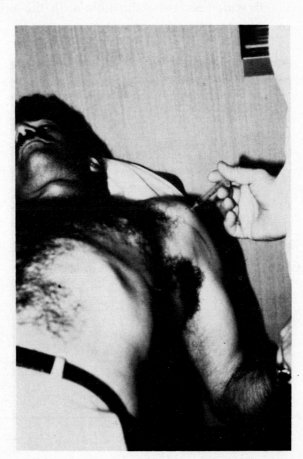

FIGURE 12–1. Position for injection in the bicipital groove area.

the shoulder extended, and the arm supinated. Then the biceps tendon is located under the examiner's finger, and a mark is made on the skin with the thumbnail. The area is prepared in a sterile fashion, and the examiner never takes his eyes off the mark made on the skin. The assistant hands the requested materials to the examiner (Fig. 12–1). In this way injection of the lidocaine and steroid mixture into the area of pathology can be assured (Fig. 12–2).

A second common entity causing pain in the throwing athlete is *rotator cuff tendinitis*. The patient usually complains of pain just prior to or after ball release and localizes the pain either generally throughout the shoulder and deep within or laterally at the insertion of the deltoid muscle. The author refers to this condition as "cuffitis," which appears to be an inflammation of the rotator cuff due to impingement. To verify that rotator cuff tendinitis is present a thorough examination and a diagnostic and therapeutic injection that is similar to that utilized in bicipital tendinitis are performed. The tender portions of the shoulder are palpated and localized on the basis of a knowledge of the anatomy.

If symptoms are compatible with the presence of a supraspinatus

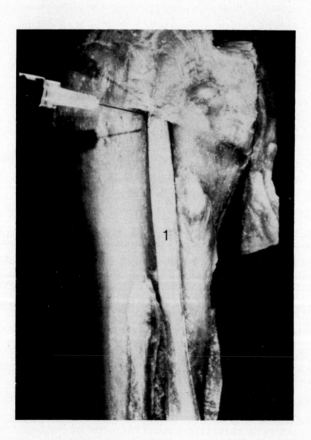

FIGURE 12–2. The optimal site of injection anatomically for the bicipital groove. (1) Long tendon of the biceps needle in the bicipital groove.

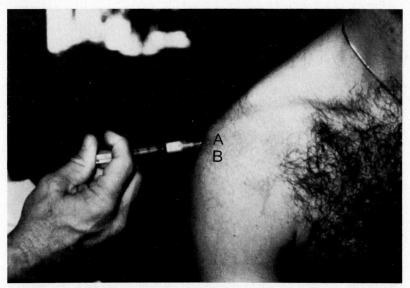

FIGURE 12–3. Position for rotator cuff bathing. *(A)* **Edge of the acromion.** *(B)* **Subacromial space.**

tendinitis, an injection into the subdeltoid bursa is made utilizing a posterior or lateral approach. The patient is seated on the end of the examining table with the arm relaxed as an assistant applies traction on the arm to open the subacromial space. The gap is marked just below the acromion with the thumbnail, and the skin is prepared in a sterile fashion. A 1.5-inch 25-gauge needle is inserted beneath the acromion and angled parallel to the under surface of the acromion for insertion of the needle into the subdeltoid bursa. The examiner's eyes should never leave the mark made on the skin. The material should flow in quite easily (Fig. 12–3). An injection into the subdeltoid bursa should provide immediate relief from the inflamed rotator cuff if the needle has been placed in the proper position (Fig. 12–4).

A common source of posterior shoulder pain is the *teres minor syndrome*. In this syndrome the patient complains of pain either at the very start or at the end of motion, and the pain is localized to the back of the shoulder. To examine the teres minor muscle the patient is placed prone on an examination table and the physician sits next to him. The patient's arm is placed forward on the examination table as he lightly grasps the forward portion of the table. The point of maximal tenderness is identified along the axillary border of the scapula (Fig. 12–5), and an injection is made into this area. The needle must contact bone. Once contact has been verified, the needle is pulled back slightly (Fig. 12–6).

Another area of the shoulder that is easily palpated and treated with injections is the acromioclavicular joint. This joint should always be evalu-

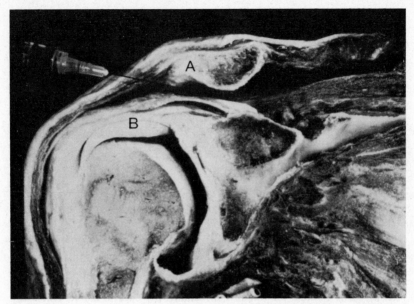

FIGURE 12–4. The optimal site of subacromial space injection for bathing the rotator cuff. *(A)* Acromion process. *(B)* Rotator cuff.

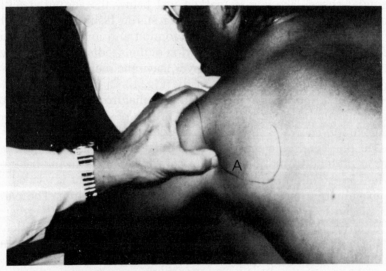

FIGURE 12–5. Preinjection identification of the anatomic site of the teres minor. *(A)* Axillary border of the scapula.

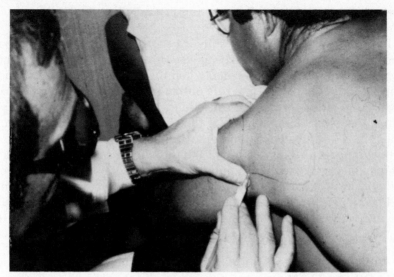

FIGURE 12–6. Injection of the teres minor insertion into the rotator cuff.

ated in a patient complaining of superior shoulder pain. If the acromiocla-vicular joint is felt to be inflamed a 5/8-inch needle connected to a tuberculin syringe can be inserted easily into the joint. A therapeutic mixture of lidocaine and steroid is injected.

Biceps tendinitis, rotator cuff tendinitis, teres minor syndrome, and lesions about the acromioclavicular joint constitute approximately 95 per cent of the inflammatory processes encountered when dealing with the throwing athlete. When combined with a thorough history, physical exam-ination, and knowledge of the anatomy of the shoulder, these areas can be successfully treated by injection for both diagnostic and therapeutic pur-poses.

Inflammatory disorders about the shoulder are quite easily diagnosed, and a reasonable differential diagnosis can be made in most cases. A more difficult diagnostic situation exists when there is a combination of mechan-ical and inflammatory processes. When there is a mechanical problem the patient has a history of feeling something slipping, moving, grinding, or popping in the shoulder. The history is extremely important, and attention to detail is crucial. A common complaint of the throwing athlete is, "My shoulder goes out of place." Frequently the cause of this complaint appears to be mechanical in origin; however, attention to detail indicates that the athlete is experiencing only pain and that he cannot throw effectively, and actually no mechanical derangement exists. The author considers that the descriptive words "goes out" are very dangerous as a basis for a diagnosis;

however, a patient may be experiencing a subluxation, dislocation, or injury to the glenoid labrum.

In examining the throwing athlete's shoulder to rule out a mechanical derangement the shoulder must be moved through a passive range of motion. Attention should be given to detail when the anterior and posterior aspects of the shoulder are palpated to rule out an anterior or posterior subluxation as well as popping or grating sensations. A grating sensation on anterior subluxation can suggest a lesion of the anterior glenoid labrum, which can be identified and treated arthroscopically.

In summary, in examination of the throwing athlete's shoulder several fundamentals are extremely important: the anatomy, the function of the shoulder, and the correct position of the patient for optimal examination and injections. Correct technique is important, since the lack of success following an injection can be related to poor technique on the part of the injector.

REHABILITATION

The objectives of a proper rehabilitation program are (1) to reduce pain, (2) to restore motion, (3) to increase strength, and (4) to improve coordination. The injection techniques described earlier are effective ways of reducing pain. Rest and occasionally oral anti-inflammatory medication are useful.

Once the pain has been reduced the next goal is to restore motion. An effective means of restoring motion to the throwing shoulder is having the patient perform the following five exercises: (1) circumduction in a clockwise direction (Fig. 12–7), (2) circumduction in a counterclockwise direc-

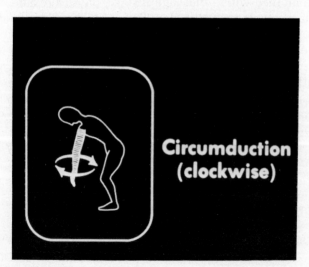

Circumduction (clockwise)

FIGURE 12–7. Forward bend. The left arm hangs, and the hand is parallel to the floor. Circles are made with a minimum of pain. The size of the circles is determined by the amount of pain and stiffness. The result is large rotational motions of the humeral head in the glenoid cavity.

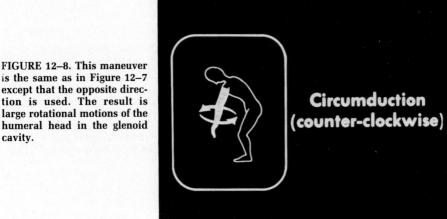

FIGURE 12–8. This maneuver is the same as in Figure 12–7 except that the opposite direction is used. The result is large rotational motions of the humeral head in the glenoid cavity.

tion (Fig. 12–8), (3) saws (Fig. 12–9), (4) cross-body movements (Fig. 12–10), and (5) rotations (Fig. 12–11). The patient performs 50 of each of these exercises in the morning and in the evening for a total of 500 repetitions.

Once motion has been restored the patient progresses to modalities intended to increase strength and improve coordination. One regimen is the "Fungo" routine, which was started 25 years ago and is still in use. The objective of this regimen is to stretch and strengthen the arm and to help the individual return to a normal throwing motion. When pain has been reduced and motion restored, the patient begins by throwing a baseball on a long easy throw from the deepest point of the outfield with the ball just barely getting back to the hitter, who is usually standing near home plate. This routine is to be performed for 30 minutes on two consecutive

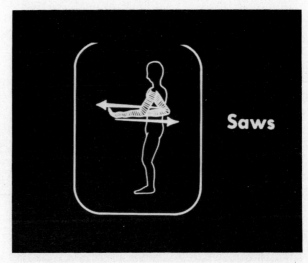

FIGURE 12–9. The elbow goes from complete flexion at the extreme of posterior shoulder motion to complete elbow extension at the extreme of forward movement of the shoulder. Smooth stretching is used, with no punching or jabbing motions. The result is flexion and extension of the humeral head in the glenoid cavity.

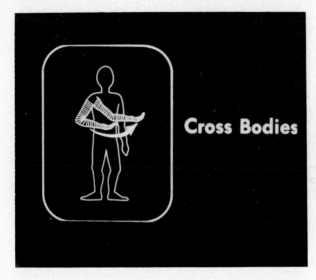

FIGURE 12–10. The body is flexed slightly forward with the elbow locked in fixed flexion. The arm moves as if in a deep trough, without rotation. The result is abduction and adduction of the humeral head in the glenoid cavity.

days. The next day the patient rests the arm for a day. The following day he progresses to stronger throws from the midoutfield, getting the ball back on five to six bounces. He performs these throws for 30 minutes on two consecutive days. The next day the patient rests the arm entirely. The following day the patient performs strong crisp throws with a relatively straight trajectory from a short outfield and returns the ball on one bouce back to the hitter. He performs this sequence for 30 minutes on two consecutive days. Once again, the following day is a rest day with no throwing at all. If the patient tolerates these activities the next day he can return to the mound or other normal positions and usual activities. He is now throwing the shortest distance, rather than working back to the mound, with repeated short throws during the rehabilitation period.

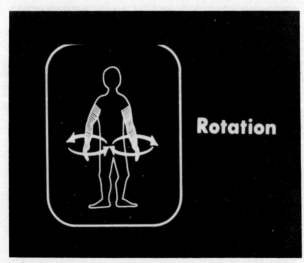

FIGURE 12–11. Simple standing with the arms hanging and the elbows moving into complete pronation and supination. The result is complete rotation of the humeral head in the glenoid cavity.

THE IMPINGEMENT SYNDROME

ROBERT E. LEACH, M.D.

During the past decade, as athletic participation by all ages and sexes has increased, a bountiful crop of informal medical-athletic terms has been garnered for certain conditions commonly seen in a variety of sports. Among these is the *impingement syndrome*.[1] The reader may recognize this as the condition formerly called the painful arc syndrome, a form of chronic rotator cuff tendinitis, and some will recognize that it has some reference to the old lay term "bursitis." What is meant by the term "impingement syndrome" is a chronic inflammatory process involving the rotator cuff and secondarily the subdeltoid bursa, as it impinges against the coracoacromial ligament and the anterior part of the acromion process.

The impingement syndrome is most commonly seen in throwing sports such as baseball, racquet sports, particularly tennis, and in swimmers. It can be seen in participants in any athletic contest in which the arm is abducted or flexed forward to 90 degrees, such as in wrestling, gymnastics, and weightlifting.

The anatomy of the shoulder with the overlying coracoacromial arch makes the impingement syndrome possible. The two tendons most involved are the supraspinatus, which is by far the most common, and the infraspinatus. Together these tendons compose a major portion of the rotator cuff. Overlying these tendons and their attachment to the greater tuberosity of the humerus is the subdeltoid bursa, which is normally a thin sheet of tissue providing a gliding mechanism between the rotator cuff and the coracoacromial arch plus the anterior aspect of the acromion. In some people with constant repetitive use there is a gradual impingement of the

121

rotator cuff against the unyielding coracoacromial ligament and the anterior aspect of the acromion process. Occasionally the distal portion of the clavicle with a protruding osteophyte on the under surface is involved.

Impingement usually takes place as the arm is either abducted or flexed forward to between 85 and 120 degrees and in particular with internal rotation of the arm. Repetitive use of the shoulder in this manner can cause chronic inflammation of the rotator cuff and a secondary inflammation of the bursa as it attempts to cushion and protect the rotator cuff. As the supraspinatus tendon becomes more inflamed, its muscle tendon unit becomes weaker, and the supraspinatus and the other cuff muscles may work inefficiently. As the arm abducts, these muscles do not depress the head into the glenoid cavity, and the head may ride up, increasing pressure on the chronically inflamed rotator cuff.

As has been shown by the detailed studies of Rathbun and Macnab,[2] there is a portion of the rotator cuff near its distal attachment that is relatively avascular and that when subjected to constant stress can deteriorate and be subject to fibrinous degeneration. This in turn can lead to calcium deposition much less commonly than to fibrinous degeneration. Over a period of time with repetitive use and more fibrinous degeneration, this process leads to small attritional tears and eventually to large tears of the rotator cuff. The latter outcome is more likely to occur in the 35- to 55-year-old athletic person than in the younger age group.

The pain is produced by elevation of the arm, usually with an element of rotation, which causes impingement of the chronically inflamed tissues against the coracoacromial ligament and bony arch of the acromion. The chronically inflamed tissues are painful with use and can even produce pain at rest. Night pain is not infrequent and can be produced by elevation of the arms during sleep or by the formation of small adhesions that set up overnight and that with motion of the arms are torn and cause pain. The more the patient tries to use the arm, the more pain there is, and so the inflammatory process continues. While pain is the major complaint, in some instances there is an element of adhesive capsulitis with decreased range of motion. Frequently the external rotators of the shoulder, particularly the supraspinatus muscle, are quite weak and may further lessen athletic prowess.

The physical examination should always be performed with the patient disrobed from the waist up. The author prefers to stand behind the patient and to watch the shoulder through its range of motion. In some instances there is a loss of abduction or forward flexion, loss of internal rotation, and more rarely, loss of external rotation. As the examiner stands behind the patient and watches him elevate the arm, an asynchrony is frequently noticed between the painful and the nonpainful shoulders. The patient attempts to duck the humeral head underneath the acromion process. This maneuver may be perceived as a slight hitch in scapulothoracic motion as the patient attempts to control the scapula and thus the position of the acromion process. There can be visible atrophy of the supraspinatus or infraspinatus muscle. Usually there is weakness of these muscle groups, and an attempt should be made to isolate the supraspinatus muscle by having the patient abduct the arm to 90 degrees, flex it forward 20 degrees, and internally rotate and then elevate it against resistance (Fig. 13–1). This is a relatively specific test for supraspinatus function, and almost invariably weakness is noted if the supraspinatus is torn or involved in a chronic disease process.

Depending on the age of the patient and his complaints, there can be an associated rotator cuff tear. In the younger patients this is less likely, although a small tear of the rotator cuff can be seen. In patients 35 to 55 years of age a small rotator cuff rupture is more common, and while the symptoms are similar to that of chronic tendinitis, a small rotator cuff rupture can lead to further degeneration and a subsequent full rupture of the rotator cuff.

Routine radiography taken with the arm in neutral, internal, and external rotation can show calcification in the cuff, but this is an infrequent finding. An axillary radiograph should be obtained routinely. The greater tuberosity should be examined carefully to see any sign of sclerosis (Fig. 13–2), erosion (Fig. 13–3), or cysts. These are changes of chronic tendinitis and should be recognized as such. Particularly when there is erosion of this area, a small rotator cuff rupture must be suspected. If a rotator cuff rupture is suspected, a shoulder arthrogram or arthroscopy should be performed to see the size of the rupture. Sometimes there can be a small flap tear of the rotator cuff, and the dye will not escape from the flap. A positive arthrogram is of value. A negative arthrogram must be interpreted with caution.

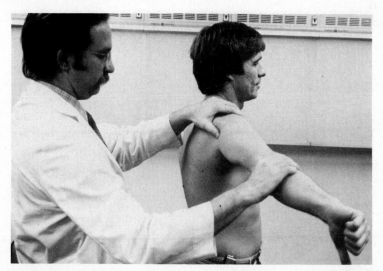

FIGURE 13–1. Testing for strength of the supraspinatus muscle with arm abduction, forward flexion, and internal rotation.

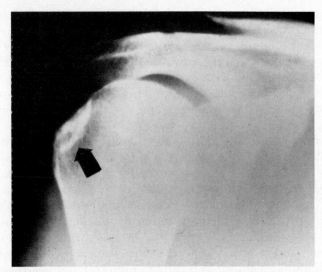

FIGURE 13–2. A sclerotic area in the greater tuberosity often indicates chronic tendinitis.

The first step in conservative treatment of the impingement syndrome is to have the person decrease the precipitating activity. For the competitive athlete this is difficult. Sometimes a modification can be made in the throwing motion, or swimmers can use a different stroke. Practically this proves difficult, and a period of decreased activity or full rest is needed if the athlete has major symptoms. The author prescribes pendulum exercises

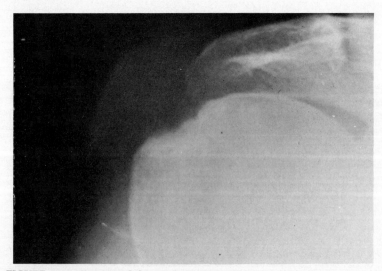

FIGURE 13–3. Erosion of the greater tuberosity seen with chronic tears of the rotator cuff.

in which the athlete leans far forward at the waist while holding a three-pound weight. The athlete is asked to do these exercises frequently during the course of the day. The concept is to restore the gliding mechanism of the bursa and the rotator cuff. With the patient leaning far forward the humeral head is brought forward away from the coracoacromial arch. Oral anti-inflammatory agents are effective, and the author frequently gives a three- to four-week course of an oral anti-inflammatory medication that can be used as necessary should symptoms return. The patient should begin with strengthening exercises for the muscles of the rotator cuff, but these should be performed against resistance with the arm at the side so that there is no further irritation of the rotator cuff during the time of performing the exercises. Surgical tubing or a bungee cord has proved to be an adequate means of providing resistance. The patient simply ties the tubing to a fixed position, puts a loop in it, and performs internal and external rotation of the shoulder against the tubing resistance with the elbow at the side (Fig. 13–4).

The condition of the majority of patients with chronic tendinitis who follow a program such as this improves greatly and can become asymptomatic. Some continue to have symptoms, and in this particular group a steroid injection into the subdeltoid bursa can decrease the inflammatory process and shrink the tissues, thus helping to control symptoms. This treatment should be combined with all the measures that have already been

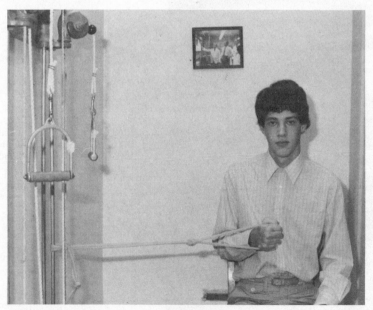

FIGURE 13–4. An exercise to strengthen internal rotators of the shoulder. The sequence is reversed to strengthen the external rotators.

instituted, and there should be a rest period of 10 to 14 days following the injection of the steroid into the subdeltoid bursa. The author makes it a policy to not make injections into the shoulder more than two times unless there has been a long interval between the period of symptoms.[3]

When conservative treatment of the symptoms of an impingement syndrome fail, the options are either to have the athlete give up the activity that is causing him pain or to consider surgery. For some people changing sports or giving up a particular sport can be a viable option. For many others it is not. Thus, surgery becomes a major consideration.

The primary goal in surgery is to decompress the tissues of the rotator cuff and thus decrease pain. This can be done in a variety of ways. The surgical procedures presently used include resection of the corcoacromial ligament,[4] the anterior acromioplasty of Neer,[1] which includes a resection of the coracoacromial ligament, the partial acromionectomy of Leach,[5] resection of the distal end of the clavicle, or resection of osteophytes on the distal end of the clavicle. The obvious aim of these various surgical procedures is to decompress the portion of the coracoacromial roof that appears to be causing symptoms.

In the author's practice in young athletes resection of the coracoacromial ligament alone (Fig. 13–5) or in combination with the Neer anterior

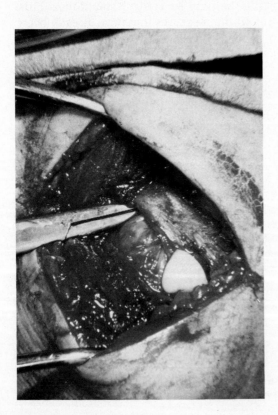

FIGURE 13–5. A hemostat under the coracoacromial ligament with a large white fibrin "rice" body to the right.

acromioplasty has been sufficient. After this procedure patients have been able to return to sports such as swimming, tennis, and throwing activities. In patients who have stage-two changes of the rotator cuff, as described by Neer[1] and by Hawkins and Kennedy,[6] the coracoacromial ligament resection is not enough but must be combined with a Neer anterior acromioplasty or in some instances with a partial acromionectomy. These patients generally are in their 30s and 40s. In patients who have stage-three changes in the rotator cuff, which can include degenerative or attritional tears, the author has found the best procedure to be a partial acromionectomy combined with whatever surgery is needed on the rotator cuff. In all of these operations the under surface of the distal end of the clavicle should be examined for any osteophytes, which should be resected.

The major problem with partial acromionectomy is the fact that the patient must be immobilized for several weeks in order to allow reattachment of the deltoid muscle before a strong rehabilitation program can be started. Unlike the total acromionectomy of Hammond,[7] partial acromionectomy does not leave a cosmetic defect. Also, strength returns to normal, although this can take six months. The author finds that the partial acromionectomy is needed most commonly for those who are over 40 and who have stage-three changes in the rotator cuff. Most others can be handled either by the resection of the coracoacromial ligament, which is best in the very young patients, or by the Neer anterior acromioplasty.

After this discussion of surgical treatment, it is important to remind the reader that the vast majority of people with an impingement syndrome can be treated by conservative measures, which usually allow the patient to return to sporting activities.

REFERENCES

1. Neer, C. S.: Anterior acromioplasty for the chronic impingement syndrome in the shoulder. J Bone Joint Surg 54A:41–50, 1972.
2. Rathbun, J. B., and Macnab, I.: The microvascular pattern of the rotator cuff. J Bone Joint Surg 52B:540–553, 1970.
3. Kennedy, J. C., and Willis, R. B.: The effects of local steroid injections on tendons: A biomechanical and microscopic correlative study. Am J Sports Med 4:11–21, 1976.
4. Jackson, D. W.: Chronic rotator cuff impingement in the throwing athlete. Orthop Trans 1:24, 1977.
5. Leach, R. E., O'Connor, P., and Jones, R. P.: Acromionectomy for tendinitis of the shoulder in athletes. Physician Sportsmed 7:96–107, 1979.
6. Hawkins, R. J., and Kennedy, J. C.: Impingement syndrome in athletes. Am J Sports Med 8:151–158, 1980.
7. Hammond, G.: Complete acromionectomy in the treatment of chronic tendinitis of the shoulder. J Bone Joint Surg 53A:173–180, 1971.

THE ACROMIOCLAVICULAR JOINT IN THE THROWING ARM

MARCUS J. STEWART, M.D.

ANATOMY OF THE ACROMIOCLAVICULAR JOINT

The acromion process occupies the highest point of the shoulder. Its upper surface, which is continuous with the crest of the spine of the scapula, is subcutaneous. The medial border of the acromion process is short and continuous with the upper lip of the crest. The anterior and lateral part of the medial border is occupied by an oval facet for articulation with the lateral end of the clavicle, and this forms the acromioclavicular joint. The clavicle is an elongated slender curved bone in the shape of the italic letter *F*. It derives its name from the Greek word meaning key or bolt. The lateral end of the clavicle articulates with the medial margin of the acromion process and is occupied by an oval articular facet. The junction of the clavicle with the acromion is not a direct articulation because there is an articulate disc of fibrous cartilage between these two bones. However, its articular surface is oblique when it is viewed looking downward, as well as laterally, so that when the bone articulates with the acromion it is placed so that if its ligaments are torn and dislocated it overrides the acromion and may be difficult to keep in place even after reduction (Fig. 14–1).

The primary stabilizer of the acromioclavicular joint is the coracoclavicular ligament, which is composed of two bands, the conoid or lateral

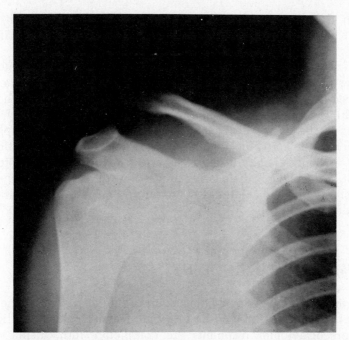

FIGURE 14–1. Nineteen-year-old male with Type III acromioclavicular separation incurred while playing football his sophomore
year. (Reprinted with permission, from Smith, M. J., and Stewart,
M. J., "Acute acromioclavicular separations," *American Journal
of Sports Medicine* 7:65, 1979. ©1979 American Society for Sports
Medicine.)

portion of the ligament and the triangular medial portion known as the
trapezoid ligament. These very strong structures prevent the clavicle from
riding upward and dislocating over the acromion process. Forward and
backward movement of the clavicle at the acromioclavicular joint is controlled to a great extent by the coracoacromial ligament, often referred to as
the acromioclavicular capsular ligament.

The coracohumeral ligament is an accessory ligament on the upper
aspect of the glenohumeral joint. This ligament extends from the lateral
side of the base of the coracoid process along the capsular ligament in a
lateral direction as a portion of the capsule and reaches the neck of the
humerus opposite the greater tuberosity. This connection strengthens the
upper part of the capsular ligament that arches over the upper aspect of the
shoulder and is under tension when the arm hangs by the side.

The coracoacromial ligament is triangular and horizontally placed.
Superiorly, it is covered by the deltoid muscle; inferiorly, it is separated by
the subacromial bursa from the supraspinatus tendon. Its primary function
is to provide an extension of the socket over the head of the humerus.
Occasionally this ligament alone has been found to cause symptoms in the
throwing motion, and its presence must not be forgotten or neglected.

Although this ligament helps to support the anterior joint, it is often necessary to resect the ligament to give relief of shoulder pain in certain athletes.

The acromioclavicular joint has a very important function in supporting the upper part of the shoulder. Stability of the acromioclavicular joint is maintained by ligaments. Injury usually occurs by direct trauma that results in stretching these ligaments. The injuries are graded as Grade I, II, or III according to the degree of ligament tear and the amount of displacement that occurs at the acromioclavicular joint.[1] The common description of the shoulder as being "knocked down" is erroneous because the deformity is the result of the clavicle dislocating upward over the acromion. Dislocation of the acromioclavicular joint is commonly referred to as "separation" of the shoulder.

ACUTE DISLOCATION OF THE ACROMIOCLAVICULAR JOINT

The amount of superior displacement of the lateral end of the clavicle is determined by the degree of the injury to the coracoclavicular ligaments. If the coracoclavicular ligaments are completely torn, displacement is maximal, and thus the acromioclavicular joint has a third-degree dislocation. If the coracoclavicular ligaments are intact, the joint can be no more than slightly subluxated. Horn[2] noted that in third-degree dislocations the deltoid and trapezius muscles are usually injured as well. According to Horn, the deltoid muscle can be avulsed from the lateral end of the clavicle for a distance of 1 to 2 inches, and the trapezius muscle can be split in line with its fibers above the acromioclavicular joint.

In complete acromioclavicular separation the lateral end of the clavicle is most often displaced superiorly. Based on a study of 41 patients, Urist[3] made the following observations. First, when the lateral end of the clavicle has not been displaced superiorly, an increase in width of the joint space, as seen in anteroposterior roentgenograms, indicates that it has been displaced posteriorly. Second, when the lateral end of the clavicle has been displaced posteriorly or has been abnormally mobile for three weeks, conservative treatment is likely to fail. According to Urist,[3] and to Jacobs and Wade,[4] the chief reason for failure of conservative treatment is that the articular disc, frayed capsular ligament, or flake of articular cartilage has been caught between the clavicle and the acromion in a way that prevents adequate reduction of the displacement. To obtain good results following surgical repair of a dislocation, the coracoclavicular ligaments must be adequately repaired and the acromioclavicular joint reduced and held in position until the repaired ligaments have healed. Merely reducing the joint and holding it reduced by internal fixation is usually insufficient; conversely, repairing or reconstructing the coracoclavicular ligaments alone is insufficient, since the ligament will stretch and the joint again subluxate unless it has been held in a reduced position.

Murray[5] and Phemister[6] were early advocates of transfixing the acromioclavicular joint using wires after reduction. Because the acromion and clavicle are small in cross section, the wires should not be any larger than 3/32 of an inch. It is best to use two unthreaded pins, each the size of a guide wire, and to bend their lateral ends to prevent them from migrating medially. Unthreaded wires are much easier to remove later than are threaded ones. Henry[7] held the acromioclavicular joint with a loop of wire. Alldredge[8] used a wire loop around the clavicle and the coracoid process. Independent of one another, Bosworth[9] in this country and Vere-Hodge[10] in England used a screw inserted through the clavicle and into the base of the coracoid process to hold the reduction. Theoretically this procedure would prevent rotation of the clavicle, which is necessary during some motions of the shoulder girdle. Kennedy and Cameron,[11] however, showed that such fixation does not prevent the clavicle from rotating; rather, it causes a synchronous rotation of both the scapula and the clavicle. The authors recommend using this fixation, especially in people under 50 years of age. In older people the shoulder girdle can fail to adapt itself to this synchonous rotation.

Horn[2] recommended that any tear of the trapezius and deltoid muscles must also be repaired, in addition to repair of the acromioclavicular joint and coracoclavicular ligaments. He believed that failure to repair these muscle tears was the chief reason for persistent pain and weakness after surgery. Jacobs and Wade[4] agreed that failure to repair these muscles was at least one cause of such symptoms. Avulsion of the deltoid muscle can be repaired by passing interrupted mattress sutures through the muscle and either around or through the clavicle. A tear in the trapezius muscle can be closed by passing similar sutures across its tear.

Many surgeons repair most acute Grade III dislocations of the acromioclavicular joint. The author usually repairs such separations in the young and middle-aged. However, Urist,[3, 12] Mumford,[13] and others believe that most such cases can be treated without surgery. In fact, Urist has listed 32 different methods of conservative treatment.[3, 12]

Depending on the circumstances, the author uses one of four operations for dislocation of the acromioclavicular joint: (1) a modified Phemister technique,[6] in which the acromioclavicular joint is reduced and transfixed with Kirschner wires and the coracoclavicular ligaments are sutured; (2) the Stewart technique,[14] in which the lateral 1 cm of the clavicle is resected obliquely, the remaining end of the clavicle is fixed to the acromion with Kirschner wires, and the coracoclavicular ligaments are sutured; (3) a modified Henry technique,[7] in which the acromioclavicular joint is reduced and transfixed with Kirschner wires and the coracoclavicular ligaments are reconstructed with fascia; and (4) resection of the lateral end of the clavicle. The modified Phemister technique is used for patients under 40 or 45 years of age whose dislocation is less than two weeks old. The Stewart technique is used for young patients whose dislocation is less than two weeks old and who plan to return to vigorous activities such as contact sports. However, resection of the lateral clavicle must not be done in patients whose epiphyseal plate at the lateral end of the clavicle is open. The modified Henry technique is used for patients under 40 to 45 years of age whose dislocation is more than two weeks old. Resection of the lateral end of the clavicle is used to treat acute or chronic separations in elderly patients or chronic dislocation in young patients.

Stewart Technique

Resection of the outer centimeter of the clavicle should be done in an oblique manner as illustrated in Figure 14–2A. The acromioclavicular joint, the lateral end of the clavicle, and the coracoid process are exposed through

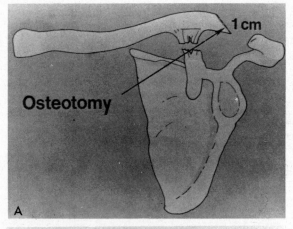

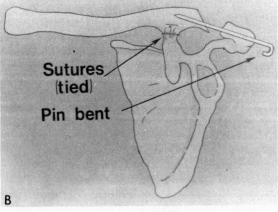

FIGURE 14–2. *A*, Oblique osteotomy of the distal clavicle, with 1 cm removed, measured from the tip of the clavicle to the acromion. *B*, K-wires bent and rotated 180 degrees. (Reprinted, with permission, from Smith, M. J., and Stewart, M. J., "Acute acromioclavicular separations," *American Journal of Sports Medicine* 7:64, 1979. ©1979 American Society for Sports Medicine.)

a curved anterior incision. Next the lateral 1 cm of the clavicle is resected subperiosteally, and an oblique osteotomy is performed through the bone from a supermedial to inferolateral direction. With a file the superior subcutaneous edge of the remaining end of the bone is smoothed. Mattress sutures are placed in the ruptured coracoclavicular ligaments but not tied. Two Kirschner wires—each the size of a guide wire—are inserted about 3 inches apart through the lateral border of the acromion process so that they enter the middle of the articular facet of the acromion process. While holding the lateral end of the clavicle reduced, the wires are advanced into the cancellous portion of the clavicle for 1 to 1.5 inches.

It is advisable at this time to take a roentgenogram of the acromioclavicular joint to determine whether the wires are well placed. The lateral tip of the pin must be bent into a 90-degree hook or it will migrate medially into the clavicle (Fig. 14–2B). The pin must be placed into the cancellous part of the clavicle and not into the cortex, since motion can cause the pin to break at the joint. This will result in loss of the stability that is needed during healing of the ligaments. The sutures that were previously placed in the coracoclavicular ligaments are tied, and the capsule and ligaments of the acromioclavicular joint are repaired. The articular disc should be used to reinforce the acromioclavicular ligaments. Any tear of the deltoid and trapezoid muscles must be repaired, and the limb should be immobilized in a sling.

The patient is encouraged to use the limb immediately, but raising the arm above the horizontal level is not permitted for three or four weeks. At eight to ten weeks after surgery the wires are removed under local anesthesia, and normal activities by the patient are gradually resumed.

It is common practice to resect the outer end of the clavicle, according to the so-called *Mumford*[13] or *Gurd*[15] procedure in cases of chronic acromioclavicular separation or degenerative joint disease. The author has been resecting the distal clavicle in acute injuries for more than 20 years and has had many athletes continue athletic activity after surgery without impairment of function. The author believes this procedure does not interfere with strength or stability of the throwing arm and that there is less chance of pain in the joint because the clavicle no longer abuts against the acromion.

Results of Treatment

One hundred and twenty-two acromioclavicular separations treated by surgery at the Campbell Clinic from 1956 to 1976 were studied.[14] The average age of patients was 27 years (range 12 to 64 years). The average time of follow-up was 4.4 years (range 1 to 16 years). There were 10 females and 112 males. The most common cause of injury was football, followed by motor vehicle accidents (Table 14–1).

TABLE 14–1. CAUSE OF INJURY*

Football	46
High school (24)	
College (20)	
Professional (2)	
Automobile accident	21
Motorcycle accident	18
Water skiing	2
Snow skiing	1
Baseball	1
Basketball	1
Racquetball	1
Miscellaneous falls	31
Total	122

*Table adapted from Smith, M. J., and Stewart, M. J., "Acute acromioclavicular separations," *American Journal of Sports Medicine* 7:68, 1979. © 1979 The Williams & Wilkins Co. Reproduced by permission.

Primary excision of the distal clavicle combined with repair of the torn ligaments was performed in 44 patients (Table 14–2). This group was compared with the 78 patients who had primary repair of the torn ligaments only. There were 34 Type II and 64 Type III separations. Twenty-four injuries were not classified. No patient with a Type I injury was treated by surgery. Both groups had the shoulders immobilized for an average of nine weeks. In the group treated by excision of the distal clavicle, internal fixation using smooth Kirschner wires was performed in 40 patients. No internal fixation was used in four patients. In the other group, internal fixation using smooth Kirschner wires was employed in 59 patients, threaded Kirschner wires in 2, Knowles pins in 3, and nonabsorbable sutures through holes drilled in the clavicle in 7. No internal fixation was used in 7 patients (Table 14–3).

Of the 122 patients treated, 86 were reexamined to evaluate results of treatment. At the time of follow-up, both groups were asked to evaluate the

TABLE 14–2. EXCISION OF THE DISTAL CLAVICLE*

	EXCISION AND REPAIR	LIGAMENT REPAIR ONLY
Average age	26 years	27 years
Number of patients	44	78
Grade of injury		
I	0	0
II	14	20
III	24	40
Unknown	6	18
Average postoperative immobilization	9 weeks	9 weeks

*Table adapted from Smith, M. J., and Stewart, M. J., "Acute acromioclavicular separations," *American Journal of Sports Medicine* 7:68, 1979. © 1979 The Williams & Wilkins Co. Reproduced by permission.

TABLE 14-3. INTERNAL FIXATION*

	EXCISION AND REPAIR	LIGAMENT REPAIR ONLY
Internal fixation		
Smooth Kirschner wires	40	59
Threaded Kirschner wires	0	2
Knowles pins	0	3
Nonabsorbable suture through drill holes	0	7
No internal fixation	4	7

*Table adapted from Smith, M. J., and Stewart, M. J., "Acute acromioclavicular separations," *American Journal of Sports Medicine* 7:68, 1979. © 1979 The Williams & Wilkins Co. Reproduced by permission.

results subjectively and to comment on shoulder pain, weakness, throwing or serving motions, and cosmetic appearance. A result was termed excellent if the patient had no pain, no limitation of motion, and was able to return to participation in sports or physical activity. A result was called good if the patient had minimal pain and mild limitation of motion that did not interfere with return to the physical activity. A result was called poor if the patient has enough pain or limitation of motion to prevent participation in previous physical activities.

The physical examination included a range-of-motion evaluation of strength in the throwing motion, tenderness, and position and stability of the distal clavicle.

Finally, radiographs were obtained to determine whether there was any residual subluxation or degenerative change.

Table 14–4 presents the subjective results of the patients who were evaluated. Primary excision of the distal end of the clavicle produced the best results; there was only one poor result in the group.

There was no significant difference in the amount of residual shoulder weakness when the two operations were compared. Fewer patients treated

TABLE 14-4. SUBJECTIVE EVALUATION*

	EXCISION AND REPAIR	LIGAMENT REPAIR ONLY
Number	32	54
Results		
Excellent	24	33
Good	7	13
Poor	1	8
Shoulder weakness	2	4
Difficulty with throwing	2	6
Dissatisfaction with cosmesis	1	2

*Table adapted from Smith, M. J., and Stewart, M. J., "Acute acromioclavicular separations," *American Journal of Sports Medicine* 7:68, 1979. © 1979 The Williams & Wilkins Co. Reproduced by permission.

with excision of the distal clavicle had difficulty with throwing a ball or with overhand serves as in tennis than with ligament repair only. No real difference in cosmetic appearance was noted between the groups.

On physical examination, no difference was found between the two groups in range of motion or weakness (Table 14–5). The only patient who had weakness in the group treated with excision of the distal clavicle had had 4 cm of the clavicle removed. (This finding is in agreement with Gillespie,[16] who found weakness in shoulders if 5 cm of the clavicle was excised.)

Fewer patients had acromioclavicular tenderness following primary excision. Two patients had prominence of the distal clavicle following ligament repair only, but without internal fixation.

Degenerative changes, visible on radiographs, ranged from mild irregularity of the acromioclavicular joint to gross changes that included calcification and ossification of the surrounding soft tissues. In 33 patients ossification between the coracoid process and the clavicle was observed. However, no symptoms could be ascribed to this ossification.

An enlargement or "bossing" of the distal end of the clavicle was occasionally associated with mild symptoms (Fig. 14–3). Presumably this enlargement is caused by a tear of the periosteum or a fracture in the cortex of the distal clavicle at the time of injury. Although this injury may not be recognized on the original radiograph, it may lead to altered congruity of the acromioclavicular joint and subsequent arthralgia. This condition occurred in three of the author's patients, but symptoms were mild and all had good results.

There was no correlation between degenerative changes in the acromioclavicular joint and the patient's symptoms. Some patients had minor degenerative changes but severe symptoms, while others had extensive degenerative changes but no symptoms.

Patients treated by excision of the distal end of the clavicle had less degenerative joint disease than those treated by ligament repair only (5 versus 24 per cent). Only two patients had degenerative joint disease in the group treated by excision of the end of the clavicle. One was a 16-year-old boy in whom the distal end of the clavicle completely reformed, and

TABLE 14–5. PHYSICAL EXAMINATION*

	EXCISION AND REPAIR	LIGAMENT REPAIR ONLY
Loss of motion		
> 10 degrees	1	2
Shoulder weakness	1	3
Acromioclavicular tenderness	1	4
Clavicle prominence	0	3

*Table adapted from Smith, M. J., and Stewart, M. J., "Acute acromioclavicular separations," *American Journal of Sports Medicine* 7:68, 1979. © 1979 The Williams & Wilkins Co. Reproduced by permission.

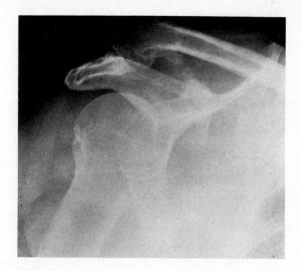

FIGURE 14–3. Excess callus and bossing of distal clavicle.

degenerative changes occurred. For this reason, it is recommended that excision of the distal clavicle not be performed if the epiphyses are open. The other patient had only the distal 5 mm of the clavicle excised and developed degenerative changes within one year of surgery.

A graph (Fig. 14–4) depicting the time of onset of the first degenerative changes showed a peak within the first year and a second peak five to six years later.

FIGURE 14–4. Time of appearance of first degenerative changes. This suggests that clinical studies should have at least a six-year follow-up. (Reprinted, with permission, from Smith, M. J., and Stewart, M. J., "Acute acromioclavicular separations," *American Journal of Sports Medicine* 7:70, 1979. ©1979 American Society for Sports Medicine.)

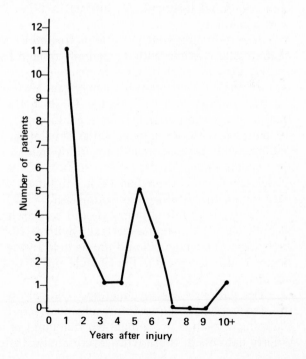

DISCUSSION

Excision of the outer end of the clavicle for derangement of the acromioclavicular joint was first described independently by Gurd[15] and Mumford.[13] Gurd[15] believed that the main function of the clavicle is to act as a point of attachment of the important shoulder muscles. Therefore, he reasoned that patients would do well even if the outer end of the clavicle was removed. He reported on three patients with complete chronic separations treated with excision of the distal end of the clavicle, and all had good results. Mumford[13] reported on four patients with chronic subluxations (not separations) who were treated with excision of the outer end of the clavicle, and they also had good results.

Moseley[17] reported on the treatment of acute and chronic acromioclavicular disruptions by excision of the outer end of the clavicle plus fascial repair of the coracoclavicular ligaments.

Urist[3] recommended excision of the distal clavicle and repair of the deltoid and trapezius muscle attachments for old injuries. However, a weakness of the shoulder muscles was noted.

Gillespie[16] reported on the treatment of 30 complete acromioclavicular dislocations by excision of the outer end of the clavicle. He found that weakness occurred if more than 5 cm of the clavicle was excised.

Weaver and Dunn[18] reported on 15 patients with acute and chronic acromioclavicular dislocations treated by excision of the outer end of the clavicle and reconstruction of the coracoclavicular ligaments using the coracoacromial ligament. No internal fixation was used, and good results were obtained.

Browne[19] compared 13 patients treated by primary excision and repair of the distal calvicle with 12 patients treated by only primary repair. In a short follow-up period, no significant difference was found between the two groups, but treatment by primary repair was favored over excision.

The author does not propose to solve the controversy over the best treatment for acromioclavicular separations and does not recommend that all patients with acromioclavicular separation have surgery. However, in patients who have residual pain following acromioclavicular joint injury, the recommended treatment is excision of the outer end of the clavicle. Distal clavicle excision has been combined with primary repair by the author, and the results are encouraging.

The grade of initial injury should be classified accurately. Radiographs of both shoulders should be taken with a 10-lb. weight suspended from each wrist; the weight should not be held in the hands. This maximizes the degree of displacement of the clavicle and gives clues as to which ligaments are torn.

The patient's age, occupation, medical condition, psychologic make-up, and expectations for future physical activity should be considered in planning a treatment regimen. No treatment at all should be performed in elderly patients or those with severe medical problems.

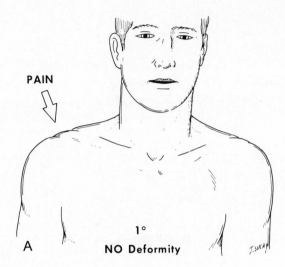

PAIN

1°
A   NO Deformity

FIGURE 14–5. Grade I partial tear of acromioclavicular ligament, no displacement.

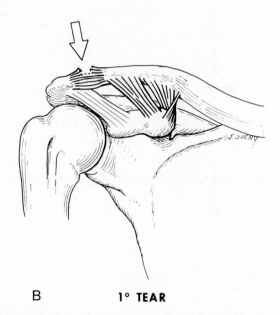

B   1° TEAR

Type I injuries (see Fig. 14–5A,B) are best treated with ice and mild analgesics followed by a muscle rehabilitation program. No "contact" is permitted in athletes for three to four weeks.

Type II injuries (see Fig. 14–6A,B) can be treated either with nonoperative methods or by surgery. The treatment must be individualized, but exact repair of the torn ligaments and muscles is usually recommended for a person engaged in contact sports or heavy manual labor. In cases of posterior subluxation, there is a greater tendency for future problems to develop than with Type I injuries.

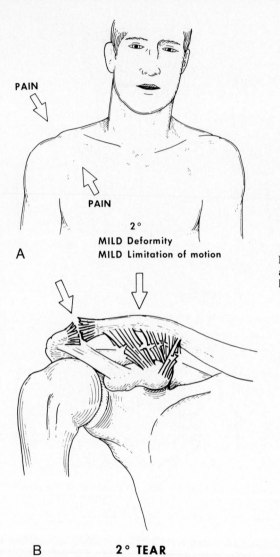

PAIN

PAIN

2°

MILD Deformity

A   MILD Limitation of motion

FIGURE 14–6. Grade II partial tear of acromioclavicular and coracoclavicular ligaments with mild displacement.

B   **2° TEAR**

The treatment of Type III injuries (Fig. 14–7A,B) also must be individualized. In the active individual engaged in contact sports or heavy labor, repair of the coracoclavicular and acromioclavicular ligaments with a beveled excision of the distal 1 cm of the clavicle is the author's treatment of choice.

In mild cases, treatment includes rest and ice application for the first 24 to 36 hours, then gradual resumption of motion and stretching; antiinflammatory drugs such as cortisone may be injected into the joint once or twice. Supportive splinting may be necessary. The Kenny Howard sling, as illustrated in Figure 14–8, properly applied and used, gives very satis-

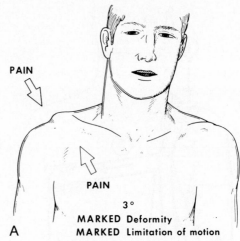

PAIN

PAIN

3°
MARKED Deformity
MARKED Limitation of motion

A

FIGURE 14–7. Complete tear of acromioclavicular and coracoclavicular ligaments with marked displacement.

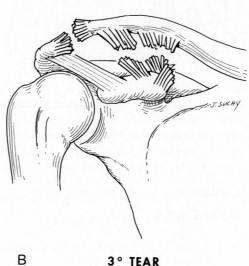

B   3° TEAR

factory immobilization. However, it is often difficult to prevail upon a patient to wear this sling for a sufficient length of time for all the ligaments to heal. It is an excellent method of immobilization for Grades I and II and is sufficient for some Grade III injuries only if the patient is willing to wear the sling for eight to ten weeks and to keep it snug at all times. Another immobilization method uses a plaster body cast that includes a support of the arm that attaches to the body jacket; a suspender strap goes over the shoulder and fastens with a buckle. When the patient lies down at night he can tighten this suspender strap to keep the clavicle in the reduced position.

The main function of the clavicle is to maintain the proper spread of the shoulders and to provide attachments for the shoulder girdle muscles and ligaments. A shoulder that has had excision of the distal clavicle can

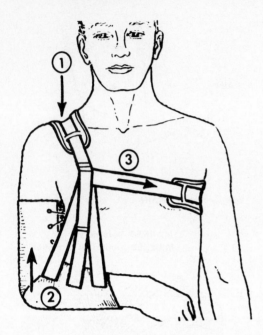

FIGURE 14–8. Kenny Howard sling in place holding the clavicle reduced.

function normally. If too much clavicle is removed, not enough anchor is left for the shoulder muscles, and therefore weakness can result. If too little clavicle is removed, the acromioclavicular joint can still articulate. Excision of the proper amount prevents the clavicle from impinging against the acromion, yet retains maximal muscle support for the shoulder.

REFERENCES

1. Allman, F. L., Jr.: Fractures and ligamentous injuries of the clavicle and its articulation. J Bone Joint Surg 49A:774, 1967.
2. Horn, J. S.: The traumatic anatomy and treatment of acute acromio-clavicular dislocations. J Bone Joint Surg 36B:194, 1954.
3. Urist, M. R.: Complete dislocation of the acromioclavicular joint: The nature of the traumatic lesion and effective methods of treatment, with an analysis of 41 cases. J Bone Joint Surg 28:813, 1946.
4. Jacobs, B., and Wade, P. A.: Acromioclavicular-joint injury: An end-result study. J Bone Joint Surg 48A:475, 1966.
5. Murray, J. W. G.: Reconstruction of the dislocated acromioclavicular joint: A simplified method. Orthop Rev 2:55, 1973.
6. Phemister, D. B.: The treatment of dislocations of the acromioclavicular joint by open reduction and threaded-wire fixation. J Bone Joint Surg 24:166, 1942.
7. Henry, M. O.: Acromio-clavicular dislocation. Minn Med 12:131, 1929.
8. Alldredge, R. H.: Surgical treatment of acromioclavicular dislocations. J Bone Joint Surg 47A:1278, 1965.
9. Bosworth, B. M.: Acromioclavicular separation: A new method of repair. Surg Gynecol Obstet 73:866, 1941.
10. Vere-Hodge, N.: Coraco-clavicular fixation by screw. In Watson-Jones, R. Fractures and Joint Injuries. 3rd ed. Baltimore, Williams & Wilkins, 1943, p. 434.

11. Kennedy, J. C., and Cameron, H.: Complete dislocation of the acromioclavicular joint. J Bone Joint Surg 36B:202, 1954.
12. Urist, M. R.: Complete dislocation of the acromioclavicular joint. J Bone Joint Surg 45A:1750, 1964.
13. Mumford, E. B.: Acromioclavicular dislocation. J Bone Joint Surg 23:799, 1941.
14. Smith, M. J., and Stewart, M. J.: Acute acromioclavicular separations: A twenty-year study. Am J Sports Med 7:62, 1979.
15. Gurd, F. B.: The treatment of complete dislocation of the outer end of the clavicle: An hitherto undescribed operation. Ann Surg 113:1094, 1941.
16. Gillespie, H. S.: Excision of the outer end of the clavicle for dislocation of the acromioclavicular joint. Can J Surg 7:18, 1964.
17. Moseley, H. F.: Athletic injuries to the shoulder region. Am J Surg 98:401, 1959.
18. Weaver, J. K., and Dunn, H. K.: Treatment of acromioclavicular injuries, especially complete acromioclavicular separation. J Bone Joint Surg 54A:1187, 1972.
19. Browne, J. E., Stanley, R. F., and Tullos, H. S.: Acromioclavicular joint dislocations: Comparative results following operative treatment with and without primary distal calvisectomy. Am J Sports Med 5:258, 1977.

SUGGESTED READING

1. Inman, V. T., Saunders, J. B., and Abbott, L. C.: Observations on the function of the shoulder joint. J Bone Joint Surg 26:1, 1944.
2. Nicol, E. E.: Miners and mannequins. J Bone Joint Surg 36B:171, 1954.

ANTERIOR SUBLUXATION OF THE THROWING SHOULDER

CARTER R. ROWE, M.D.

Recurrent anterior transient subluxation of the shoulder should be considered as the diagnosis in the athlete who experiences a forceful overextension of his arm and subsequently finds that he is unable to throw hard, serve in tennis, swim overhand, or use his arm in elevation and external rotation because of a sudden sharp pain in his shoulder. In throwing sports such as baseball a common complaint is the inability to throw in from the outfield. If he is a pitcher, his arm "goes dead" in the cocked position, eliminating the ability to come forward with the arm in the throwing motion (Fig. 15–1A). The quarterback of a football team finds that he is no longer able to throw the "long bomb" because of a paralyzing pain in the shoulder. The tennis player avoids the serving position (Fig. 15–1B) and has to serve underhanded. The volleyball player complains that he is unable to "spike" the ball. The free-style swimmer is unable to forcefully carry his arm overhead in the crawl stroke.

During the 1950s the author examined several athletes who had suddenly lost the power and function of their throwing arms because of sudden shoulder pain and who had failed to respond to the usual treatment for bursitis, tendinitis, and impingement syndrome. These cases were puzzling because the athletes' shoulders did not respond to the usual conservative measures. In the early 1960s a jockey was referred to the author because of inability to whip his horse in races. This patient had seen a number of qualified orthopaedic surgeons, who were unable to make a definite diag-

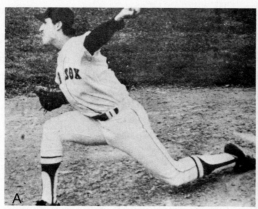
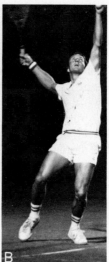
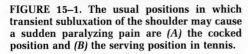

FIGURE 15–1. The usual positions in which transient subluxation of the shoulder may cause a sudden paralyzing pain are *(A)* the cocked position and *(B)* the serving position in tennis.

nosis. The results of all routine studies were normal. He had not responded to treatments such as injections, ultrasound, diathermy, heat, rest, and physical therapy. In desperation, the jockey asked that his shoulder be examined surgically, since he was convinced that "something was wrong." At surgery a severe Bankart lesion was found. After this had been repaired, the jockey was completely relieved of symptoms and returned to competitive racing. He had not been aware of instability of his shoulder, only of severe pain when he attempted to swing his arm around to whip his horse.

In the late 1960s Blazina and Satzman[1] reported on a series of patients with recurrent anterior subluxation of the shoulder with the same "dead arm" syndrome. The patients in his series had been *aware* of the shoulder slipping out when they attempted to throw or to forcefully use the arm in elevation and external rotation. This study increased the recognition that instability of the shoulder can be a cause of a painful throwing arm. Remembering the case of the jockey who was *not aware* of his shoulder subluxation the author recognized two groups of patients with subluxating shoulders:

1.   Those who were aware that their shoulders were "slipping" or popping out

2.   Those who were not aware of shoulder instability and who experienced only the paralyzing pain

In 1981 the author together with Dr. Bertram Zarins reported on 60 shoulders with the "dead arm" syndrome caused by transient anterior subluxation.[2] Twenty-six of the patients (27 shoulders) were aware of the shoulder subluxation, whereas 32 patients (33 shoulders) were not aware that subluxation had occurred. It was interesting that the mechanism of injury, clinical symptoms, pathology, and response to treatment were the same in both groups.

Fifty-eight per cent of the shoulders had been subjected to forceful external rotation of the arm in positions of abduction or elevation of the arm. Twenty-eight per cent had been injured by a direct blow, whereas in 14 per cent the injury was produced by excessive throwing or pitching or hard serving in tennis.

The "dead arm" syndrome caused by transient subluxation of the shoulder is being more generally identified and reported today[3-11] and should be considered in the diagnosis of a painful disabling throwing arm in the young adult athlete. The significant diagnostic features of recurrent transient subluxation of the shoulder are:

1.   A sudden forceful hyperextension injury of the arm such as an arm tackle in football, sliding into a base with arms outstretched, or a direct blow to the shoulder.

2.   The inability to forcefully use the arm in positions of elevation and external rotation, or extension caused by sudden pain and weakness of the arm. The patient finds that he is unable to throw hard, to extend his arm upward for a lay-up in basketball, or to serve in tennis. "I can't even play catch with my kids," is a common complaint.

3.   The "apprehension test" result is consistently positive. As a rule, the patient avoids raising his arm in elevation and external rotation as in throwing. When pressure is applied posteriorly to the humeral head when the patient is standing (Fig. 15–2) or when lying in a supine position the pain and apprehension are reproduced.

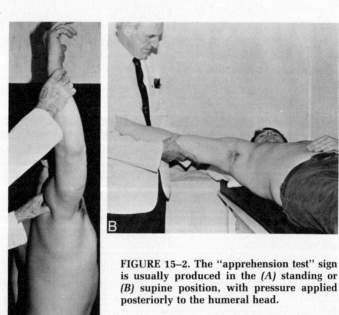

FIGURE 15–2. The "apprehension test" sign is usually produced in the (A) standing or (B) supine position, with pressure applied posteriorly to the humeral head.

4.   Radiographic findings can be helpful. Forty per cent of the author's series had Hill-Sachs lesions (mild in 19, moderate in 3, and severe in 2). Changes along the anterior glenoid rim were present in 45 per cent and consisted of spur formation, flattening of the anterior glenoid rim, and in one shoulder a fracture of the anterior rim. Axillary views should be taken routinely.

5.   Arthrotomograms and arthroscopy can be helpful in identifying trauma to the capsular attachment to the rim of the glenoid cavity.

Differential diagnosis is important, especially in the group of patients who are not aware of the shoulder slipping out. The previous diagnoses of patients in the author's series were interesting. Fifty-five per cent of patients had been diagnosed as having some condition other than subluxation when they were first seen by the author. Surgical procedures had been performed on seven patients—including "decompression" of the shoulder (sectioning of the coracoacromial ligament and anterior acromioplasty) in three patients and tenodesis of the long head of the biceps in three patients—all without relief of symptoms.

TREATMENT

Treatment consists of a period of specific resistive exercises for at least a two-month period (Fig. 15–3). Ten of the 60 (17 per cent) shoulders in the author's series responded to resistive exercises. Surgical exploration of the shoulder was carried out in the remaining 50 shoulders.

Bankart lesions (avulsion of the labrum and capsule from the anterior glenoid rim) were present in 64 per cent of the shoulders, excess laxity of the capsule in 26 per cent, and excessive opening of the interval between the subscapularis and supraspinatus tendons in 40 per cent. Capsular laxity was the only lesion in eight of the 50 shoulders (16 per cent).

Surgical Treatment

When a Bankart lesion was present repair by a routine Bankart procedure was performed (Fig. 15–4). When a Bankart lesion was not present, a modified capsulorrhaphy was carried out (Fig. 15–5). When a large opening of the interval between the subscapularis and supraspinatus tendons was present, it was partially closed with interrupted sutures, with care being taken not to limit the division of the two tendons around the coracoid process. The advantage of the Bankart procedure was that it allowed clear identification of the subscapularis tendon, the capsule in its entirety, the degree of laxity of the capsule with the arm in complete external rotation, the rim of the glenoid cavity, and the humeral head.

Postoperative management was similar to that used after repair of a recurrent anterior dislocation of the shoulder.[12] A sling is used for a few

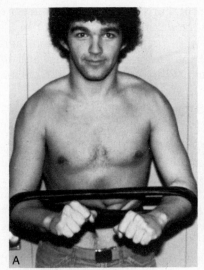
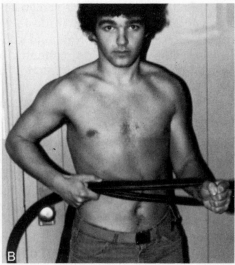
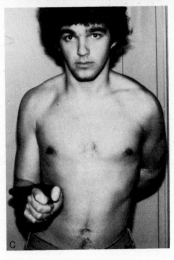

FIGURE 15–3. Resistive exercises are carried out with the use of an elastic belt in *(A)* abduction to 50 degrees, *(B)* external rotation, and *(C)* internal rotation.

days only, after which the arm is free. Exercises and use of the arm are increased gradually as they can be tolerated. Pendulum exercises are begun on the third or fourth day. Light work is tolerated usually within four to six weeks after surgery, and by three months patients are allowed to swim, row, and take part in light sports. By six months contact sports, throwing, and heavy labor are permitted.

RESULTS

Of the ten shoulders treated with only resistive exercises, five were graded as excellent, three as good, and two as fair results.

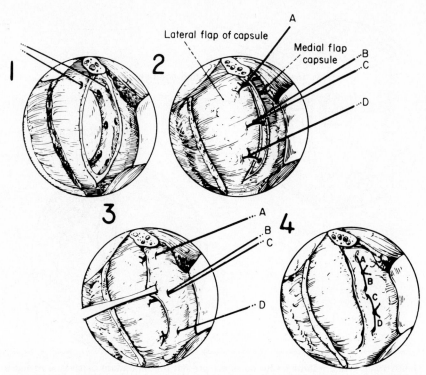

FIGURE 15–4. When a Bankart lesion is present, the lateral capsule is reattached to the rim of the glenoid cavity and reinforced by overlapping with the medial capsule. (Reprinted, with permission, from Rowe, C. R., and Zarins, B., "Recurrent transient subluxation of the shoulder," *Journal of Bone and Joint Surgery* 63A:863, 1982.)

Of the fifty shoulders that were treated with surgical procedures, 70 per cent were graded as excellent, 24 per cent as good, and 6 per cent as fair.

Thirty-three dominant shoulders were operated on. Sixty-four per cent of these patients could throw hard, were able to return to throwing sports, and were not limited in other sports or work. Of the eight patients whose injuries were produced by hard pitching, results in four were graded as excellent (they could throw hard but not pitch consistently). Four had good results; these patients could play tennis, serve hard, and play football. The patients in the author's series were not professional baseball players and consequently lacked the demands of rotation pitching. However, one patient returned to pitching for a large state university after his "dead arm" condition, which had disabled him for two years, was relieved.

Of the 15 nondominant shoulders, 87 per cent had no limitations in sports or work, and the patients returned to the sports in which they had participated prior to injury.

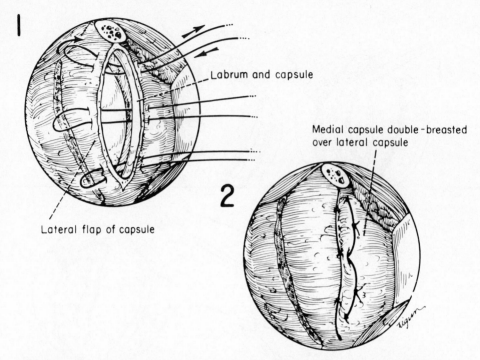

Labrum and capsule

Medial capsule double-breasted over lateral capsule

Lateral flap of capsule

FIGURE 15–5. When a Bankart lesion is not present the redundant capsule is reefed in a double-breasted manner. (Reprinted, with permission, from Rowe, C. R., and Zarins, B., "Recurrent transient subluxation of the shoulder," _Journal of Bone and Joint Surgery_ 63A:863, 1982.)

DISCUSSION

Although there are many causes for the lame painful arm in throwing sports, in the young athlete who had experienced an injury to the arm (usually a severe hyperextension of the arm in elevation or external rotation) and who is disabled subsequently by a sharp paralyzing pain in the shoulder when throwing, recurrent transient subluxation of the shoulder should be suspected. The athlete may drop the object he is throwing or holding. The pain soon disappears but returns again when he forcefully uses his arm in the throwing position.

The "apprehension test" is routinely positive in anterior shoulder subluxation. This test can be carried out most effectively with the patient standing, by elevating and externally rotating his arm in the sensitive position and applying pressure posteriorly to the humeral head.

Impingement syndromes usually are produced by rotation of the arm at 90 degrees of abduction in the impingement position. The pain is not as severe as transient subluxation and is not relieved as rapidly. The author has not found transient subluxation of the biceps tendon in the young healthy athlete. This also has been the experience of other orthopedic surgeons.[13]*†‡

Emphasis must be placed on the difficulty of arriving at the correct diagnosis of the patient, who is not aware that his shoulder is subluxating. In the author's series six patients had previously been operated on, three had undergone "decompression" surgery for an impingement syndrome, and three had had transplantations of the long head of the biceps tendon, all without relief of symptoms. These findings attest to the difficulty of diagnosis in this group.

CONCLUSIONS

1. In the young adult athlete, recurrent transient subluxation of the shoulder may be the case of the "dead arm" syndrome.

2. While many patients are aware of a momentary slipping out of the shoulder, an equal number of patients are not aware of subluxation of the shoulder.

3. Diagnosis in the latter group may be very difficult. A careful history and physical examination are most important. A positive "apprehension test" is a consistent physical finding.

4. Response to nonoperative and operative treatment has been very encouraging, with good to excellent results in 94 per cent of patients.

REFERENCES

1. Blazina, M. E., and Satzman, J. S.: Recurrent anterior subluxation of the shoulder in athletics—a distinct entity. In Proceedings of the American Academy of Orthopaedic Surgeons. J Bone Joint Surg 51A:1037, 1969.
2. Rowe, C. R., and Zarins, B.: Recurrent transient subluxation of the shoulder. J Bone Joint Surg 63A:863, 1981.
3. Bateman, J. E.: The Shoulder and Neck. 2nd ed. Philadelphia, W. B. Saunders Company, 1978, p. 506.
4. DePalma, A. F.: Surgery of the Shoulder. 2nd ed. Philadelphia, J. B. Lippincott Company, 1973, pp. 83, 355, 408, 417.
5. LeClerc, J.: Chronic subluxation of the shoulder. In Proceedings of the Dewar Orthopaedic Club. J Bone Joint Surg 51B:778, 1969.
6. Morton, K. S.: The unstable shoulder: Recurrent subluxation. In Proceedings of the Canadian Orthopaedic Association. J Bone Joint Surg 59B:508, 1977.
7. Neer, C. S., II, and Foster, C. R.: Inferior capsular shift for involuntary inferior and multidirectional instability of the shoulder. A preliminary report. J Bone Joint Surg 62A:897, 1980.
8. Norwood, L. A., DelPizzo, W., Jobe, F. W., and Kerlan, R. K.: Anterior shoulder pain in baseball pitchers. Am J Sports Med 6:103, 1978.

---

*DePalma, A. F., 1980: Personal communication.
†Neer, C. S., 1980: Personal communication.
‡Rockwood, C. A., Jr., 1980: Personal communication.

9. O'Donoghue, D. H.: Treatment of Injuries to Athletes. 3rd ed. Philadelphia, W B. Saunders Company, 1976, p. 211.
10. Protzman, R. R.: Anterior instability of the shoulder. J Bone Joint Surg 62A:909, 1980.
11. Rockwood, C. A., Jr.: Subluxation of the shoulder—the classification, diagnosis, and treatment. Orthop Trans 4:306, 1979.
12. Rowe, C. R., Patel, D., and Southmayd, W. W.: The Bankart procedure. A long-term end-result study. J Bone Joint Surg 60A:1, 1978.
13. Warren, R. F., Dines, D. M., and Inglis, A. E.: Surgical treatment of the long head of the biceps. Orthop Trans 4:90, 1980.

16

POSTERIOR SHOULDER INSTABILITY

LYLE A. NORWOOD, M.D.

The throwing athlete places unique stresses on the shoulder joint during the throwing act. In the cocking position of throwing, the abducted arm is in marked external rotation with the humeral head against the anterior capsule and the subscapularis tendon. In the follow-through phase the abducted arm is in forward flexion with the humeral head resting against the posterior capsule and the infraspinatus and teres minor tendons. The motion from cocking to follow-through takes the arm through acceleration, release, and deceleration; the humeral head moves from external rotation and anterior glenoid position to the internal rotation and posterior glenoid position.

Posterior shoulder instability occurs in throwing when motion places the humeral head against the posterior capsule and the cuff tendons. The throwing athlete places his arm in this position during deceleration and follow-through phases. Injuries associated with throwing, training, lifting, or trauma that affect the posterior shoulder (glenoid cavity, labrum, capsule, infraspinatus tendon, teres minor tendon, and humeral head) can lead to posterior instability and symptoms during throwing. This chapter focuses on the diagnosis and treatment of posterior shoulder instability. The causes of instability are discussed elsewhere.[1]

The most common symptoms of posterior subluxation associated with throwing are discomfort and soreness. Experienced throwers can appreciate abnormal humeral head motion and identify the throwing motion phase that produces symptoms; younger athletes with less sophistication cannot identify the specifics. The diagnosis is established by shoulder examination

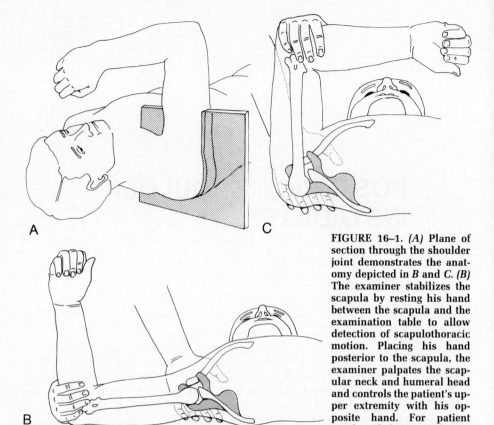

FIGURE 16–1. *(A)* Plane of section through the shoulder joint demonstrates the anatomy depicted in *B* and *C*. *(B)* The examiner stabilizes the scapula by resting his hand between the scapula and the examination table to allow detection of scapulothoracic motion. Placing his hand posterior to the scapula, the examiner palpates the scapular neck and humeral head and controls the patient's upper extremity with his opposite hand. For patient comfort, balance, and control, the examiner controls the patient's arm at the olecranon and proximal forearm. The examiner moves the extremity to 90 degrees of abduction and external rotation. The patient's arm rests in the neutral position between flexion and extension. The examination begins with the humeral head resting in the normal position in the glenoid cavity. The examiner then brings the arm into forward flexion. *(C)* If posterior subluxation is present, the examiner can feel the humeral head slip posteriorly to the glenoid cavity. The patient verifies the familiar sensation and associated discomfort experienced during athletics. The arm is then returned to the neutral position in 90 degrees of abduction. Both the patient and the examiner feel the humeral head relocate to the reduced position. Some patients are more uncomfortable when the humeral head leaves the glenoid cavity, others when the humeral head relocates. If the initial examination does not indicate subluxation, the humeral rotation and degree of abduction are changed, and the examination is repeated. (From Norwood, L. A., and Terry, G. C., "Shoulder posterior subluxation," *American Journal of Sports Medicine* 12:25, 1984.)

in the symptomatic position, usually in abduction and forward flexion (Fig. 16–1). Supine examination helps to calm apprehension, eliminate active muscle contraction, and control the effects of gravity. The examiner can detect the abnormal humeral motion as the humeral head leaves the glenoid cavity or as it returns. The most reassuring examination technique begins with the abducted arm in the neutral position. The examiner brings the arm into forward flexion. Posterior subluxation can be felt by the patient and the examiner as the humeral head moves posteriorly. The patient and the examiner can detect the abnormal motion as the humeral head relocates itself when the examiner brings the arm from forward flexion into a neutral position.

Different shoulders subluxate at different levels of abduction, depending on the exact arm position during trauma or the degree of arm abduction during symptomatic activities. Placing the arm into different degrees of abduction increases the chance of detecting posterior subluxation. The examiner must also detect motion of the scapulothoracic joint during the examination. The hand of the examiner that controls the scapulothoracic motion also palpates the scapulohumeral joint to detect subluxation or relocation motion.

The athlete's age and the mechanism of injury help the physician to direct the treatment of posterior shoulder instability. Roentgenograms of adolescents rarely show humeral head or posterior glenoid findings. Most of the instability in adolescence is a developmental laxity, and adolescent athletes should exercise to strengthen and tighten the posterior shoulder. These athletes respond well to exercises for strengthening the posterior cuff; healing is also aided by growth, time, and physical maturity. In the author's experience, no thrower in this young age group has remained symptomatic after performing strengthening exercises.

Teenagers are more skeletally mature than adolescents and have more force and bone mass, which might lead to fractures of the humeral head or glenoid cavity. Exercises are prescribed for these athletes only if there are no fractures. Expectations for full recovery are not as great as for adolescents because older shoulders cannot tighten with growth and maturity.

Older teenagers and adults are skeletally mature. Posterior discomfort may decrease or disappear with exercise; however, symptoms frequently recur if the athlete resumes throwing.

The mechanism of injury is important for athletes. Falls, blows to the shoulder, or heavy lifting can produce changes of the glenoid cavity or humeral head. Roentgenograms of the shoulder should be taken prior to treatment and exercise. For all shoulders an axillary lateral roentgenogram is needed to show the posterior glenoid cavity. This permits detection of posterior glenoid fractures. Shoulders with displaced posterior glenoid fractures have posterior instability and remain unstable while the bone is displaced. Detection of displaced posterior glenoid fracture may lead to reduction, proper healing, and a stable and asymptomatic shoulder.

Strengthening of the posterior rotator cuff should be accomplished without placing the shoulder in the subluxated position. As the loaded shoulder ranges through the subluxation position during exercise, the humeral head may subluxate. This subluxation further irritates the joint, establishes apprehension, and prevents strengthening and tightening. To avoid this kind of subluxation, the author prefers exercise with the wall pulley, performed with the elbow at the side. The athlete is instructed to

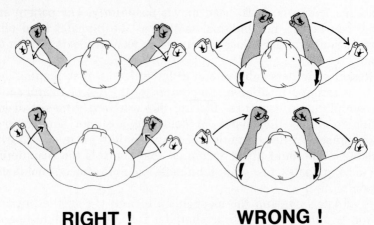

RIGHT !   WRONG !

FIGURE 16–2. Exercise position. The elbows are kept at the side. Forward flexion is specifically avoided to keep the humeral head in the center of the glenoid cavity and to keep the head away from the posterior aspect of the glenoid labrum and cuff. The arm does not return to neutral position, and this also avoids the posterior instability position. Wall pulleys are preferred over free weights for this exercise.

have the arm at 45 degrees of external rotation at the start of the exercise and not to return the arm to the neutral position. Thus the subluxated position is avoided (Fig. 16–2). While specific attention is directed to the supraspinatus, infraspinatus, and teres minor muscles, the trapezius and deltoid muscles should not be overlooked. Supraspinatus muscle strengthening exercises are added to the shoulder shrugs as well as other exercises that strengthen abductor muscles. These exercises strengthen the shoulder for possible throwing.

Certain exercises are performed to increase strength and stability; however, other exercises and arm positions should be avoided. Since the most frequent nonthrowing cause of posterior subluxation is "bench pressing," this is contraindicated while the arm is symptomatic. Heavy pushing or pulling is also avoided.

Surgical treatment is necessary only in approximately 20 per cent of older teenagers and adults with recurrent posterior subluxation. Increased skeletal maturity eliminates the need for surgery in many patients. Adults who do not throw for a living can alter their daily routines and avoid recurrent subluxation by avoiding certain arm positions and activities. The patients who most frequently require surgery are the older teenagers and the young adults who lift, push, or pull heavy weights. If these shoulders do not respond to protective motion or rehabilitation, posterior shoulder reconstruction can be indicated; however, careful preoperative analysis of the causes of injury is mandatory to assure satisfactory results. The prognosis is not good for individuals with congenitally loose shoulders or for patients with habitual dislocation. Although posterior reconstruction in appropriately selected athletes prevents recurrence of subluxation, ability to throw competitively is probably not restored. The author tells athletes that they will not be able to throw on a professional level or at a highly competitive level after posterior reconstruction. Return to contact sports, however, would be expected among patients whose shoulders are neither congenitally loose nor habitually dislocated.

REFERENCES

1. Norwood, L. A., and Terry, G. C.: Shoulder posterior subluxation. Am J Sports Med 12:25, 1984.

SUGGESTED READING

1. Bloom, M. H., and Obata, W. G.: Diagnosis of posterior dislocation of the shoulder with use of Velpeau axillary and angle up roentgenographic views. J Bone Joint Surg 49A:943, 1967.
2. Boyd, H. B., and Sisk, T. D.: Recurrent posterior dislocation of the shoulder. J. Bone Joint Surg 54A:779, 1972.
3. Dimon, J. H.: Posterior dislocation and posterior fracture dislocation of the shoulder. South Med J 60:661, 1967.
4. Dorgan, J. A.: Posterior dislocation of the shoulder. Am J Surg 89:890, 1955.
5. Greenhill, B. J.: Persistent posterior shoulder dislocation: Its diagnosis and treatment by posterior Putti-Platt repair. J Bone Joint Surg 54B:763, 1972.
6. McLaughlin, H. L.: Posterior dislocation of the shoulder. J Bone Joint Surg 34A:584, 1952.
7. McLaughlin, H. L.: Locked posterior subluxation of the shoulder. Surg Clin North Am 43:1621, 1963.
8. Neviaser, J. S.: Posterior dislocations of the shoulder. Surg Clin North Am 43:1623, 1963.
9. Nobel, W.: Posterior traumatic dislocation of the shoulder. J Bone Joint Surg 44A:523, 1962.
10. Samilson, R. L., and Miller, E.: Posterior dislocations of the shoulder. Clin Orthop 32:69, 1964.
11. Scott, D. J.: Treatment of recurrent posterior dislocations of the shoulder by glenoplasty. J Bone Joint Surg 49A:471, 1967.
12. Wilson, J. C.: Traumatic posterior (retro-glenoid) dislocation of the humerus. J Bone Joint Surg 31A:160, 1949.

IMPINGEMENT, BICEPS, AND ROTATOR CUFF LESIONS

FRED ALLMAN, M.D.

CONSERVATIVE TREATMENT

Shoulder impingement syndrome is a very common lesion with well understood biomechanical and pathophysiologic bases. The early stages are seen frequently among athletes involved in throwing, racquet sports, or swimming because each of these acts requires forward flexion, abduction, and internal rotation.

The injury is usually a result of force overload, and unless this can be corrected progression to other more severe stages is likely to occur.

The overhead motion required of certain athletes creates a force overload to the biceps brachii tendon and the rotator cuff. This overload is likely to result in injury owing to several factors.

The normal anatomy of the shoulder makes possible the impingement syndrome. The roof of the shoulder, the acromion process and the coracoacromial ligament form a potential barrier for passage of the rotator cuff and biceps tendon. The subdeltoid bursa acts to cushion and lubricate the cuff and tendon, but when inflamed and thickened may contribute to the impingement syndrome. As the arm elevates to 80 degrees, the greater tuberosity and attached tendons come closer to the anterior edge of the acromion process and the coracoacromial ligament. At this point, through 125 degrees of forward flexion or abduction, contact is possible. As the arm elevates higher, the humeral head drops down in the glenoid, helping to clear the greater tuberosity.[1]

158

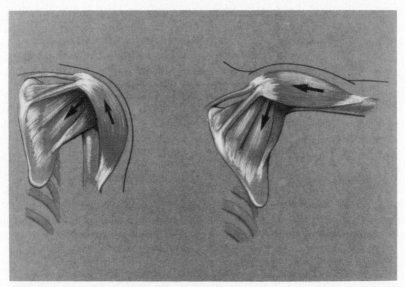

FIGURE 17–1. The rotator cuff and deltoid muscle forces at the onset of abduction (zero degrees) and with the arm elevated 90 degrees. The deltoid force changes from a shear to a compressive force. Thus, a damaged or weakened supraspinatus muscle causes loss of counterbalance and allows the vertical force of the deltoid muscle to compress the tissue more.

Also, many years ago Codman noted that the final one-half inch of the supraspinatus portion of the rotator cuff is the area of relative hypovascularity. This area has since been called the "critical zone of Codman."

Emphasis in conditioning drills and other activities often overdevelops the internal rotator muscles of the shoulder while neglecting the external rotators. This situation most frequently leads to an imbalance between the external-internal rotators with resultant weakness and pain from force overload in the external rotators. The anatomic sketch (Fig. 17–1) shows the rotator cuff and deltoid muscle forces at the onset of abduction (zero degrees) and with the arm elevated 90 degrees. The deltoid force changes from a shear to a compression force. Thus, a damaged or weakened supraspinatus muscle causes loss of counterbalance and allows the vertical force of the deltoid muscle to compress the tissue more. The result is the cycle of pain inhibiting muscle action, rotator cuff weakness, cuff contracture, greater loss of counterbalance, and further damage.[2]

Neer[3] has classified impingement lesions into three stages. The author has added another important stage, *Prestage I*. Prevention of impingement lesions is possible if the condition is recognized in this stage and if appropriate measures are taken, namely to decrease the force overload.

If appropriate corrective measures are not taken, edema and hemorrhage are likely to occur, and *Stage I* impingement will follow as a result of overuse and myostatic contracture. Even in Stage I, however, if the force overload is recognized early and reduced and the biomechanics are improved, the condition is fully reversible, and complete healing is possible.

However, if the trauma is repeated without correction of the imbalance, the condition in time will progress to *Stage II* or over a longer period to *Stage III*, with or without a tear of the rotator cuff. See Figure 17–2 for an outline of the progression from Stage I to Stage III.

It must be emphasized that the treatment of choice for all stages of impingement is conservative even when there is a small tear in the rotator cuff, as may be found in Stage III. Conservative treatment should be tried for all patients initially regardless of sex, age, sport, profession, or avocation.

Surgery should be reserved for those unresponsive to conservative treatment and for those with a complete tear of the rotator cuff, usually the size of a nickel or larger. If the tear is small enough so that the fibers of the rotator cuff are abutting, with proper treatment healing can occur without surgery. Neer,[3] Jobe,[4] and others have stated that over 90 per cent of impingement lesions respond to conservative management with proper treatment.

The ARISE Program

Proper conservative treatment for impingement lesions is provided by a program that can be remembered by the acronym ARISE.

A—Analgesics and Anti-Inflammatories. These two can usually be combined into one medication, depending on the degree of involvement. Medications used range from aspirin to phenylbutazone. Two aspirin tablets are taken four times daily; phenylbutazone, 100 mg, is taken four times a day with milk or food.

R—Rest. This does not mean total rest but avoidance of painful activity. Slings should not be used, and there should be no significant decrease in function, only an alteration of activity, to prevent more damage. Initially overhead activity should be restricted. The pitcher can be switched to another position on the team while undergoing treatment, the throwing mechanism can be altered, or a swimmer can continue to train with a kick board.

I—Ice. Ice decreases the inflammatory reaction. It is most beneficial after the workout. Ice massage to the involved area is usually quite helpful. Some patients prefer heat (but heat may cause increased vascularity).

S—Specific Stretching and Strengthening. These activities improve the quality of muscle function.

E—Evaluation. Almost on a daily basis the response of the individual to the treatment program must be evaluated, and treatment should be adjusted accordingly. If there is increased pain, soreness, and stiffness the treatment may be too aggressive. If there is little soreness, pain, and stiffness the program can usually be accelerated. It should be remembered that no two people respond to a given treatment program at the same rate; therefore

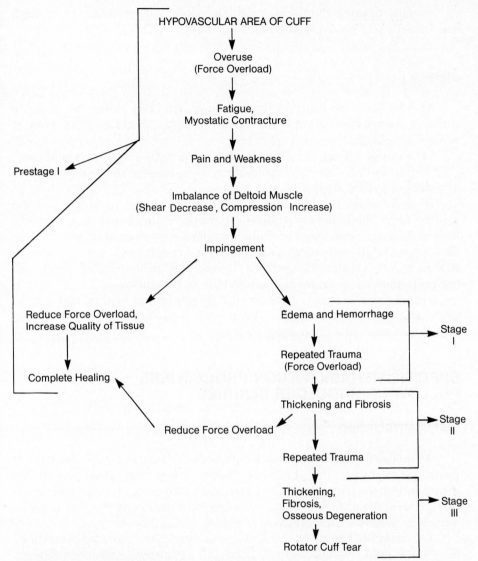

FIGURE 17–2. Stages of impingement lesions indicating reversibility of prestage I, stage I, and early stage II if appropriate measures are taken (such as a reduction in force overload and an increase in quality of tissue).

modalities, exercises, medications, and procedures must be adjusted according to the response of the individual.

Evaluation should also include an analysis of the biomechanics involved in the patient's particular activity. Faulty posture, improper technique, lack of coordination and skill should be evaluated along with improved quality of muscle function.

Aerobic training should be continued along with training for strength and flexibility of uninvolved parts of the body.

Steroids

The injection of steroids into tendons has been shown to produce collagen necrosis and diminished tensile strength. Therefore steroids must be used sparingly, if at all.

When used, 40 mg of methyl prednisolone with lidocaine is preferred. This is injected into the subdeltoid bursa in an attempt to shrink the bursa and decrease inflammation.

In conclusion, the importance of prevention must be stressed when dealing with impingement lesions. If properly diagnosed and properly treated Prestage I and Stage I lesions are completely reversible. Stage II and III lesions, while not always completely reversible, can nevertheless be treated by conservative measures in a very high percentage of cases with the individual's safe return to the previous activity level.

Proper warm-up and "cool-down," proper biomechanics, and a good stretching and strengthening program with well coordinated movements are all essentials of a prevention program.

SPECIFIC REHABILITATION PROCEDURES FOLLOWING SHOULDER INJURIES[4]

Early Rehabilitation

At this early stage the rotator cuff is compromised by its subacute or postsurgical status. The shortness of the rotator cuff muscles and the disproportionate strength of the other musculature of the pectoral girdle make conventional full-range exercise inappropriate even if active range of motion is possible. The following exercises are indicated:

1. **Gripping Exercises.** A hand dynamometer or tennis ball is gripped at several points along the arc from full (pain-free) abduction-flexion-external rotation to full adduction-extension-internal rotation. This action brings the rotator cuff into synergistic (fixative) contraction and also conditions forearm muscles that have probably atrophied if inactivity has been of long duration (Fig. 17–3).

2. **Codman (Pendulum) Exercise.** This exercise increases the range of motion while stimulating contraction of the rotator cuff owing to the gentle traction applied to the muscles (Fig. 17–4).

3. **Bench Press Supports.** The patient lies in a supine position on the bench and holds the barbell in a "locked-out" position. A freely held barbell or dumbbell is preferable to a statically held weight machine, since four-

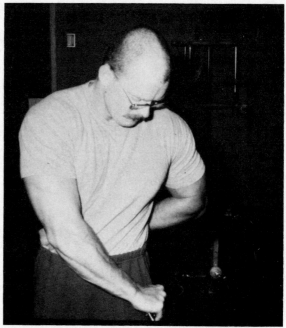

FIGURE 17–3. Gripping exercise. A hand dynamometer or tennis ball is gripped at several points along the arc from full (pain-free) abduction-flexion-external rotation to full adduction-extension-internal rotation. This action brings the rotator cuff into synergistic (fixative) contraction and helps condition forearm muscles.

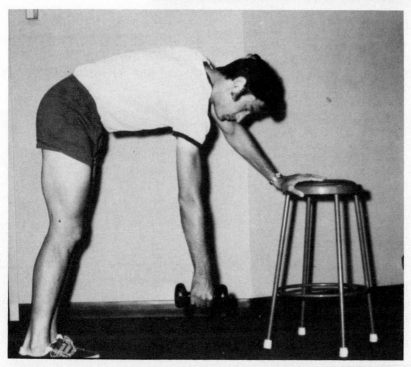

FIGURE 17–4. Codman (pendulum) exercises. The athlete uses a slow progressive clockwise and counterclockwise circular motion while holding a light dumbbell with the trunk flexed forward. This exercise increases the range of motion while stimulating contraction of the rotator cuff, owing to the gentle traction applied to the muscle.

way control is stimulated by the free barbell and not by the weight machine. The weight should be only heavy enough to stimulate fixation of the cuff gently. Progression is accomplished by widening the grip gradually from about 20 to 30 inches (to pain tolerance). This procedure increases the external rotation gradually. The weight is also increased gradually (Fig. 17–5).

4. **Deadlift Supports.** The barbell or corresponding lever of the multi-station weight training apparatus is held with an overhand grip at the front of the thighs. The shoulders are held in a shrug position. Single efforts lasting ten seconds are performed. Progression is attained by widening the grip and increasing the weight (Fig. 17–6).

5. **Hanging from a Chinning Bar.** A bench or chair is used to elevate the body so that the bar can be grasped regardless of a limited range of motion. The bar is gripped, but no effort is made to support full or partial weight until the arms can be painlessly held over the head. The patient merely grips the bar and isometrically sets the latissimus muscles in a comfortable range. Once full weight-bearing is possible, progression is attained by widening the grip.

Intermediate Rehabilitation

At this stage the rotator cuff should be able to contract fully without pain, but full range of motion is not present and strength is not yet fully

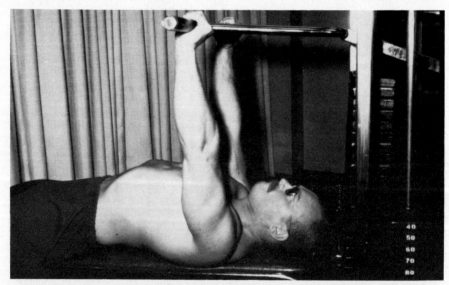

FIGURE 17–5. Bench press supports. The patient lies in a supine position and holds the barbell in a "locked-out" position. The weight should be only heavy enough to stimulate fixation of the cuff gently.

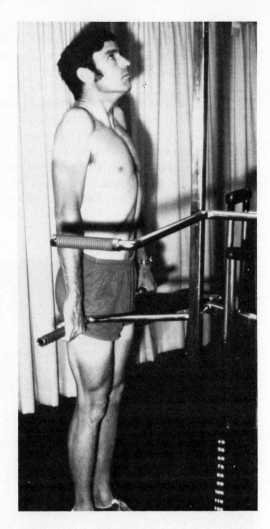

FIGURE 17–6. Deadlift supports. The barbell or corresponding lever of the multistation weight training apparatus is held with an overhand grip at the front of the thighs. The shoulders are held in a shrug position. Single efforts lasting ten seconds are performed.

developed. The rotator cuff, however, is adequate to take on conventional shoulder conditioning exercises that develop strength and further increase range of motion. The following exercises are performed:

1. **Light Dumbbell Circles.** This is a progression from the pendulum exercises. While the patient stands upright the dumbbell is directed upward and outward in a rotary manner and then upward and inward in the opposite direction. These exercises progress by widening the excursion of the circle and increasing the weight.

2. **Bench Presses.** Progressing from supports, the patient gradually adds bending to the movement until a full-range bench press is possible. Additional weight is added. Once again, because of the need to support the weight in all directions, freely held weights are preferable to weight

machines. Dumbbell bench exercises, or "flies," while they may present a safety problem, offer a wider range of motion.

3. **Upright Rowing.** This is a progression from the deadlift supports, in which the same grip is used and the weight is raised to a position high on the chest. Varying the width of the handgrips is desirable (Fig. 17–7).

4. **"Lat" Machine Pull-downs to the Rear of the Neck.** A shoulder-width grip is used at first, with later progression to a wider grip. Weight is added until the patient is able to progress to behind-the-neck pull-ups (only if a minimum of six pull-downs can be performed) (Fig. 17–8).

5. **Dumbbell Resistive Exercises for the Supraspinatus Muscle.**[5] The rotator cuff in the shoulder needs to be strengthened separately from the other shoulder muscles. With the elbow straight and the thumb turned toward the floor, the arm is slowly raised in a plane about 30 degrees

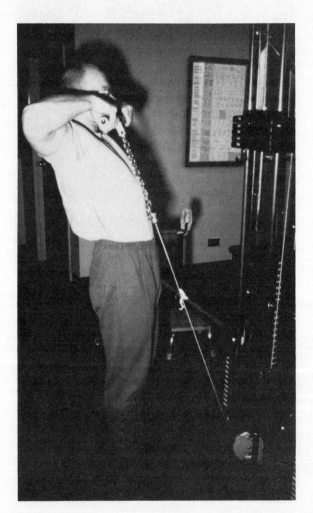

FIGURE 17–7. Upright rowing. This is a progression from the deadlift supports, in which the same grip is used and the weight is raised to a position high on the chest.

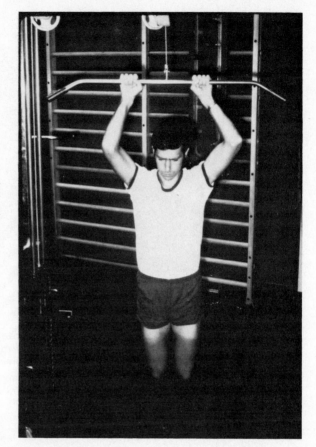

FIGURE 17–8. "Lat" machine pull-downs to the rear of the neck. A shoulder-width grip is used at first, with later progression to a wider grip. Weight is added until the patient is able to progress to behind-the-neck pull-ups.

forward of that posture. The arm must not be lifted higher than just below shoulder level. Finally the arm is slowly lowered to the starting position, and the exercise is repeated (Fig. 17–9).

Advanced Rehabilitation

The progress within the intermediate stage has probably brought the athlete to a nearly normal level of development. To develop extra strength of the shoulder, along with increased flexibility, the following program can be utilized:

1. **Alternate Dumbbell Presses or Presses Behind the Neck**

2. **Dumbbell Bench Presses, Incline Presses, "Flies" or Parallel Bar Dips.** See Figure 17–10.

3. **Bent-Arm Pull-Overs**

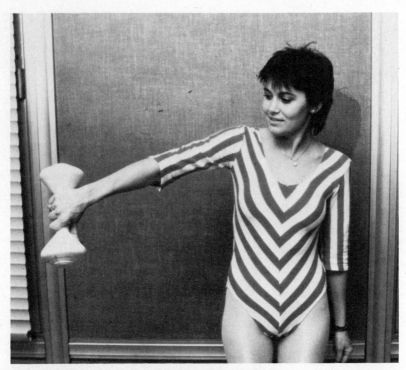

FIGURE 17–9. Dumbbell resistive exercises of the supraspinatus muscle. With the elbow straight and the thumb turned toward the floor, the arm is slowly raised in a plane about 30 degrees forward of the coronal plane.

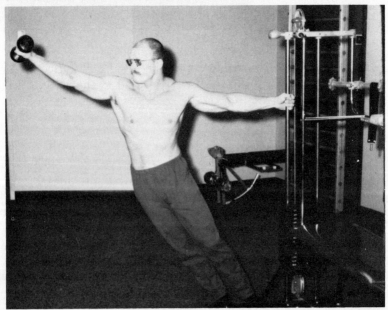

FIGURE 17–10. Light dumbbell "flies" for stretching the pectoral girdle and rib cage.

4. High Pulls. These are performed with a snatch grip or repetition "cleans."

All of these exercises are done for strength at a level of weight, repetitions, and number of sets to assure maximal development in accordance with the individual's potential. The exercises are done to the extremes of motion so that flexibility is improved. If these exercises are properly done in this manner, no specific flexibility exercise is needed.

5. Straight-Arm Pull-Overs Across the Width of a Bench. These are performed using a progressively wider grip. The weight is kept at a constant light level (30 pounds).

6. Light Dumbbell "Flies." These are performed with a medicine ball between the shoulder blades or with an elastic cable stretching of pulley weights. In the latter situation, the cable is held in back of the shoulders with the palms facing forward at shoulder height, and the cable is worked forward and backward, stretching the pectoral girdle and rib cage.

Stretching of the Rotator Cuff[6]

Stretching should be an integral part of each exercise session and should be continued after return to full sports activity.

1. Shoulder Stretch at 90 Degrees. The capsule around the shoulder

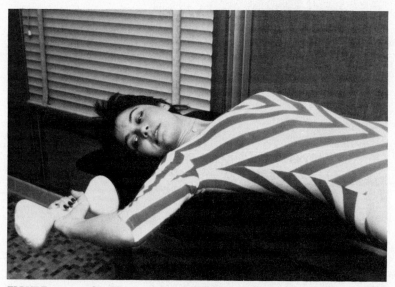

FIGURE 17–11. Shoulder stretch at 90 degrees. Exercises are begun on a table by holding a small weight. The shoulder should be over the table edge and the elbow bent to 90 degrees. The weight is just allowed to pull the arm down gently in this position.

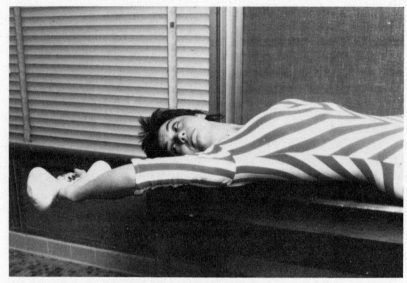

FIGURE 17–12. Shoulder stretch with the arm at 135 degrees. This is a progression of the previous exercise (Fig. 17–11), but with the arm at 135 degrees.

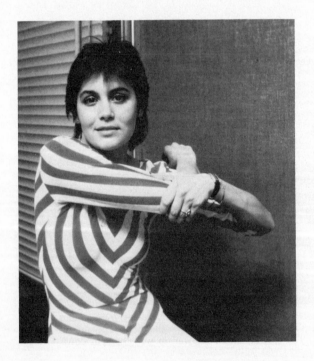

FIGURE 17–13. Posterior shoulder stretch. The arm is gently pulled across the body to stretch the back portion of the shoulder joint.

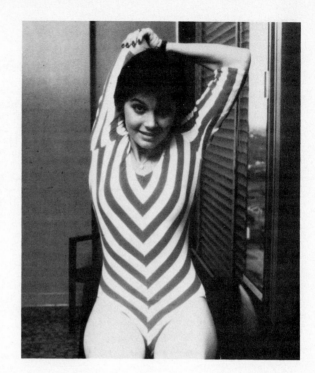

FIGURE   17–14.   Inferior shoulder stretch. The patient reaches overhead and gently pulls on the elbow with the opposite hand to slowly stretch the inferior cuff.

joint needs to be stretched before maximal movement can be obtained. Exercises are begun on a table by holding a small weight. The shoulder should be over the table edge and the elbow bent to 90 degrees. The weight is just allowed to pull the arm down gently in this position (Fig. 17–11).

2.   **Shoulder Stretch with the Arm at 135 Degrees.** During static flexibility exercises a particular position is held for a period of time. Static stretching is the best way to initiate a sequence. After stretching, a muscle can be gently moved through the range of motion. In this exercise, raising the arm another 35 degrees stretches more of the tissue surrounding the shoulder (Fig. 17–12).

3.   **Shoulder Stretch with Arm Overhead.** This exercise should be repeated with the arm as far overhead as possible. The head should remain supported while the shoulder itself is over the table edge. Again, the weight is allowed to pull the arm down gently.

4.   **Posterior Shoulder Stretch.** The back portion of the shoulder joint can be stretched by gently pulling the arm across the body (Fig. 17–13).

5.   **Inferior Shoulder Stretch.** The other portions of the can be stretched by reaching overhead and gently pulling on the elbow with the opposite hand (Fig. 17–14).

REFERENCES

1. Leach, R., 1984: Personal communication.
2. Perry, J.: Anatomy and biomechanics of the shoulder in throwing, swimming, gymnastics and tennis. Clin Sports Med 2, July 1983.
3. Neer, C. S.: Impingement lesions. Clin Orthop 173:70–77, 1983.
4. Jobe, F. W., and Moynes, D.: Delineation of diagnostic criteria and a rehabilitation program for rotator cuff injuries. Am J Sports Med 10:336–339, 1982.
5. Allman, Fred L., M.D. "Sports Medicine—Therapeutic Exercise." *Therapeutic Exercise,* Fourth Edition, Williams & Wilkins: Baltimore, MD, 499–501.
6. Moynes, D.: Prevention of injury to the shoulder through exercises and therapy. Clin Sport Med 2, July 1983.

SUPRASCAPULAR NERVE ENTRAPMENT

ROBERT WELLS, M.D.

The source of shoulder pain in the throwing athlete is commonly difficult to locate. Accuracy in determining the anatomic site of the pain is most important in planning effective treatment. Suprascapular nerve entrapment may be an obscure and infrequent source of pain and can occasionally lead to confusion in the diagnosis.

Shoulder pain and limited shoulder function in the throwing athlete originate from one of four types of problems:

1. Shoulder cuff tendinitis or impingement syndrome beneath the coracoacromial arch, or both
2. Instability of the glenohumeral articulation
3. Biceps tendon inflammation or instability
4. A variety of scapular problems secondary to one of the other three

Problems affecting the scapula are usually secondary to other conditions, which may include:

1. Restricted range of glenohumeral motion
2. Inflammation or entrapment of cervical nerve roots
3. Brachial plexitis or other forms of thoracic outlet syndrome
4. Muscular atrophy related to disuse

One of these scapular problems is suprascapular neuropathy. It is not uncommon in the pitcher with recurrent or long-term shoulder pain to see muscle atrophy in the infraspinatus and the supraspinatus fossae of the scapula. This condition is thought to result from impingement and traction to the suprascapular nerve.

The origin of this nerve is at the upper trunk of the brachial plexus immediately distal to its formation by coalition of the roots of C5 and C6. The nerve passes distally behind the plane of the plexus to the upper border of the scapula. There it passes through the scapular notch in a foramen completed by the transverse scapular ligament, which bridges the opening of the notch. At this location the nerve innervates the supraspinatus muscle, sends branches to the posterior aspect of the shoulder joint, and passes around the lateral edge of the base of the scapular spine to innervate the infraspinatus muscle.

The suprascapular nerve is a motor nerve only. Any pain associated with its irritation is deep and poorly localized.

The common point of impingement of the suprascapular nerve is at the scapular notch. The cross-sectional area of the nerve is close to that of the notch, and in some individuals there may be a scant fit.

The author believes that the common atrophy in the supraspinatus and infraspinatus muscles is a result of such nerve entrapment and not simply of disuse. The nerve pinch occurs if motion in the glenohumeral joint becomes restricted by either contracture or muscle spasm.

Sequentially, for instance, the development of anterior or superior tendinitis of the shoulder cuff may be followed by (1) restricted excursion of tendon motion beneath the coracoacromial arch, (2) posterior tightening of the capsule and cuff, (3) limited internal rotation, (4) a resultant greater range of scapular motion for a desired degree of shoulder motion, and (5) traction entrapment of the suprascapular nerve at the notch.

Other predisposing conditions may lead to a similar sequence—the end result being atrophy and further diminution of the stabilizing effect of the shoulder cuff muscles.

Diagnosis depends on maintaining an "index of suspicion" and knowledge of the anatomy and function of the shoulder joint. After observation of supraspinatus or infraspinatus muscle atrophy in association with vague posterior and lateral shoulder pain, a suprascapular nerve block with a local anesthetic and steroid preparation can be a valuable diagnostic as well as therapeutic aid. A decrease in pain when the shoulder is at rest and a greater range of permitted adduction without reproducible discomfort confirms the source of the problem.

Usually one or two such blocks in a patient whose primary glenohumeral joint motion is improving results in resolution of the problem.

When the benefit of nerve blocks is repeatedly transient, operative release of the nerve by section of the transverse scapular ligament may be needed. In the author's experience this procedure has not been found necessary for the athlete, since youthful condition results in the self-limited form of the condition. Suprascapular nerve release in two older individuals has produced dramatically good results, however.

When treating long-term shoulder pain the physician should look for atrophy in the supraspinatus and infraspinatus muscles. Suprascapular nerve blocks may be a helpful part of treatment.

SUGGESTED READING

1. Kopell, H. P., and Thompson, W. A. L.: Peripheral Entrapment Neuropathies. Baltimore, Williams & Wilkins, 1963.
2. Thompson, R. C., Jr., Schneider, W., and Kennedy, T.: Entrapment neuropathy of the inferior branch of the suprascapular nerve by ganglia. Clin Orthop 166:185, 1982.

NEUROVASCULAR
SYNDROMES

CHAMP L. BAKER, M.D. / ROBERT THORNBERRY, M.D.

INTRODUCTION

Disability resulting from compression on neurovascular structures in the shoulder and arm of the throwing athlete rarely has been diagnosed in the past. With increasing awareness of subtle symptoms and signs related to abnormalities in the shoulder girdle and rotator cuff, problems related to compression of both nerves and vascular structures are becoming increasingly recognized. Diagnostic evaluation of the throwing athlete with shoulder pain should include identification of a neurologic or vascular origin for the pain.

HISTORY

Prior reports of neurovascular problems in the shoulder have dealt primarily with compromise of the thoracic outlet caused by a variety of anatomic structures. There is very little in the literature specifically directed toward neurovascular problems of the throwing athlete.

The first mention of neurovascular compromise in the shoulder was related to cervical ribs as described by Hunald in 1743. Coote later recommended cervical decompression for supernumerary ribs in 1861. Murphy reported compression on the subclavian artery by the cervical rib in 1905, and Halsted reported 27 cases with significant dilatation of the subclavian artery distal to the rib in a series of 716 patients with radiographic evidence of cervical ribs. Brickner in 1927 and Telford in 1937 and 1948 mentioned compression related to thoracic ribs.

Adson and Coffey in 1927, with later reinforcement by Ochsner, Gage, and DeBakey in 1935, popularized the idea of production of the *thoracic outlet syndrome* by compression of the scalene muscles. Naffziger,[1] however, is given credit for the importance of scalene compression as a result of his work on brachial plexus neuritis, which was published in 1938.

Costoclavicular compression of the vessels at the level of the first rib secondary to hyperabduction of the arm was suggested by Lewis and Pickering in 1934 and again by Edon in 1939. Falconer and Weddel coined the term *costoclavicular syndrome* in the early 1940s to denote any compression in this space that produces vascular syndromes. Wright[2] investigated vascular compression caused by hyperabduction of the arm in military recruits and published his results in 1945. Tullos[3] and others have brought awareness of the occlusion of the axillary artery during the pitching act secondary to this hyperabduction. Recently there has been renewed recognition of the so-called *effort thrombosis*[4-6] in throwing athletes. This thrombosis of the axillary subclavian vein, occurring after trauma or an unusual forceful effort, had been described by Sir James Paget in 1875 and by Von Schroetter in 1884 and was previously known as the Paget-Schroetter syndrome.

ANATOMY

The passage through which the great vessels reach the axilla from the neck and chest is the thoracic outlet. The floor is formed by the upper border of the first rib, and the roof is formed by the inferior border of the clavicle. The scalene muscles further divide the space into compartments, with the anterior scalene muscle originating from the transverse process of the third, fourth, fifth, and sixth cervical vertebrae and inserting into the border of the first rib. The middle scalene muscle originates from the transverse process of all vertebrae and inserts into the first rib behind the subclavian artery. Therefore, the subclavian artery and the brachial plexus enter between the scalenus anticus and scalenus medius muscles. The neurovascular bundle, including the axillary artery, passes at a more distal location underneath the tendinous portion of the insertion of the pectoralis minor muscle into the coracoid process of the scapula.

On the basis of these anatomic relationships there are therefore several sites that can cause compression of neurovascular structures. These include (1) compression of the subclavian vein between the anterior scalene muscle, clavicle, and rib, (2) compression of the subclavian artery and brachial plexus between the anterior and middle scalene muscles, (3) compression of the neurovascular bundle between the clavicle and first rib, and (4) compression of the axillary artery under the insertion of the pectoralis minor muscle.

CLINICAL PRESENTATION

Compromise of the neurovascular supply of the upper limb produces a myriad of signs and symptoms. Because of this, clinical pictures can be confusing and include nonspecific complaints and vague physical findings. Different symptoms develop depending on the anatomic structure that is constricted—nerve or vessels—and also depending on the site of constriction. Pain and paresthesia from the neck and shoulder down to the hand are common and particularly involve the medial aspect of the elbow and the ulnar aspect of the forearm to the small and ring fingers. This involvement is due to the compromise of the ulnar nerve originating from C7–8 and T1 and forming the medial trunk of the brachial plexus. There can be weakness of grasp and difficulty with fine manipulation of the fingers of the hand. Patients can complain of weakness and numbness in the arm as well as pain, particularly with any use of the arm raised above the head. There can be nocturnal paresthesia caused by movement of the arm above the head.

Throwing athletes can complain of easy fatigability and muscle ache after throwing, which could be secondary to vascular symptoms. These symptoms could be caused by obstruction from the subclavian vein with stiffness, venous congestion, edema, coolness, pallor, and claudication resulting if there is thrombophlebitis. Arterial pulses are usually present; however, they can be absent if the axillary artery is compromised.

CLINICAL TESTS

The diagnosis of compromise to the neurovascular supply to the upper extremity is often made only after exhaustive noninvasive and invasive studies. A detailed history of the symptoms of the athlete, with particular emphasis on the precipitating causes, is extremely important along with a detailed clinical examination, with emphasis on the cervical spine and the entire shoulder girdle. Three clinical tests are important in helping to elucidate the site of compression in the cervical area.

Adson's test, as first described by Alford Adson in 1927, is used to determine the presence or absence of subclavian arterial constriction caused by the scalene anticus muscle (Fig. 19–1). As described by Doctor Adson, "The test consists of having the patient take a deep breath, elevate his chin and turn it to the affected side. This is done as the patient is seated upright with his arms resting on his knees and alteration or obliteration of the radial pulse or change in blood pressure is a pathognomonic sign of scalene anticus syndrome."[7]

The *costoclavicular maneuver* or the so-called *military brace position* (Fig. 19–2) reduces the space between the clavicle and the first rib, thus compromising the structures in that area. This maneuver is performed with

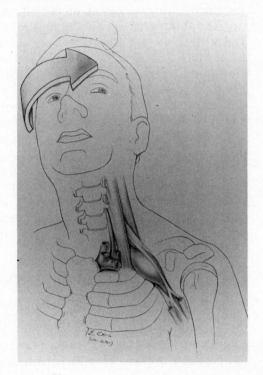

FIGURE 19–1. Adson's test. With the neck extended and on deep inspiration the chin is turned toward the affected side. Constriction by the scalene muscles on the subclavian artery can cause a diminished or obliterated distal radial pulse.

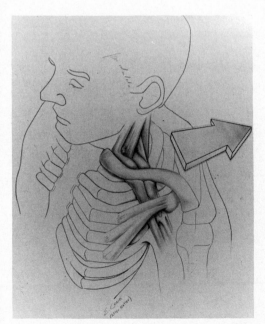

FIGURE 19–2. Costoclavicular maneuver. With the shoulders thrust back in an upright position the neurovascular bundles can be compressed between the clavicle and first rib to cause a distal diminution or obliteration of pulse.

the patient sitting upright, with the hands resting on the thighs and the shoulders thrust back in an erect posture.

The third maneuver is the *hyperabduction maneuver* as described by Wright (Fig. 19–3).[2] The patient sits upright and the arm is abducted from 90 to 180 degrees and externally rotated to cause compression of the neurovascular bundle, particularly of the axillary artery, as it passes underneath the insertion of the pectoralis minor muscle and the coracoid process. As Tullos[3] has pointed out, this maneuver actually consists of extension and then abduction and external rotation rather than hyperabduction and is a common movement found in the wind-up or cocking phase of the pitching act.

Each of these maneuvers can have both false-positive and false-negative results, and it is important to evaluate the patient's normal as well as symptomatic side. A true positive test result should involve reproduction of some of the presenting symptoms and complaints and can serve as a useful diagnostic tool in helping to locate the site of compression.

ANCILLARY DIAGNOSTIC TESTS

There are several additional studies that can be performed after the history and physical examination to help elucidate the cause of the patient's complaints. Radiographs of the cervical spine should be taken to rule out the presence of cervical or first thoracic ribs. Cervical ribs (Fig. 19–4) are

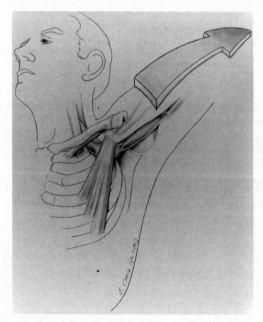

FIGURE 19–3. Wright's maneuver. With the arm extended, abducted, and externally rotated the middle portion of the axillary artery can be constricted under the insertion of the pectoralis minor muscle.

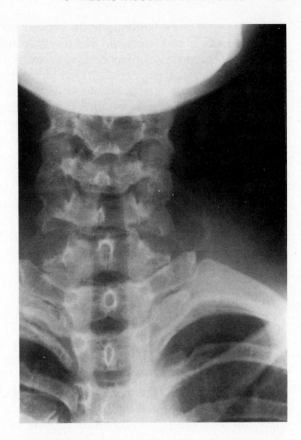

FIGURE 19–4. Radiograph of a cervical rib.

the most common bony abnormalities associated with neurovascular compression, although fewer than 10 per cent of patients with radiographic findings of extra ribs have symptoms. The ribs originate from the transverse process of C7 and usually attach directly or by ligaments to the first rib. Radiographs are also important to determine abnormalities or fractures of the clavicle or first rib, which may cause constriction by their position. Cervical radiographs can also reveal arthritic changes that can cause nerve root compression and that could cause similar symptoms, as found in neurovascular compromise. Other radiographs that can be useful include chest films, which can show a superior sulcus tumor—Pancoast's tumor—as the precipitating cause of pain referred to the shoulder, although this is an unusual finding in the young adult population.[8]

Electromyographic studies and nerve conduction velocity studies are somewhat controversial as diagnostic aids in delineating a thoracic outlet syndrome. They can best be used as a means of eliminating the possibility of more peripheral lesions such as in carpal tunnel syndrome or ulnar nerve neuropathy at the elbow or wrist. Such studies are also useful in differential diagnosis of cervical radiculopathy with referred shoulder pain.

There is some work being done on evoked potentials and F-waves, but at present nerve conduction and electromyographic studies are helpful only as an indirect means of diagnosing neurovascular compromise.

Doppler measurements of arterial blood flow in the arm of the throwing athlete can be quite useful and have been employed by physicians treating some baseball teams to screen their pitchers. Digital subtraction angiography may be of some help in individual cases rather than arteriographs. For true determination of vascular compromise, however, both phlebograms and angiographic studies of the subclavian vessels are indicated. It is important to remember to perform the test in both anatomic and abducted positions. Cahill[9] stresses the importance of having a subclavian arteriogram done according to the Seldinger technique, which puts emphasis on the external rotated abducted position of the arm as well as on allowing the dye to flow distally enough to examine the posterior humeral circumflex artery.

SPECIFIC SYNDROMES

Axillary Artery Occlusion. The axillary artery is the chief artery of the upper limb and begins as a continuation of the subclavian artery at the outer border of the first rib as it leaves the axilla and becomes the brachial artery. The axillary artery is arbitrarily divided into three parts, first, second, and third, with the second part lying behind the pectoralis minor muscle. As Wright demonstrated in 1945, the second part can become occluded by pressure from the pectoralis minor muscle as the arm is brought overhead in extension, abduction, and external rotation (Fig. 19–3). Tullos has described this occlusion in throwing athletes and finds that the abduction occurs during the wind-up or cocking phase in the baseball pitcher. He considers that transient occlusion of the artery caused by the outstretched pectoralis minor muscle is likely and that with repeated local trauma intimal arterial damage can occur with development of subsequent thrombosis.

Symptoms can include pain and tenderness over the supraclavicular space with associated symptoms of claudication and fatigue and diminished or absent distal pulses, cyanosis, and decreased skin temperature. Symptoms are usually exacerbated when the arm is placed in the positions of hyperabduction and external rotation.

Noninvasive studies such as Doppler studies can be diagnostic, but arteriograms are often necessary for a complete diagnosis. Arteriographic studies can demonstrate thrombosis with complete occlusion of the artery or aneurysmal dilatation of the artery caused by partial occlusion.

Treatment of this vascular condition is usually surgical and ranges from sympathectomy to thrombectomy to excision of the thrombosed area with either reanastomosis or bypass with vascular grafts. Professional baseball pitchers have returned to professional baseball after vascular reconstruction with minimal adverse effects, although there have been instances of propagation of thrombus resulting in cerebral vascular accidents and partial paralysis.

Effort Thrombosis. Although axillary artery occlusion is somewhat rare, thrombosis of the axillary venous system is not nearly as uncommon. Initial descriptions by Sir James Paget in 1875 and by Von Schroetter in 1884 are still valid today. The condition is often called *effort thrombosis* because of its frequent association with a forceful event that produces direct or indirect injury to the vein. The axillary vein begins at the lower border at the teres major muscle as a continuation of the basilic vein and becomes the subclavian vein on the outer margin of the first rib. The axillary vein lies on the medial side of the axillary artery, and constriction can occur at several points along its anatomic course, with the most severe compression occurring in the costoclavicular space after hyperextension of the neck, hyperabduction of the arm, or the assumption of the "military brace position" with a backward thrust of the shoulders. Constriction often occurs between the costocoracoid ligament and the first rib or the subclavian muscles and the first rib, or more commonly between the clavicle and the first rib.

The condition occurs in young athletic and active men and usually involves the right side and is usually preceded by strenuous effort or repetitive action. Symptoms usually develop within the first 24 hours with either pain or swelling or both and are confined to the upper extremity. Cyanosis secondary to venous congestion may occur, or a prominent venous distension pattern may be developing over the shoulder as a result of the collateral vein distension. A tender cordlike structure at times may be palpable in the axilla.

The diagnosis of deep vein thrombosis is usually made on the basis of symptoms and signs alone, with venous pressure measurements increased on the involved side as compared with the contralateral side. Final confirmation is made by phlebographic demonstration of occlusion of the deep veins with either nonvisualization of a short segment of the vein seen as a result of acute thrombi (Fig. 19–5) of a late study demonstrating well developed collaterals and recanalization of the thrombosed segment with so-called first rib bypass collateral (Fig. 19–6) as a result of the increase in collateral venous network bypass. Initial treatment is often related to the initial signs and symptoms. In most cases rest and elevation of the arm are the only treatment methods and lead to resolution of symptoms. Anticoagulation therapy is often used in the acute phase to prevent progression of the thrombus. Some surgeons have resorted to initial venous thrombectomy because of the residual complaints following conservative and anticoagulation therapy. Local thromboembolic therapy using either streptokinase or urokinase has been employed with some success.[5] This technique involves changing and advancing the tip of the infusion catheter proximally to the remaining unlysed thrombus to avoid poor diffusion of the thrombolytic medication as a result of collateral pathways.

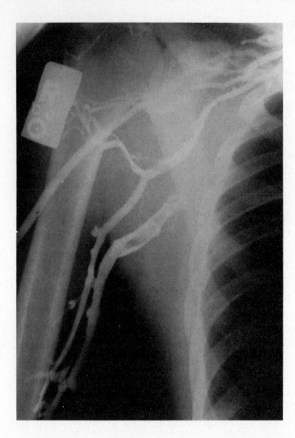

FIGURE 19–5. Venogram demonstrating an acute subclavian thrombosis.

Complications include mild chronic residual complaints of exertional claudication of the arm in 60 to 75 per cent of the patients. Previously it was thought that pulmonary embolus rarely occurred in primary deep vein thrombosis of the upper extremity. However, Barnett and Levitt in 1951[10] presented a well documented case showing pulmonary embolus following an upper extremity thrombosis, and it is now believed that this may be a more common complication.

Quadrilateral Space Syndrome. Cahill and Palmer in 1967[9] described compression of the posterior humeral circumflex artery and axillary nerve or one of its major branches occurring in the quadrilateral space in 18 patients. The quadrilateral space is formed by the teres minor, the teres major, the long head of the triceps, and the surgical neck of the humerus with the axillary nerve and the posterior humeral circumflex vessels passing backward through the space below the capsule of the shoulder. Compression can occur because of fibrous bands within this space with the arm abducted and externally rotated.

Symptoms are usually nonspecific, with pain and paresthesia in the upper extremity not associated with trauma. Symptoms are aggravated by

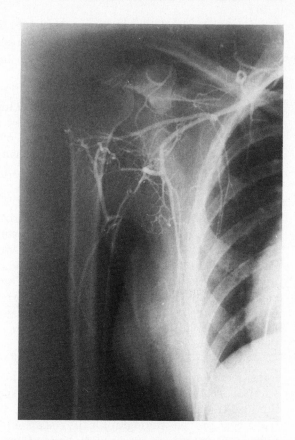

FIGURE 19–6. Increased collateral venous bypass after thrombosis of the subclavian vein.

abduction external rotation of the humerus. The other results of the physical examination are usually essentially normal except for findings of discrete point tenderness posteriorly in the quadrilateral space. Results of neurologic examination usually are normal as are those of nerve conduction and electromyographic studies. Confirmation of diagnosis is based on the subclavian arteriogram done according to the Seldinger technique, which allows for the dye to be followed distally so that the posterohumeral circumflex artery can be examined with the arm in abduction external rotation. The artery can be patent with the humerus at its side with a positive study result but can occlude with abduction and external rotation. Surgical decompression of the quadrilateral space through a posterior approach is recommended, and although this syndrome has not been previously described in throwing athletes, it should be considered in the differential diagnosis of pain and paresthesia in the upper extremity.

Thoracic Outlet Syndrome. Thoracic outlet syndrome is an ill-defined term pertaining to the collection of signs and symptoms associated with pain and paresthesia of the upper shoulder caused by compression of the neurovascular bundle by any of the anatomic structures encountered in the thorax. Although this syndrome is classically found in middle-aged women with drooping of the shoulders and large bosoms, it has been described in well conditioned muscular male athletes and in particular in baseball pitchers who have pain while throwing.[11]

The signs and symptoms are similar to those of any compression of the artery, veins, or nerves in the thorax that include stiffness, venous engorgement, coolness, claudication, and/or numbness and tingling in the extremity. Adson's maneuver can show obliteration of the radial pulse, although Wright's position or the military brace position or both can also reveal compression. Any of the previously described ancillary tests can give positive results, including radiographic evidence of cervical ribs.

Once the diagnosis has been established through diagnostic studies and elimination of other more specific syndromes the initial treatment is nonoperative, consisting of postural improvement and shoulder strengthening exercises as well as avoidance of precipitating symptoms. Any patients with complicating vascular problems should have appropriate invasive studies and follow-up treatment. The majority of patients usually can be treated well by this exercise program, which includes rest, local injection at the trigger areas or anti-inflammatory medication, and range-of-motion and pendulum exercises as well as specific shoulder girdle exercises that have been proposed.[12]

Surgical treatment[13] is recommended for those patients whose symptoms persist after an appropriate time of rest and an exercise program with surgical treatment directed toward the precipitating site of constriction. Surgical treatment usually involves excision of a cervical rib if its presence has been proved radiographically, scalenotomy of the scalene anticus muscle, or release of constricting bands found in the thorax at the site of occlusion.

DIFFERENTIAL DIAGNOSIS

There are other sites in the shoulder and arm that can produce a myriad of symptoms that can mimic compression of neurovascular structures and which should be included for completeness of evaluation. These include (1) cervical disc protrusion, (2) brachial neuritis, particularly with involvement of the ulnar nerve at the elbow or wrist, (3) carpal tunnel syndrome, (4) suprascapular nerve syndrome, and (5) neurologic entrapment of specific peripheral nerves, including (a) dorsal scapular nerves, (b) long thoracic nerves, (c) involvement of pronator teres muscle and entrapment of the median nerve, (d) radial nerves, and (e) cubital tunnel syndrome.

SUMMARY

Injuries to the neurovascular supply of the upper extremity and particularly the shoulder can occur as a result of local trauma or repetitive minor trauma such as that found in the throwing athlete. Owing to the unusual demands placed on the throwing athlete specific normal anatomic structures can become pathologic and cause compression of neurovascular entities to produce distal symptoms that are either neurologic, arterial, or venous in nature. The symptoms range from subtle fatigability to frank anesthesia and loss of blood supply. Symptoms are usually determined by the vessel or nerve that is compromised and also by where the occlusion occurs. Specific syndromes can occur because of compression of certain anatomic structures. These include (1) arterial occlusion by the pectoralis minor muscle, (2) venous thrombosis of the subclavian or axillary vein as a result of constriction of the clavicle or first rib, (3) occlusion of posterohumeral circumflex artery or axillary nerve caused by constrictive bands in the quadrilateral space, and (4) compression of any neurovascular structures in the shoulder associated with a variety of constricting areas, including the clavicle and first rib or scalene anticus and/or the first rib.

Diagnostic evaluation of these compressive symptoms of the upper extremity should include (1) thorough and accurate history and physical examination with emphasis on Adson's test, Wright's maneuver, and the military brace position, (2) diagnostic studies including cervical radiographs, chest films, Doppler measurements, electromyograms, and nerve conduction studies and vascular studies, including venography and arteriography to determine the status of vascular supply. Cervical myelograms can be indicated at times. Relief is usually obtained with nonoperative treatment for the more common constrictions with emphasis on postural and shoulder girdle strengthening exercises and avoidance of precipitating factors. Vascular occlusion can be treated with anticoagulants or surgical methods, including thrombectomy, sympathectomy, and/or vascular bypass grafts. Surgical release of the anterior scalene muscles and removal of the cervical rib are usually performed through a transaxillary approach with removal of the first rib to enlarge the floor of the thoracic outlet. This technique has been well described by Roos.[13]

Suspected compromise of any of the neurovascular structures in the shoulder and axilla should be considered in the differential diagnosis of a throwing athlete with neck, shoulder, or elbow pain or a combination of these symptoms.

REFERENCES

1. Naffziger, H. C., and Grant, W. T.: Neuritis of the brachioplexus mechanical in origin: the scalenous syndrome. Surg Gynecol Obstet 67:722, 1938.
2. Wright, I. S.: The neurovascular syndrome produced by hyperabduction of the arm. Am Heart J 29:1, 1945.
3. Tullos, H. S., Erwin, W. D., Woods, W. G., Wukasey, D. C., Cooley, D. A., and King, J. W.: Unusual lesions of the pitching arm. Clin Orthop 88:169, 1972.
4. Adams, J. T., and Deweese, J. A.: "Effort" thrombosis of the axillary and subclavian veins. J Trauma, 11:923, 1971.

5. Becker, G. J., Holden, R. W., Rabe, F., Castaneda-Zuniga, W. R., Sears, N., Dilley, R. S., and Glover, J. L.: Local thromboembolic therapy for subclavian axillary vein thrombosis. Interventional Radiography. 149:419, 1973.
6. Coone, W. W., and Park, W.: Thrombosis of the axillary subclavian veins. Arch Surg 94:657, 1967.
7. Adson, A. W.: Surgical treatment for symptoms produced by cervical ribs and scalenus anticus muscle. Surg Gynecol Obstet 85:687, 1947.
8. Spengler, D. M., Kirsch, M. M., and Kaufer, H.: Orthopaedic aspects and early diagnosis of superior sulcus tumor of lung (Pancoast). J Bone Joint Surg 55A:1645, 1973.
9. Cahill, B., and Palmer, R.: Quadrilateral space syndrome. J Hand Surg 8:65, 1983.
10. Barnett, T., and Levitt, L.: "Effort" thrombosis of the axillary vein with pulmonary embolism. JAMA 146:1412, 1951.
11. Strukel, R. J., and Garrick, J. G.: Thoracic outlet compression in athletes. Am J Sports Med 6:35, 1978.
12. Britt, L. P.: Nonoperative treatment of thoracic outlet syndrome symptoms. Clin Orthop 51:45, 1967.
13. Roos, D. B.: Transaxillary approach for first resection to relieve thoracic outlet syndrome. Ann Surg 163:354, 1966.

SUGGESTED READING

1. Brown, C.: Compressive invasive referred pain to the shoulder. Clin Orthop 173:55, 1983.
2. Leffert, R. D.: Thoracic outlet syndrome in the shoulder. Clin Sports Med 2:439, 1983.
3. Telford, E. D., and Maddershed, S.: Pressure of the cervico-brachial junction. J Bone Joint Surg 30B:249, 1948.

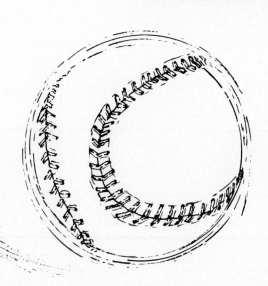

PART
THREE

THE
ELBOW
IN THE
THROWING
ATHLETE

FUNCTIONAL ANATOMY
OF THE ELBOW

HUGH S. TULLOS, M.D. / WILLIAM J. BRYAN, M.D.

A comprehensive appreciation of elbow osteology, ligamentous constraints, muscular control, and regional soft tissues is necessary to understand functional elbow anatomy.

BASIC OSTEOLOGY

The elbow is a joint involving freedom of motion about both its longitudinal and its transverse axes (Fig. 20–1). The first degree of freedom—flexion-extension—is provided by a humeroulnar joint. The distal humerus is composed of the trochlea, which articulates with the olecranon process and the trochlear notch of the ulna, and the capitellum, which is aligned to the superior surface of the radial head. The trochlea projects 45 degrees in front of the axis of the humeral shaft as does the trochlear notch of the ulna, so that this anterior projection promotes flexion to 150 degrees. Active flexion is further limited by apposition of the anterior muscles of the arm and forearm, hardened by contraction (Fig. 20–2). In passive flexion the radial head impacts against the humeral radial fossa, the coronoid process of the ulna impacts against the humeral coronoid fossa, and tension develops in the triceps muscle and the posterior elbow capsule. Elbow extension to zero degrees is facilitated by the concavity of the humeral olecranon fossa, but further elbow extension is checked by impaction of the olecranon into the olecranon fossa, by tension in the anterior capsule, and by resistance of the biceps and brachial muscles.

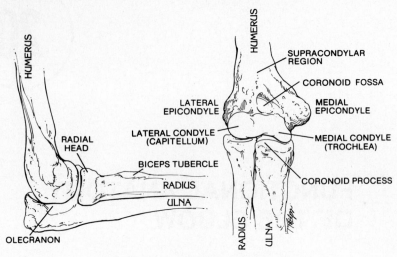

FIGURE 20–1. Basic elbow osteology.

Morrey and Chao[1] have additionally noted that there is 5 degrees of ulnar internal rotation during early elbow flexion and 5 degrees of ulnar external rotation during terminal extension. This motion is slight but could explain the findings of King, Brelsford, and Tullos[2] regarding degenerative changes in the medial side of the olecranon tip in baseball players.

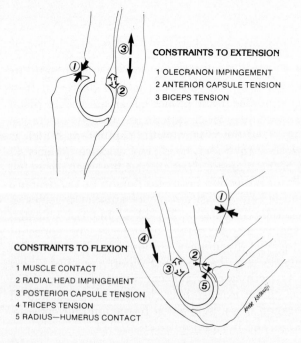

CONSTRAINTS TO EXTENSION

1 OLECRANON IMPINGEMENT
2 ANTERIOR CAPSULE TENSION
3 BICEPS TENSION

FIGURE 20–2. Constraints to elbow extension and flexion.

CONSTRAINTS TO FLEXION

1 MUSCLE CONTACT
2 RADIAL HEAD IMPINGEMENT
3 POSTERIOR CAPSULE TENSION
4 TRICEPS TENSION
5 RADIUS—HUMERUS CONTACT

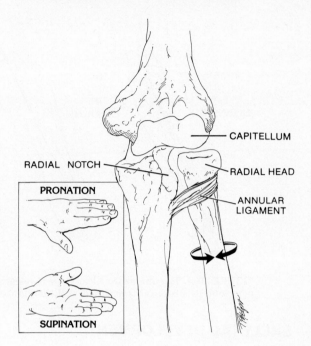

FIGURE 20–3. The proximal radioulnar articulation.

CAPITELLUM

RADIAL NOTCH

RADIAL HEAD

ANNULAR LIGAMENT

PRONATION

SUPINATION

The second degree of rotational freedom is provided by the unique articulation of the radius with the capitellar portion of the humerus, so that forearm pronation and supination are allowed (Fig. 20–3).

The proximal radioulnar articulation is made up of the radial head, the radial notch of the ulna, and the annular ligament. The annular ligament makes up four fifths of the fibro-osseous ring, which retains the head but allows for rotational movement. The remaining one fifth is composed of the radioulnar notch. The concave radial head glides on the spheroidal capitellum and simultaneously rotates about its vertical axes during pronation and supination, allowing the forearm to rotate through 150 degrees.

It should be noted that the patterns of motion for the humeroulnar and proximal radioulnar joints are separate, although the joints are effectively one, being invested by a common synovial membrane.

There is a valgus "carrying angle" at the elbow (Fig. 20–4) that is determined by the articulation of the ulna and the radius with the humerus. This angle is best visualized with the forearm supinated and the elbow extended. The carrying angle in adults varies from 10 to 15 degrees and is greater in women. The varying depth of the inner lip of the trochlea accounts for the fact that the "carrying angle" diminishes with elbow flexion so that in full flexion the elbow is in a varus position.

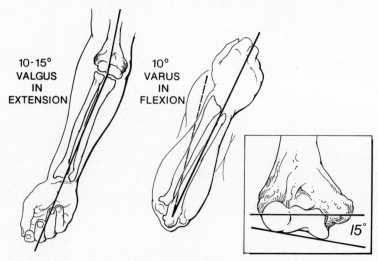

10-15°
VALGUS
IN
EXTENSION

10°
VARUS
IN
FLEXION

15°

FIGURE 20–4. The unique trochlear slope (15 degrees) allows the elbow to pass from valgus to varus positions as flexion proceeds.

SKELETAL DEVELOPMENT

Skeletal development of the elbow revolves around the primary ossification centers of the humerus, ulna, and radius with six distinct centers of secondary ossification. The ages of appearance and closure of these centers are shown in any standard anatomy text. A single bony center is the usual radiographic appearance for secondary ossification centers. When variation is noted in the size and density of a secondary ossification center in a comparative extremity radiograph (especially with fragmentation), the presence of osteochondritis dissecans must be considered. An intimate knowledge of these ossification centers is also necessary in the growing athlete for appraisal of possible avulsion fracture. Figure 20–5 demonstrates the centers most frequently involved in throwing injuries to the elbow in childhood and adolescence.

THE ROLE OF COLLATERAL LIGAMENTS IN MEDIOLATERAL STABILITY

Since valgus stress plays an important role in throwing injuries, it is critical to examine the determinants of medial and lateral elbow stability. The medial and to a lesser degree the lateral collateral ligaments act as stays to keep the articular surfaces in close apposition and to prevent sideways motion. They do not normally stretch. The so-called lateral collateral ligament (Fig. 20–6), however, is a true collateral ligament. It originates from the lateral epicondyle and has its primary insertion on the

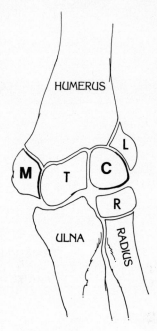

FIGURE 20–5. The key secondary growth centers involved in childhood and adolescent throwing arm injuries; M = medial epicondyle; C = capitellar; R = radial head; T = trochlear; and L = lateral epicondyle.

annular ligament with only a few nonfunctional weak fibers being attached to the margins of the radial notch of the ulna. More importantly, the anconeus muscle appears to provide lateral support as does the forearm extensor muscles, which arise from the lateral epicondyle.

In contrast, there is a well developed ligament on the medial side (Fig. 20–7) that is formed by three distinct bands that are continuous with one another: the anterior oblique, a small transverse nonfunctional ligament,

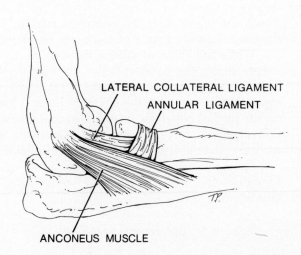

FIGURE 20–6. Lateral elbow stability. The lateral collateral ligament does not run from the humerus to the ulna.

LATERAL COLLATERAL LIGAMENT

ANNULAR LIGAMENT

ANCONEUS MUSCLE

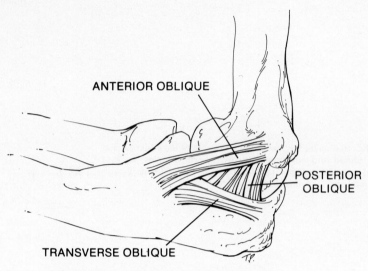

FIGURE 20–7. The elbow medial collateral ligament.

and the posterior oblique ligament. The anterior oblique ligament is band-shaped, extremely robust, and runs from the undersurface of the medial epicondyle to a point in the medial aspect of the ulnar surface just below the coronoid process. This ligament is taut throughout the entire arc of elbow flexion owing to its unique anatomic attachment. Functioning through the entire elbow range of motion, the anterior oblique ligament is therefore the primary constraint to valgus stress at the elbow. The characteristics of the posterior oblique ligament are quite different, being taut in flexion and lax in extension. Indeed, if the posterior oblique ligament in cadaveric specimens is sectioned and the anterior oblique ligament is left intact, the elbow does not become unstable.* Thus, the posterior oblique ligament does not play a primary role in elbow stability.

While the anterior oblique ligament is the first line of defense against valgus stress, the radiocapitellar joint on the lateral side of the elbow is also important in this respect. If the radial head or a portion of the capitellum is removed, the lateral buttress is lost and stresses are increased on the medial collateral ligament so that attenuation or rupture can occur. Conversely, if forces acutely or repetitively exceed the capacity of the medial collateral ligament the radiocapitellar joint is subjected to compressive forces, often leading to radial head or capitellar fractures or the formation of intra-articular loose bodies from the articular cartilage fragmentation.

---

*Tullos, M. S., 1984: Personal communication.

DETERMINANTS OF ANTEROPOSTERIOR STABILITY

In that there is no basic ligamentous support posteriorly, the stability of the elbow in terms of anterior stress depends on the integrity of the collateral ligaments, the joint capsule, and surprisingly little on the trochlear-olecranon articulation. Anatomic studies indicate that when the olecranon process has been removed but the anterior oblique ligament is intact, the elbow remains stable.[3]* Irrespective of whether the olecranon process is intact or not, if the anterior oblique ligament is severed the elbow becomes unstable under anterior stress.

Posterior displacement is checked by the anterior capsule, the abutment of the radial head against the capitellum, and the abutment of the ulnar coracoid process against the trochlea.

MUSCULAR CONTROL

The three primary flexor muscles of the elbow are the biceps brachii, the brachoradialis, and the brachialis (Fig. 20–8). The biceps is by far the most important and plays a secondary role in supinating the forearm and coapting the glenohumeral joint by means of its long head. The pronator teres and flexor carpi radialis longus are secondary flexors.

The triceps is the only effective extensor of the elbow, with some feeble assistance provided by the anconeus muscle. The triceps is most powerful in a position of shoulder flexion and when the elbow and shoulder are simultaneously extended from this position. The primary muscles of supi-

---

*Tullos, M. S., 1984: Personal communication.

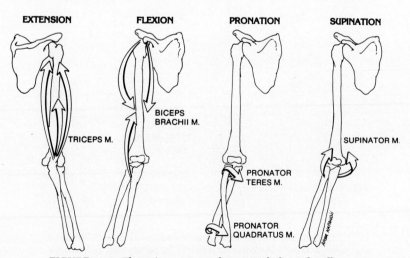

FIGURE 20–8. The primary muscular control about the elbow.

nation are the supinator and the biceps, the latter muscle being the most powerful rotator muscle of the forearm.

The important pronator muscles are the pronator teres and the pronator quadratus.

The superficial flexor forearm muscles arise from a common origin on the medial epicondyle. Forceful muscle contraction or repetitive valgus stress in the act of throwing in the skeletally developing athlete can result in separation of the secondary ossification center from the underlying bone. In the adult athlete such stresses can result in strains, sprains, or frank flexor muscle belly tears.

The extensors, carpi radialis brevis, digitorum communis, digiti minimi, and carpi ulnaris share a common tendon or origin that is attached to the front of the lateral epicondyle. All four muscles aid in elbow extension in addition to their more distal function. Repetitive stress on the lateral epicondyle-extension tendon junction can give rise to lateral epicondylitis or "tennis elbow."[4]

NERVE RELATIONSHIPS

The radial nerve (Fig. 20–9) approaches the elbow from the anterior compartment after passing from the spinal groove through the lateral intermuscular septum. After passing close to the lateral epicondyle, the radial nerve terminates by dividing into the posterior interosseous nerve

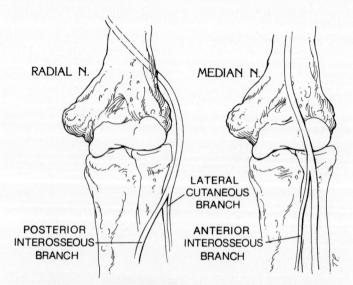

RADIAL N.

MEDIAN N.

LATERAL
CUTANEOUS
BRANCH

POSTERIOR
INTEROSSEOUS
BRANCH

ANTERIOR
INTEROSSEOUS
BRANCH

FIGURE 20–9. The radial nerve courses posteriorly to the humerus and gains access to the anterior forearm by passing the radial neck. The median nerve stays anterior.

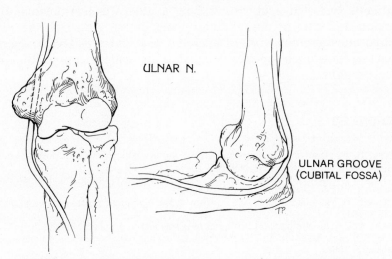

ULNAR N.

ULNAR GROOVE
(CUBITAL FOSSA)

FIGURE 20–10. The course of the ulnar nerve around the medial elbow.

and the lateral cutaneous nerve of the forearm. The important branches are well catalogued in most anatomy texts.

The median nerve (Fig. 20–9) remains anterior to the elbow in its course, lying on the surface of the brachialis and passing between the two heads of the pronator, at which location its anterior interosseous branch may become trapped with undue athletic activity, thus leading to the anterior interosseous syndrome.[5, 6]

The ulnar nerve (Fig. 20–10) exits the anterior arm, piercing the triceps fascia as it approaches the cubital tunnel. Careful attention must be paid to releasing this fascia with anterior ulnar nerve transposition lest a new compression syndrome be created. The ulnar nerve gives off no branches until it reaches the all-critical cubital fossa. As the nerve passes through the tunnel it gives off branches to the flexor carpi ulnaris and the medial half of the flexor digitorum profundus. The accompanying ulnar collateral artery provides critical blood supply and is closely approximated. Proximally and distally the nerve is protected by muscle, but within the cubital tunnel it is relatively unprotected and is especially vulnerable to compression. The floor of the tunnel is formed by the medial collateral ligament and the roof of the arcuate ligament, which extends from a fixed point on the medial epicondyle to a ·movable attachment at the olecranon. This ligament is taut at 90 degrees of flexion and therefore compresses the nerve as elbow flexion increases. Any deficiency in the anterior oblique portion of the medial collateral ligament allowing the elbow to open in valgus places undue stress on the ulnar nerve and at times may lead to "tardy ulnar nerve palsy."[7, 8]

As techniques of elbow examination expand to include radiographs, arthrograms, computed axial tomographic scans, and high-speed cinematography the basics of elbow anatomy are sometimes forgotten. Nevertheless, an intimate knowledge of gross elbow anatomy is instrumental in the evaluation and care of any athletic elbow injury. Although the idea of spending an afternoon with an anatomy text and a cadaveric specimen sounds unappealing, it can greatly enhance the reader's appreciation of this fascinating joint.

REFERENCES

1. Morrey, B. F., Askew, L. J., and Chao, E. Y.: Biomechanical study of normal functional elbow motion. J Bone Joint Surg 63A:872, 1981.
2. King, J. W., Brelsford, H. J., and Tullos, H. S.: Analysis of the pitching arm of the professional baseball pitcher. Clin Orthop 67:116, 1969.
3. McKeever, F. M., and Buck, R. M.: Fracture of the olecranon process of the ulna. JAMA 135:1, 1947.
4. Nirschl, R. P.: The etiology and treatment of tennis elbow. J Sports Med 2:308, 1974.
5. Farber, J. S., and Bryan, R. S.: The anterior interosseous nerve syndrome. J Bone Joint Surg 50A:521, 1968.
6. Spinner, M.: The anterior interosseous nerve syndrome. With special attention to its variations. J Bone Joint Surg 52A:84, 1970.
7. Froimson, A. I., and Zahrawi, F.: Treatment of compression neuropathy of the ulnar nerve at the elbow by epicondylectomy and neurolysis. J Hand Surg 5:391, 1980.
8. Gay, J. R., and Love, J. G.: Diagnosis and treatment of tardy paralysis of the ulnar nerve. J Bone Joint Surg 29:1087, 1947.

EXAMINATION OF THE THROWING ELBOW

HUGH S. TULLOS, M.D. / WILLIAM JAY BRYAN, M.D.

INITIAL EXAMINATION

As in all orthopedic medicine, a carefully recorded history and physical examination provide most of the information that is needed to successfully treat the majority of athletes. Ancillary tests such as radiographs, isokinetic testing, and arthroscopy are discussed in this chapter, but it must be made clear that these tests play a minor role. Table 21–1 lists the pertinent questions to ask the athlete with an ailing elbow. Attention to detail cannot

TABLE 21–1. HISTORY TAKING FOR THE PATIENT WITH AN INJURED THROWING ELBOW

What and where	Location and nature of pain or restricted motion
	Associated neck, shoulder, or wrist pain or restricted motion
When	Date of onset
	Date of repeated injury
How	Caused by specific incident?
	Activities that aggravate
	Activities that relieve
	Position played
	Type of pitches thrown
	Training schedule and recent change
	Effect of treatment to date

be overemphasized, since the slightest change in training schedule and an "almost forgotten" sprain or strain can lead to the proper diagnosis and treatment.

Examination of the throwing athlete's elbow begins with unobstructed exposure of the entire upper body and both upper extremities under proper lighting in an ambient-temperature environment.

The elbow, being but one link in a kinetic chain of several joints, must be considered in context. Careful attention must be paid to problems of the cervical spine in which ligamentous sprain or degenerative disc disease with pain radiating to the elbow can simulate elbow disease. A complete shoulder examination, as discussed in Chapter 6, may reveal subtle or overt shoulder pathology affecting elbow mechanics. Wrist or hand problems can likewise adversely affect elbow function.

VISUALIZATION

Differences in limb size are often encountered and must be considered in the context of limb dominance and exercise hypertrophy as first described by King.[1] A tape measure can be used to quickly quantitate arm and forearm girth. The carrying angle varies, averaging 14 degrees in females and 11 degrees in males. Differences between left and right should be slight, although King has described the development of cubitus valgus along with forearm hypertrophy in professional pitchers. Great differences should be explored by radiographic analysis.

MOTION

Motion is measured from full extension (zero degrees) to full flexion (150 degrees). As discussed in Chapter 20, the elbow changes from a valgus to a varus angle because of the unique structure of the trochlea. If this pattern is not present, radiographic analysis is in order. Hyperextension of the elbow is usually associated with generalized ligamentous laxity and is seldom seen in the throwing athlete. On the other hand, flexion contracture is commonly encountered (Fig. 21–1). Flexion contracture can be the result of recurrent anterior capsular sprains or forearm flexor strains. Intra-articular pathology such as osteochondritis dissecans or loose bodies can also give rise to anterior elbow discomfort. The inability to fully flex the elbow (Fig. 21–2) can indicate triceps tendinitis, posterior capsule tightness from sprain, or intra-articular loose bodies.

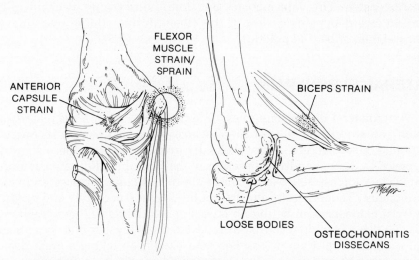

FIGURE 21–1. Causes of elbow flexion contracture (inability to fully extend the elbow).

ANTERIOR ELBOW PAIN

Anterior elbow pain can be caused by a sprain or avulsion of the biceps tendon insertion. Capsular sprain is common and is caused by elbow

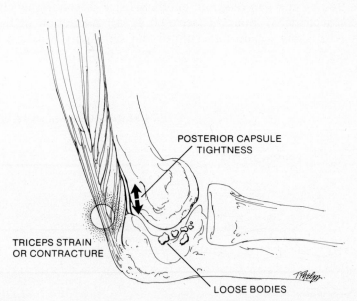

FIGURE 21–2. Causes of elbow extension contracture (inability to fully flex the elbow).

hyperextension. This injury comes not from the throwing mechanism but from untoward hyperextension of the elbow during sliding, working out with weights, or batting practice.

LATERAL ELBOW PAIN

Anterolateral elbow tenderness (Fig. 21–3) along with decreased pronation and supination suggest the diagnosis of radiocapitellar incongruity or a radial head fracture. In the skeletally immature athlete these signs can be caused by osteochondritis dissecans of the capitulum. Repeated compression of the radiocapitellar joint can injure the articular cartilage and create loose bodies. Tenderness in the area of the lateral epicondyle and origin of the wrist extensors can be due to lateral epicondylitis or "tennis elbow."[2] This condition is seldom caused by repeated throwing, but it is occasionally seen in baseball players or coaches who have been taking a great deal of batting practice or batting fungo. A bulging beneath the anconeus muscle behind the lateral epicondyle indicates elbow effusion or hemarthrosis. This is the best site for performing elbow aspiration or injection of appropriate medications.

POSTERIOR ELBOW PAIN

Olecranon bursae can arise superficially at the triceps tendon from repeated trauma and can reach an enormous size, becoming mechanically painful or secondarily infected (see Fig. 21–4). Aspiration of the bursal contents with Gram's stain and culture and sensitivity tests are in order

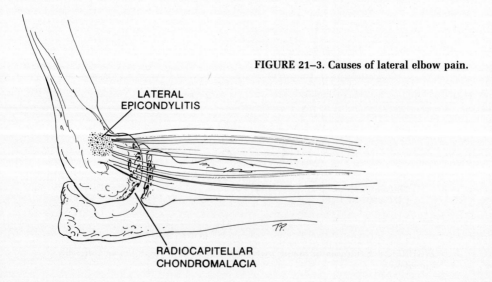

FIGURE 21–3. Causes of lateral elbow pain.

LATERAL
EPICONDYLITIS

RADIOCAPITELLAR
CHONDROMALACIA

FIGURE 21–4. Causes of posterior elbow pain.

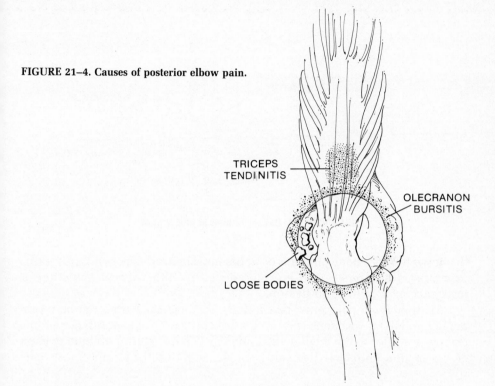

TRICEPS
TENDINITIS

OLECRANON
BURSITIS

LOOSE BODIES

when a pre-existing olecranon bursa becomes painful, red, and swollen. The medial olecranon area is often a source of pain in the throwing athlete because as the elbow extends valgus stress and slight rotation of the ulna result in medial olecranon-humeral fossa impingement. Andrews has called this the "valgus extension overload syndrome."[3] This syndrome can cause medial olecranon loose bodies in pitchers, as described many years ago by Tullos and Brelsford.[4] Tenderness in the triceps tendon is usually caused by triceps tendinitis. Rupture of the triceps muscle or tendon in throwing sports is extremely rare.

MEDIAL ELBOW PAIN

The common sites of medial elbow pain in throwing athletes are (1) the flexor muscle origin at the medial epicondyle, (2) the medial collateral ligament, and (3) the ulnar nerve (Fig. 21–5). In the skeletally immature athlete, the junction of the medial epicondyle secondary growth center with the underlying humerus is stressed in tension, leading to medial epicondylitis or a fracture through the epiphysis. In the adult, tensile stresses at

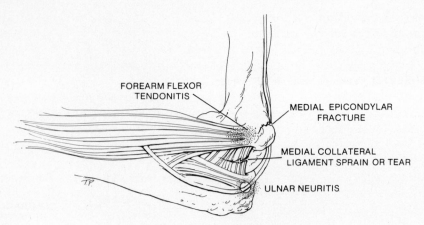

FIGURE 21–5. Causes of medial elbow pain.

the flexor tendon–bone junction or in the muscle itself may result in sprains or strains, respectively, and are reproduced by either direct palpation or resistance against forearm flexion.

Medial elbow pain must be carefully distinguished from the pain of a medial collateral ligament sprain or tear. The pain from such ligamentous tears is posterior to the medial epicondyle (over the anterior oblique portion of the medial collateral ligament) and is reproduced by applying valgus

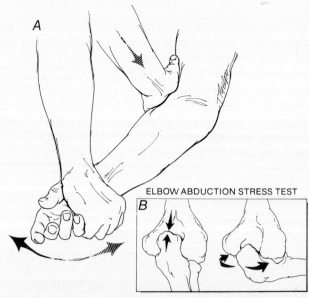

FIGURE 21–6. As the insert (B) demonstrates, the elbow should be flexed at least 30 degrees so that the olecranon will be unlocked from the olecranon fossa.

stress. To detect valgus instability (Fig. 21–6) the elbow must be flexed approximately 30 degrees to free the olecranon of its fossa. Comparisons with laxity in the opposite elbow should be performed.

Symptoms of ulnar nerve compression can arise with or without medial collateral ligament laxity. They can be reproduced by percussing the nerve in the ulnar groove. Decreased nerve conduction velocity can be measured using electromyelography to clarify the nature of pathology. Ulnar nerve transfer may be indicated in some cases.

The combination of flexor muscle sprain, medial collateral ligament tendinitis, and ulnar nerve entrapment is often encountered, since all three conditions are secondary to excess valgus stress. Each requires different medial attention, and the need to differentiate the three cannot be overemphasized.

ISOKINETIC TESTING

Isokinetic testing using the Cybex dynamometer (Fig. 21–7A) has allowed for accurate measurement of muscle power and torque around the elbow. Comparisons can be made to the opposite arm, or more significantly serial examinations can be undertaken with attention to increasing or decreasing performance.

RADIOGRAPHS

Radiographs are a vital part of examining the throwing elbow and require excellent technical standards to obtain proper views. The anteroposterior, lateral, and in selected cases gravity stress views are essential. Tomography, arthrography, and computed axial tomographic scans are playing an increasingly important role in evaluation of elbow pain or limited motion.

For the anteroposterior and lateral views (Fig. 21–8) the patient should be seated at the edge of the radiography table with the limb placed on the film. The anteroposterior film is then taken with the elbow in full extension. The forearm can be positioned at various degrees of pronation and supination if better examination of the radial head is desired. In cases of flexion contracture two views perpendicular to the humerus and two perpendicular to the radius-ulna can be taken to show the bony structure correctly.

A lateral view is best obtained by flexing the joint to 90 degrees and placing the elbow on the film. To better visualize the radial head, the pronation or supination of the forearm is varied.

In children and adolescent athletes comparison views of the opposite elbow should always be taken. Irregularities and "displacement" of the secondary growth centers may prove to be variations in normal anatomy as opposed to signs of acute or chronic abnormalities.

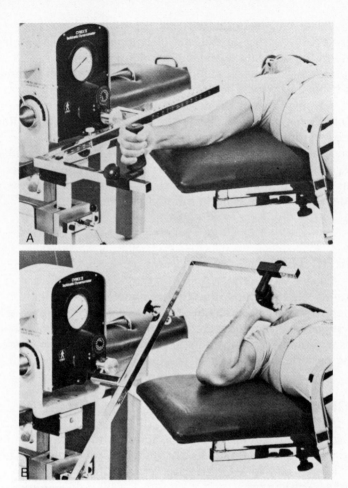

FIGURE 21–7. Isokinetic testing allows for accurate determination of muscle power and torque as the joint moves from flexion to extension.

The most useful diagnostic test for acute medial instability is the gravity stress test as described by Woods and Tullos[5] (Fig. 21–9). With the patient supine, the shoulder is externally rotated and the elbow is flexed 15 to 20 degrees in order to bring the olecranon process out of its fossa. If the elbow is unstable, the weight of the forearm and hand exerts enough valgus force to open the medial side. In large athletes one to two pounds of weight can be attached to the wrist. Excessive force is not necessary and may cause additional ligament damage.

A rather sophisticated test for demonstrating loose bodies is the arthrotomogram. A quantity of radiopaque dye in conjunction with air is used to obtain a double-contrast study. Tomograms are then obtained, and the presence of intra-articular loose bodies is better delineated.

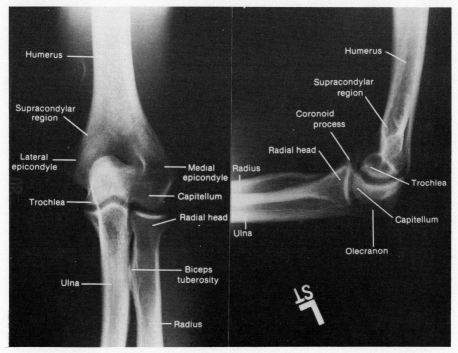

FIGURE 21–8. Key features of anteroposterior and lateral elbow radiographs.

ARTHROSCOPY

The role of arthroscopy in evaluating elbow disorders[6-7] remains somewhat controversial, since elbow congruency makes placement of instruments difficult. While the arthroscope may focus attention on intra-articular problems, it must be remembered that most intra-articular problems of the elbow are caused by extrinsic factors such as valgus instability.

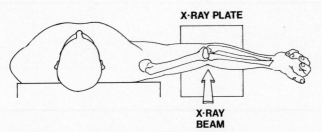

FIGURE 21–9. The gravity stress test to detect medial instability. (After Woods, W. G., and Tullos, H. S.[5])

REFERENCES

1. Tullos, H. S., and King, J. W.: Throwing mechanism in sports. Orthop Clin North Am 4:709, 1973.
2. Nirschle, R. P.: The etiology and treatment of tennis elbow. J Sports Med 2:308, 1974.
3. Wilson, F. D., Andrews, J. R., Blackburn, T. A., and McCluskey, G.: Valgus extension overload in the pitching elbow. Am J Sports Med 11:83, 1983.
4. King, J. W., Brelsford, H. J., and Tullos, H. S.: Epicondylitis and osteochondritis of the professional baseball pitcher's elbow. In Proceedings of the American Academy of Orthopedic Surgeons, Symposium on Sports Medicine. St. Louis, C V Mosby Company, 1969.
5. Woods, W. G., Tullos, H. S., and King, J. W.: The throwing arm: Elbow joint injuries. J Sports Med 1:43, 1973.
6. Andrews, J. R., Farrell, J., and Carson, W. G.: Arthroscopy of the elbow. American Academy of Orthopedic Surgeons Instructional Videotape No. VT-119, 1983.
7. Johnson, L. L.: Arthroscopy of the elbow. In Diagnostic and Surgical Arthroscopy. St. Louis, C V Mosby Company, 1981, pp. 390–399.

RADIOGRAPHIC EVALUATION OF THE THROWING ELBOW

KENNETH M. SINGER, M.D.

INTRODUCTION

Accurate radiographic evaluation of the symptomatic elbow in throwing athletes requires a combination of high-quality radiographs and knowledgable interpretation. Multiple views and tomography are often necessary. The films must then be interpreted by the clinician who has the first-hand knowledge of the patient's clinical history and physical findings and who also is experienced and knowledgable about the spectrum of injuries that can occur as a result of the throwing mechanism. Clinical correlation is essential, since radiographic findings are frequently the major determinant of the treatment method.

MEDIAL LESIONS

Radiographically detectable lesions as a result of tension overload on the medial side of the elbow may be quite subtle. Perhaps the most common finding in patients with chronic medial pain is ulnar hypertrophy or medial traction spurring (Fig. 22–1). In the skeletally immature elbow enlargement, fragmentation, and beaking of the medial epicondyle have been well described (Fig 22–2).[1,2] Because of the variation in normal anatomy, it is often necessary to have comparison views of the nonthrowing elbow to

211

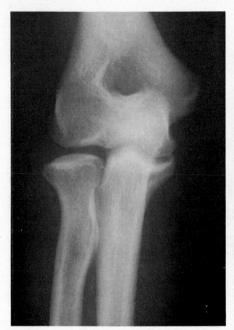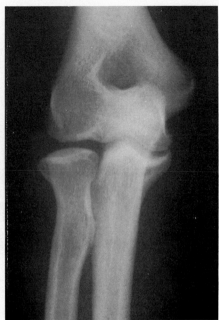

FIGURE 22–1. Traction spurring of the medial aspect of the ulna.

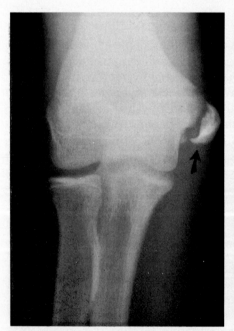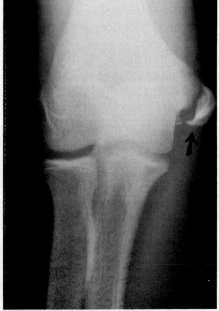

FIGURE 22–2. Chronic medial epicondylar changes in the throwing arm of a 12-year-old with four years of pitching experience.

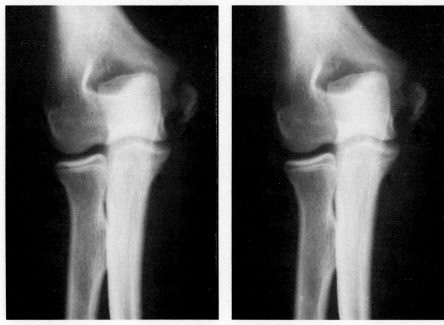

FIGURE 22–3. Acute medial epicondyle epiphyseal fracture in an 11-year-old.

determine asymmetry. While the medial lesions can be associated with symptoms, they are manifestations of extra-articular irritation, do not have long-term implications, and usually need be treated only symptomatically.[3]

Occasionally severe pain results from a single traumatic throwing act, and radiographic evaluation differentiates between medial ligamentous disruption and acute avulsion of the medial epicondyle (Fig. 22–3).

Chronic medial pain in the mature throwing elbow is more frequently the result of repetitive microtrauma to the ligamentous supporting structures. The ligament may become lax or tear as a result of previous injury and scarring, and stress radiographs sometimes can aid in diagnosis. If ulnar nerve symptoms are present, a loose body should be sought in the area of the ulnar groove (Fig. 22–4), and sometimes an ulnar groove view can be helpful.

LATERAL LESIONS

The compressive and rotatory forces occurring across the joint between the radial head and the capitellum during the acceleration phase are potentially quite stressful to the lateral side of the elbow. These strong forces occur on a repetitive basis during the throwing act and primarily affect the articular cartilage and underlying subchondral bone. This can

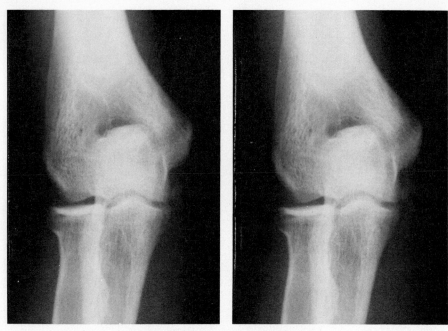

FIGURE 22–4. A loose body in the ulnar groove.

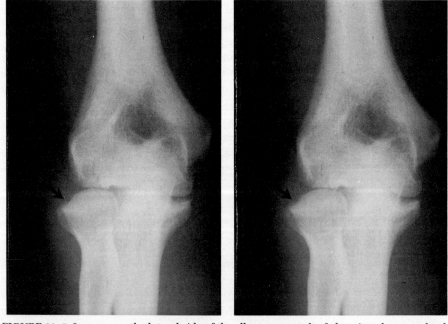

FIGURE 22–5. Lucency on the lateral side of the elbow as a result of chronic valgus overload.

produce osteochondrosis or osteochondritis dissecans of the capitellum or radial head (Fig. 22–5), which sometimes results in loose bodies (Fig. 22–6) and occasionally progresses to severe degenerative arthritis (Fig. 22–7). Lateral lesions, unlike those occurring on the medial side, can result in permanent damage to the elbow and often shorten or terminate the career of the throwing athlete.[4, 5]

In the early stages radiographs may just show a lucency in the capitellum, which is often best seen in the oblique view (Fig. 22–8) and in questionable instances can be seen more clearly with tomograms (Fig. 22–9). As the lesion progresses—sometimes without symptoms—a loose body can form and reside either in the lateral compartment or anteriorly (Fig. 22–10).

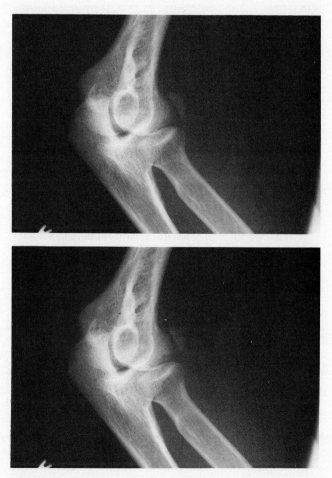

FIGURE 22–6. A loose body in the anterior aspect of the elbow.

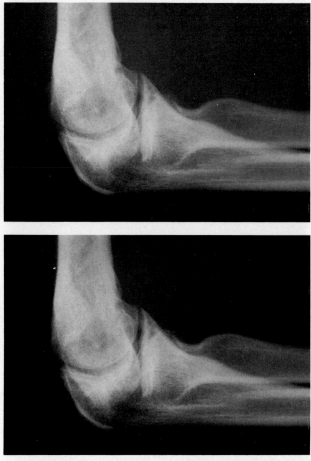

FIGURE 22–7. Degenerative arthritis of the elbow.

POSTERIOR LESIONS

Radiographic abnormalities involving extension overload usually occur as a result of chronic impingement of the olecranon tip into the olecranon fossa (Fig. 22–11). Hypertrophy of the ulna is a normal finding in the throwing athlete as a result of the strong triceps action, but occasionally a stress fracture of the olecranon develops (Fig. 22–12). Frequent impingement of the olecranon results in osteophytic enlargement and occasionally in loose bodies in the posterior fossa (Fig. 22–13).

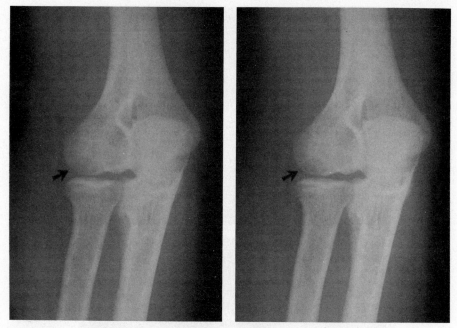

FIGURE 22–8. Oblique view of the elbow to better demonstrate the lateral compartment.

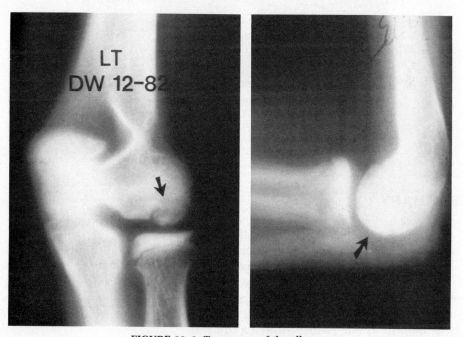

FIGURE 22–9. Tomogram of the elbow.

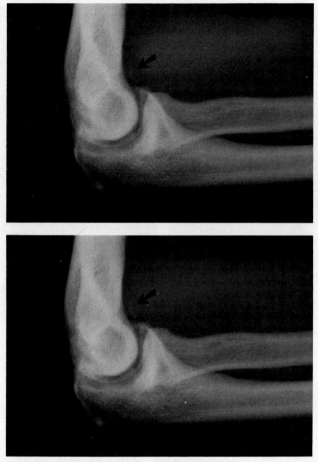

FIGURE 22–10. A loose body in the anterior compartment.

SUMMARY

Radiographic abnormalities of the throwing elbow occur in relatively predictable patterns. Standard anteroposterior, lateral, and oblique views show most abnormalities. Supplementary views such as the radial head profile, ulnar groove views, and occasionally tomography can be useful and should be considered when warranted by the clinical situation. Neither arthrography nor computed tomography of the elbow have yet been shown to be helpful in diagnosing throwing injuries.

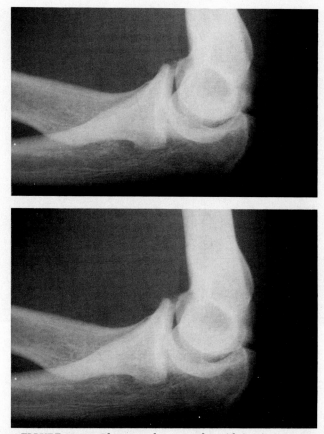

FIGURE 22–11. Olecranon hypertrophy with impingement.

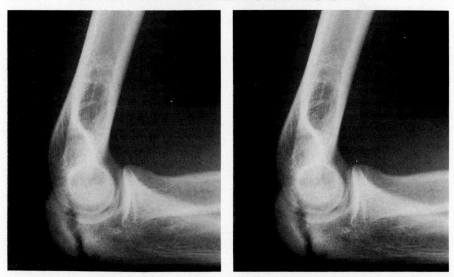

FIGURE 22–12. A rare stress fracture of the olecranon.

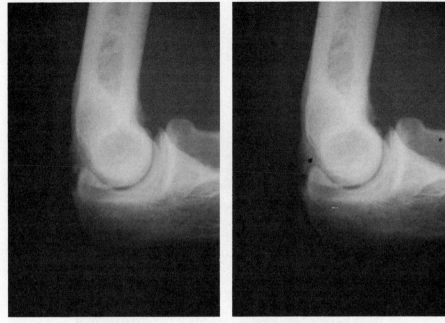

FIGURE 22–13. A loose body in the posterior compartment.

REFERENCES

1. Adams, J. E.: Bone injuries in very young athletes. Clin Orthop 58:129, 1968.
2. Brogden, B. S., and Crow, M. D.: Little Leaguer's elbow. Am J Roentgenol 83:671, 1960.
3. Micheli, L. J.: Overuse injuries in children's sports: The growth factor. Orthop Clin North Am 14:337, 1983.
4. Pappas, A. M.: Elbow problems associated with baseball during childhood and adolescence. Clin Orthop 164:30, 1982.
5. Tullos, H. S., and King, J. W.: Lesions of the pitching arm. JAMA 220:264, 1972.

ARTHROSCOPY OF THE ELBOW

WILLIAM G. CARSON, JR., M.D. / JAMES R. ANDREWS, M.D.

INTRODUCTION

The elbow joint is a common source of pain in the throwing athlete. Although most of the elbow problems encountered in a throwing athlete are related to overuse syndromes and tendinitis, occasionally a throwing athlete sustains more significant injuries, such as osteochondritis dissecans of the capitellum or loose bodies. Although utilized most commonly to diagnose and treat certain disorders of the knee, arthroscopy has also been applied to certain pathologic processes of the elbow.[1] Because the ultimate goal in treating injuries of athletes is to return the athlete to his sport as rapidly as possible and with as little surgical intervention and rehabilitation as necessary, arthroscopy is well suited for these needs.

This chapter presents a discussion of the indications for arthroscopy of the elbow as well as the technique and anatomy of the elbow seen arthroscopically.

INDICATIONS

Arthroscopy of the elbow is a relatively new advancement, and indications for its use are still being developed. At this time the authors consider that elbow arthroscopy is indicated in the following situations:

1. Extraction of loose bodies

2. Debridement of osteochondritis dissecans of the radial head and capitellum

3. Partial synovectomy in rheumatoid disease

4. Partial synovectomy and debridement of other degenerative processes about the elbow

5. To aid in the diagnosis of the chronically painful elbow when other pathologic processes have been excluded.

These indications most readily apply to chronic disorders of the elbow. Arthroscopic examination of the acute elbow injury is less clearly indicated. Theoretically, however, arthroscopy of the elbow might be utilized to evaluate fractures of the radial head, olecranon, or capitellum.

SURGICAL TECHNIQUE

Although local anesthesia has been described for elbow arthroscopy,[2] the authors think that general anesthesia is preferable for complete relaxation and comfort of the patient. With the patient supine on a standard operating table the forearm and wrist are placed in a wrist gauntlet connected to an overhead pulley that is suspended from the end of the operating table. The entire arm is allowed to extend over the side of the table, and the elbow is positioned at 90 degrees of flexion (Fig. 23–1). This position provides excellent access to both the medial and lateral aspects of the elbow, and the forearm may be freely pronated and supinated.

Another advantage of this positioning is the relaxation of the neurovascular structures in the antecubital fossa as the elbow is flexed to 90 degrees. A tourniquet is routinely used for the control of bleeding, and the entire arm, including the hand, is draped in a sterile fashion after a routine skin preparation has been performed.

Bony landmarks are outlined on the skin with a sterile marking pen prior to the initiation of the procedure. The lateral structures to be outlined are the radial head and the lateral epicondyle and the medial structure to be identified is the medial epicondyle.

The three most commonly used arthroscopic portals for examination of the elbow are the anterolateral, anteromedial, and posterolateral portals.

Anterolateral Portal. The anterolateral portal is the most commonly used portal for examination of the elbow and is frequently used as the initial entrance into the joint. When inserting arthroscopic instruments into a smaller joint such as the ankle or elbow maximal joint distension must be achieved as the instruments pass into the joint space. The distension is provided by injecting saline solution through an 18-gauge needle at the initiation of the procedure. Following the establishment of this first arthroscopic portal, fluid injection directly through the arthroscope cannula provides continued distension.

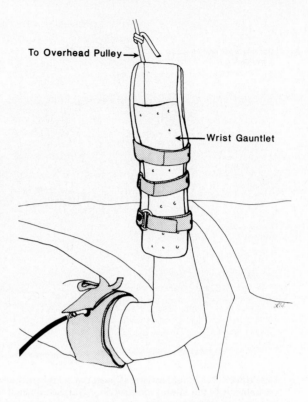

FIGURE 23–1. The arm positioned for arthroscopy of the elbow.

To Overhead Pulley→

Wrist Gauntlet

The most common location for insertion of a needle into the elbow joint and for injection of saline solution is the lateral aspect directly between the lateral epicondyle, the radial head, and the olecranon tip. This triangular area is often utilized for aspiration of the elbow, and in this area the instruments traverse only skin, a thin subcutaneous layer, the anconeus muscle, and then the capsule. Once the elbow joint is maximally distended the actual anterolateral arthroscopic portal, located somewhat anterior and distal to this location, can be established. With the elbow flexed 90 degrees an 18-gauge needle is placed approximately 2 cm distal and 1 cm anterior to the lateral epicondyle, just anterior to the radial head (Fig. 23–2). Pronation and supination of the forearm facilitate palpation of the radial head. This approach is somewhat more distal and anterior to the usual approaches used for aspiration of the elbow described earlier. The needle is aimed directly toward the center of the joint. Further distension of the joint is performed through the needle cannula with the use of intravenous connecting tubing and a 50-cc syringe.

Entrance into the elbow joint is confirmed by observing free backflow. Once this is verified and the elbow joint is maximally distended, the larger instruments such as the arthroscope and cannulas can be inserted. As previously mentioned, the 90-degree position of the elbow as well as the

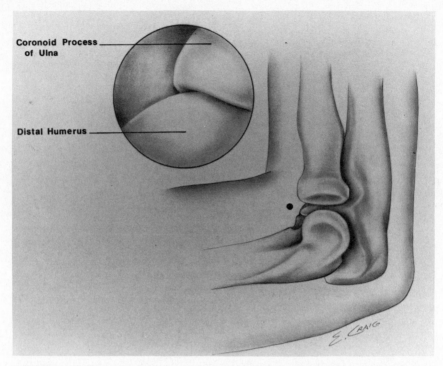

FIGURE 23–2. The anterolateral portal is established approximately 2 cm distal and 1 cm anterior to the lateral epicondyle. Arthroscopic anatomy as seen through this portal includes the distal humerus and the coronoid process of the ulna.

maximal distension displace the antecubital neurovascular structures anteriorly and provide more space above the bony epicondyles for the appropriate instruments. Athough smaller arthroscopes, such as the 2.7-mm needle scope, have been successfully utilized for arthroscopy of the elbow,[2] the authors have found that the larger 4-mm 30-degree angled arthroscopes offer superior visualization and can safely be inserted through the anteromedial, anterolateral, and posterolateral portals by the technique described here.[1] It has been found extremely helpful to connect a hand-held camera to the arthroscope for ease of visualization and documentation.

Anteromedial Portal. With the arthroscope in place through the anterolateral portal, instruments may now be placed through the anteromedial portal under direct visualization provided by the arthroscope already in place. This portal is located approximately 1 cm anterior and 2 cm distal to the medial epicondyle (Fig. 23–3). An 18-gauge needle is directed toward the center of the elbow joint, once again with the elbow flexed 90 degrees. Confirmation of the needle's entrance into the joint is provided by the arthroscope under direct visualization. Once this has been established a small skin incision is made and with careful observation of the angle of the previously placed needle larger instruments may be safely inserted through the medial portal.

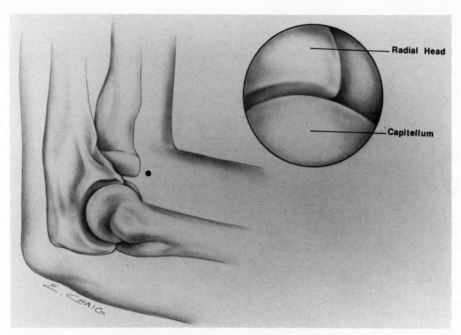

FIGURE 23–3. The anteromedial portal is illustrated. Instruments enter the skin approximately 2 cm distal and 1 cm anterior to the medial epicondyle. The arthroscopic view includes the capitellum and the radial head.

With many of the newer arthroscopic systems with interchangeable inflow and arthroscopic cannulas it is possible to freely change from the medial to the lateral portal. The majority of arthroscopic surgical procedures are performed for pathologic processes located in the lateral aspect of the elbow, such as loose body removals, osteochondritis dissecans of the capitellum, or chondromalacia of the radial head. Since the anteromedial portal provides superior visualization of these lateral structures, it is necessary to be familiar with the insertion of both anterolateral and anteromedial portals.

Posterolateral Portal. The third portal that may occasionally be required for arthroscopy of the elbow is the posterolateral portal. This portal is located approximately 2 cm proximal to the olecranon tip just posterior and superior to the lateral epicondyle over the lateral margins of the triceps muscle (Fig. 23–4). This portal is most easily established by extending the elbow to relax the triceps muscle and by inserting the instrument while aiming directly for the olecranon fossa.

The operative arthroscopic instruments commonly used for surgery of the knee may also be used in the elbow joint. These instruments include such devices as motorized suction instruments, knives, punches, and graspers. If surgery is to be performed on processes involving the lateral side of the elbow the arthroscope is usually placed through the anteromedial portal and the instrument through the anterolateral portal. Surgical proce-

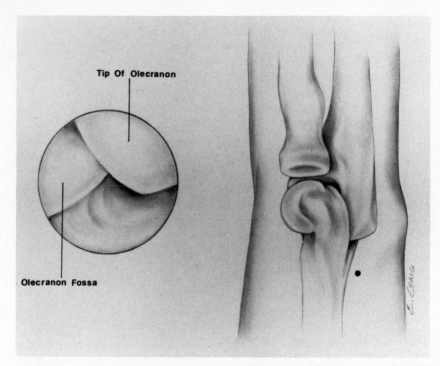

FIGURE 23–4. The posterolateral portal is established with the arm extended to visualize the tip of the olecranon and the olecranon fossa. Instruments enter the skin through the posterolateral portal approximately 2 cm proximal to the olecranon tip, just posterior and superior to the lateral epicondyle.

dures on the medial side of the elbow require that the arthroscope be placed anterolaterally and the instruments anteromedially.

Upon completion of the arthroscopic procedure a soft dressing is applied to the elbow. Immobilization is usually not required. Early range of motion of the elbow may be performed in most cases.

ARTHROSCOPIC ANATOMY OF THE ELBOW

The arthroscopic anatomy of the elbow is described as visualized through the various arthroscopic portals.

Anterolateral Portal. The structures visualized through the anterolateral portal include the distal humerus and trochlear ridges and the coronoid process of the ulna (Fig. 23–2). Extension of the elbow provides a better view of the medial and lateral trochlear ridges and the trochlear notch of the distal humerus, and flexion facilitates visualization of the coronoid process and the ulna. The radial head may occasionally be viewed from this anterolateral portal by retracting the arthroscopy posteriorly and directing the 30-degree angle lens toward the radial head.

Anteromedial Portal. The radial head and capitellum are best visualized from the anteromedial portal (Fig. 23–3). Pronation and supination of the forearm facilitate visualization of the radial head. The annular ligament occasionally can be visualized as it courses over the radial neck. If the arthroscope is retracted and directed toward the ulna the coronoid process can be visualized through the anteromedial portal.

Posterolateral Portal. Two major areas that can be visualized from the posterolateral portion are the olecranon fossa, located over the posterior aspect of the distal humerus, and the tip of the olecranon (Fig. 23–4). Flexion and extension of the elbow facilitate visualization of the distal humerus.

DISCUSSION

Arthroscopy of the elbow can be quite useful in evaluating chronic elbow complaints in the throwing athlete. In addition to establishing a definitive diagnosis, arthroscopy of the elbow can also be used to treat certain pathologic processes such as loose bodies, osteochrondritis dissecans of the capitellum, or chondromalacia of the radial head. In a preliminary study of over 40 patients who underwent arthroscopy of the elbow excellent or good results were obtained in the removal of loose bodies, partial synovectomy, and chondroplasty of the capitellum and radial head. Several of these throwing athletes were found to have advanced cartilaginous damage of the capitellum and radial head at the time of arthroscopic examination. If arthroscopic examination had been performed earlier in this patient population and a definitive diagnosis of cartilaginous damage had been established, the patients could possibly have been saved from further articular cartilage damage by discontinuing their individual sport or activity. The authors therefore consider the diagnostic portion of elbow arthroscopy to be very important in the overall treatment of certain pathologic processes about the elbow.

In order for arthroscopy of the elbow to be effective, a systematic and reproducible arthroscopic examination and technique need to be utilized. The authors believe that the technique and identification of anatomic structures described here provide a safe and reliable means of performing arthroscopy of the elbow. Attention to detail, especially to establish the various portals, is essential to perform a safe arthroscopic examination and to avoid damage to nearby neurovascular structures. The rehabilitation period following arthroscopy of the elbow is relatively short and the throwing athlete can return to his sport in a minimal amount of time.

REFERENCES

1. Andrews, J. R., Farrell, J., and Carson, W. G.: Arthroscopy of the elbow. American Academy of Orthopaedic Surgeons Videotape No. VT-119, 1983.
2. Johnson, L. L.: Arthroscopy of the elbow. In Diagnostic and Surgical Arthroscopy. St. Louis, C V Mosby Company, 1981, pp. 390–339.

LITTLE LEAGUER'S ELBOW*

STEPHEN C. HUNTER, M.D.

INTRODUCTION

The term *Little Leaguer's elbow* was initially coined by Brogden[1] in 1960 to refer to an avulsion of the ossification center of the medial epicondyle caused by the pitching act in the adolescent athlete. Since the initial description, at least a dozen pathologic conditions have been included under this general classification. These pathological entities are classified according to their anatomic location (Table 24–1).[2–9]

ETIOLOGY

The stress placed on the elbow by the pitching motion has been implicated as the cause of the multiple pathologic conditions of Little Leaguer's elbow.[6, 9] The phases of the pitching mechanism—wind-up, cocking, acceleration, release and deceleration, and follow-through—can be correlated with specific injuries.[9]

During the cocking phase, considerable distractive force is placed on the medial side of the elbow. This results in tension on tissues attached to the medial epicondyle including the flexor muscles. Consequently, the

*This work was supported in part by the Hughston Sports Medicine Foundation, Inc., 6262 Hamilton Road, Columbus, Georgia 31995.

TABLE 24–1. CLASSIFICATION OF PATHOLOGY IN LITTLE LEAGUER'S ELBOW ACCORDING TO ANATOMIC LOCATION

Medial	Avulsion of the medial ossification center
	Strain of the flexor muscles
	Traction spurs of the ulnar coronoid process
	Ulnar neuropathy
Lateral	Lateral epicondylitis
	Osteochondral fractures of the capitellum
	Deformities of the radial head
	Loose bodies
Posterior	Avulsion fractures of the olecranon
	Olecranon spurs
	Triceps strain
Anterior	Strains or spurs
	Joint degenerative changes

medial elbow ligaments can be overstretched, and traction spurs can develop on the ulnar coronoid process. The ulnar nerve can also be stretched (Fig. 24–1). Compression of the lateral compartment[8, 9] forces the radial head against the capitellum and can result in a fracture of the capitellum or deformation of the radial head. Loose bodies can break off in the joint as a result of these bone injuries.

During the acceleration phase, the tension and compression forces in

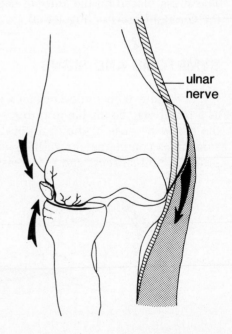

ulnar nerve

FIGURE 24–1. Forces causing injury that usually occur during the cocking phase of throwing: compression of the radiocapitellar joint laterally and tension on the flexor muscles and ulnar nerve medially.

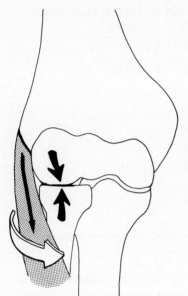

FIGURE 24–2. Forces causing injury that usually occur during the acceleration phase of throwing.

the elbow are low. However, the extreme pronation of the forearm places the lateral ligaments under tension. As a result lateral epicondylitis can occur (Fig. 24–2).

During follow-through the hyperextension of the elbow can cause injury to the olecranon process. Spurs can form as a result in the olecranon fossa. The stress placed on the anterior capsule can result in traction spurs from the coronoid process (Fig. 24–3).

SYMPTOMS AND SIGNS

A patient with Little Leaguer's elbow usually complains of pain[5] and as a result may be unable to throw.[3, 8, 10] The pain can be nonspecific about the elbow because of the multifocal nature of the pathology. The patient sometimes complains of swelling, and prolonged or extensive activity can produce joint stiffness and a decrease in range of motion.[8]

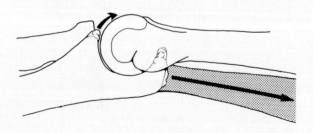

FIGURE 24–3. Forces acting on the elbow that occur during the follow-through phase of throwing.

On examination the olecranon process, the medial and lateral epicondyles,[9] or the radial head[7] can be tender. There can be a decrease in range of motion caused by soft tissue fibrosis and loss of the normal contour in the elbow.[3, 5, 9, 10] Clinical and radiographic evaluation can reveal an increase in valgus angulation of the elbow that is caused by the collapse of the lateral compartment and the bony overgrowth of the medial compartment.[9, 11]

Radiographic changes frequently are seen in elbows that have significant chemical findings (see Chapter 22). Medially there may be fragmentation or accelerated growth and separation of the epicondylar epiphysis.[12] An acute fracture of the medial epicondyle or the olecranon may also be evident. Laterally, osteochondritis of the capitellum and the radial head can occur accompanied by loose bodies.[8] Adolescent baseball pitchers who are asymptomatic can also have radiographic findings of bone hypertrophy, enlargement of the medial epicondyle and the secondary ossification centers, or a lateral compression sign.[5, 10]

EPIDEMIOLOGY

Concern about the risk of significant injury has prompted several studies of the prevalence and severity of injury to the elbow in adolescent pitchers.[5, 7, 10] Approximately 20 per cent of the athletes studied had complaints of elbow pain, but most had lost no time from pitching. Over the last ten years, the incidence of significant pathology, such as degenerative change in the lateral compartment, has been only 1 in 10,000. Thus, the incidence of debilitating injury to the adolescent pitcher's elbow is small. Some of these young athletes may develop problems later, however, if they continue to pitch.[3]

TREATMENT

Most cases of elbow pain caused by excessive pitching can be treated successfully by rest.[11] Avulsion fractures of the medial epicondyle are best treated by splinting and rest, but a complete separation of the bony metaphysis may require surgical repair if treatment by rest fails. Compression of the ulnar nerve should be treated by operative decompression if symptoms are severe and treatment by rest has failed.[2, 4]

Degenerative changes in the lateral compartment are associated with a poor prognosis. Although the osteophytes and loose bodies can be removed surgically,[8] ankylosis may remain, and the young athlete may be unable to throw. Children with this problem should discontinue throwing sports.

Prevention, of course, is the best treatment. The Little League has rules that limit the amount a child may pitch during a game (see the Appendix at the end of this chapter). Recommendations have been made to further limit the amount of throwing allowed and to prohibit curve ball pitching.[12]

Unfortunately, however, there are no limitations on pitching at home or during practice. The education of parents and coaches on the signs and symptoms of elbow problems improves the chances of early diagnosis and treatment. An informed coach who is alerted to the early signs and symptoms of problems in the adolescent pitcher's elbow can use good judgment and conservative measures to prevent lifelong deformity and impairment of function.

REFERENCES

1. Brogden B. S., and Crow, M. D.: Little Leaguer's elbow. Am J Roentgenol 83:671, 1960.
2. Godshall, R. W., and Hansen, C. A.: Traumatic ulnar neuropathy in adolescent baseball pitchers. J Bone Joint Surg 53A:359, 1971.
3. Grana, W. A., and Rahskin, A.: Pitcher's elbow in adolescents. Am J Sports Med 8:333, 1980.
4. Hang, Y. S.: Tardy ulnar neuritis in a Little League baseball player. Am J Sports Med 9:244, 1981.
5. Larson, R. L., Singer, K. M., Bergstrom, R., and Thomas, S.: Little League survey—the Eugene study. Am J Sports Med 4:201, 1976.
6. Limpscomb, A. B.: Baseball pitching injuries in growing athletes. J Sports Med 3:25, 1975.
7. Micheli, L. J., and Smith, A. D.: Sports injuries in children. Curr Probl Pediatr 12, 1982.
8. Pappask A. M.: Elbow problems associated with baseball during childhood and adolescence. Clin Orthop 164:30, 1982.
9. Tullos, H. S., and King, J. W.: Lesions of pitching arm. JAMA 220:264, 1972.
10. Gugenheim, J. J., Stanley, R. F., Woods, G. W., and Tullos, H. S.: Little League survey: The Houston Study. Am J Sports Med 4:189, 1976.
11. Micheli, L. J.: Overuse injuries in children's sports: The growth factor. Orthop Clin North Am 14:337, 1983.
12. Adams, J. E.: Bone injuries in very young athletes. Clin Orthop 58:129, 1968.

Little League Pitching Rules*

1. Any player on a team roster may pitch.

2. If a player pitches in less than four (4) innings, one calendar day of rest is mandatory. If a player pitches in four (4) or more innings, three (3) calendar days of rest must be observed. A player may pitch in a maximum of six (6) innings in a calendar week, Sunday through Saturday. Delivery of a single pitch constitutes having pitched in an inning.

Example

If a player pitched in four or more innings on	and is still eligible, that player can pitch again on the following
Sunday	Thursday
Monday	Friday
Tuesday	Saturday
Wednesday	Sunday
Thursday	Monday
Friday	Tuesday
Saturday	Wednesday

3. Only two players of League age 12 may be used as pitchers during a calendar week. Either or both may pitch in one or more games, but each is limited to a total of six (6) innings within the calendar week and subject to rest periods described in section 2.

4. Once removed as a pitcher a player may not pitch again in the same game.

5. Not more than five (5) pitchers per team shall be used in one game.
Exception: In the case of the injury to a fifth pitcher an additional pitcher may be used.

6. Violation of any section of this Regulation can result in protest of the game in which it occurs. Protest shall be made in accordance with Playing Rule 4.19.

Notes

A. The withdrawal of an ineligible pitcher after that pitcher is an-

---

*Adapted from *Little League Baseball, Official Regulations and Playing Rules*, Section VI, "Pitchers," 1984, pp. 12–13.

nounced, but before a ball is pitched, shall not be considered a violation. Litle League officials are urged to take precautions to prevent protests. When a protest situation is imminent, the potential offender should be notified immediately.

B. Innings pitched in games declared "no contest" or "regulation drawn games" shall be charged against the pitcher's eligibility for that week. If pitching is resumed in the following week or weeks the pitcher of record may continue up to six (6) innings or to the extent of remaining eligibility for the calendar week.

Minor League. A player who has attained League age of 12 is not eligible to pitch.

SURGICAL MANAGEMENT OF ACUTE AND CHRONIC ELBOW PROBLEMS

MICHAEL E. BERKELEY, M.D. / JAMES B. BENNETT, M.D. /
G. WILLIAM WOODS, M.D.

INTRODUCTION

The physician who is concerned with the elbow of the throwing athlete faces a spectrum of problems ranging from acute valgus injuries in the adolescent to the advanced degenerative changes in the arm of the professional. In evaluating these injuries, more than the usual amount of caution must be exercised when surgery is recommended as an appropriate treatment. Many acute elbow injuries respond to surgery, but unfortunately much of the pathology seen in throwing athletes is degenerative in nature. Our surgical procedures are often not adequate to alter the effects of repetitive stress on a joint that clearly is not designated to sustain these types of forces. Consequently surgery is palliative at best in these cases, and a realistic assessment of an athlete's future may dictate that he decrease his level of play rather than undergo an operative procedure and a long rehabilitation period with little or no improvement.

MEDIAL EPICONDYLE FRACTURES

The medial epicondyle may be avulsed by either its ligamentous or its muscular attachments as a result of valgus stress, massive muscular contraction, or posterior dislocation of the elbow. Traditionally, satisfactory results have been obtained by nonoperative treatment, and surgery has been reserved for those cases in which the epicondylar fragment is excessively displaced or trapped within the joint.[1] Some authors have stated that open reduction in displaced fractures reduces the incidence of joint stiffness.[2] Woods and Tullos reported that satisfactory results occurred after conservative treatment even with displaced fractures. However, they stated that fibrous or bony union of the medial epicondyle in a nonanatomic position can produce valgus instability and an inability to throw effectively.[3]

The treatment of medial epicondyle fractures should be based on an accurate assessment of elbow instability if the patient is to participate in throwing sports. Determination of instability by clinical examination is difficult because the humerus tends to externally rotate when valgus stress is applied to the elbow. Plain radiographs can be unreliable, since they do not indicate the amount of fragment displacement that has occurred at the time of injury. Also the epicondylar fragment may appear to be in a satisfactory position but can be rotated as much as 90 degrees with functional lengthening of the medial collateral ligament (Fig. 25–1). Assessment of valgus instability is best made using the gravity stress test. With the patient in a supine position the shoulder is externally rotated and the elbow is flexed 15 to 20 degrees in order to bring the olecranon clear of the fossa. If the elbow is unstable the weight of the forearm opens the medial side (Fig. 25–2). Regional block or general anesthesia may be necessary in the apprehensive patient.

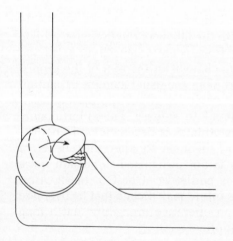

FIGURE 25–1. Forward rotation of the medial epicondyle fragment may lead to impairment of the collateral ligament function.

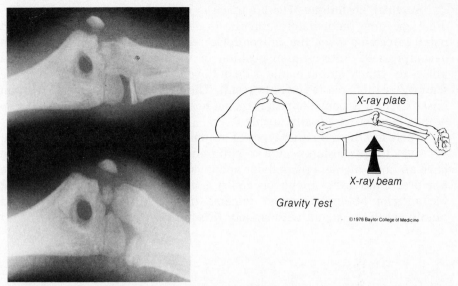

FIGURE 25–2. Gravity stress x–ray. *Above left:* Plain view of the elbow. *Below left:* The gravity stress test demonstrates displacement of the epicondylar fragment. *Right:* Technique for obtaining a gravity stress view. Fifteen to 20 degrees of flexion is necessary to unlock the olecranon from its fossa. Gravity alone is sufficient to demonstrate medial instability.

TREATMENT

Stable Nondisplaced Fractures

Medial epicondylar stress fractures and minor avulsions associated with throwing that are found to be stable on valgus stress should be immobilized at 90-degree flexion for three to four weeks, with subsequent active protected range of motion.

Stable Displaced Fractures

The authors recommend that medial epicondylar fractures displaced more than 1 cm in elbows that are stable to valgus stress be treated with open reduction.

Unstable Medial Epicondyle Fractures

Elbows that are unstable to valgus stress warrant open reduction of the medial epicondylar fragment and, if necessary, repair of the anterior oblique ligament.

Surgical Technique. The approach is made through a curved longitudinal incision immediately anterior to the medial epicondyle to avoid painful scarring over the epicondylar region. The ulnar nerve is then decompressed. Anterior transposition of the nerve is not recommended unless the injury on the medial side of the elbow is extensive and excessive scarring in this area is likely to result. The incision usually heals with an unsatisfactory widened appearance, but fortunately scars on the medial side of the elbow are not easily visible.

There are three distinct types of lesions that require surgical treatment.

TYPE I. This lesion occurs in children under the age of 14 years who have an open medial epicondylar apophysis (Fig. 25–3A). The epicondyle fractures through the apophysis and is avulsed by the forearm flexors, and the anterior oblique ligament remains intact. Anatomic reduction and pinning of the fragment with smooth Kirschner wires are performed.

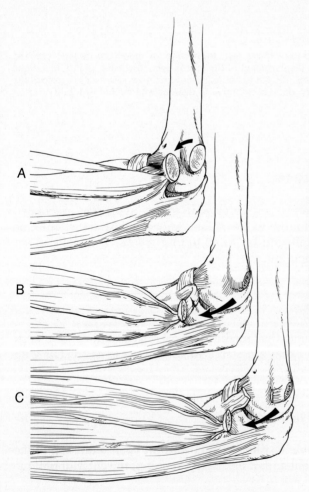

FIGURE 25–3. *(A)* A Type I fracture demonstrates fracture through physis; a large epicondylar fragment with an attached anterior oblique ligament and flexor muscles are displaced distally. *(B)* A Type II fracture demonstrates avulsion of the epicondylar fragment and possible injury to the anterior oblique ligament. *(C)* A Type III fracture demonstrates avulsion of the flexor mass with a small epicondylar fragment and rupture of the anterior oblique ligament.

TYPE II. This lesion occurs in children over the age of 15 in whom the medial epicondylar apophysis already has been closed (Fig. 25–3B). In this type the fragment is large and contains the insertion of the anterior oblique ligament. Occasionally the ligament may be torn within its substance. During open reduction the fragment should be everted and the ligament inspected. If a tear is present it should be repaired with nonabsorbable suture prior to fixation of the epicondyle with Kirschner wires.

TYPE III. The fracture fragment is small and does not contain the origin of the anterior oblique ligament, indicating that the flexor mass has avulsed the fragment while the ligament has torn, usually in its middle area (Fig. 25–3C). The ligament should be repaired with nonabsorbable suture and the flexor muscles reattached to the epicondyle. Small fragments may need to be excised, and the flexor origin may have to be sutured to the bone using drill holes.

With internal fixation, protected motion of the elbow can begin three weeks postoperatively. The pins are removed five or six weeks after surgery. Six months are usually required to regain full extension.

ACUTE MEDIAL INSTABILITY

Acute valgus instability of the adult elbow has been reported following contact injuries such as falls on the outstretched arm or rarely as a result of throwing, specifically javelin throwing.[4-6] This is a serious injury in the throwing athlete because valgus instability is usually incompatible with a high level of performance.

Unfortunately, the diagnosis of acute medial instability is often not made in the acute stage. The athlete may complain only of acute medial pain and have signs of ulnar nerve irritation. Ecchymosis on the medial aspect of the elbow may be delayed for as long as 72 hours. Acute medial ligament damage must be differentiated from forearm flexor muscle rupture. In the former condition valgus stress applied to the elbow with the forearm muscles relaxed produces pain, while in the latter resistive flexion of the wrist is painful. A valgus stress view should be obtained for all patients suspected of having a significant valgus injury. If the elbow is very painful regional or general anesthesia may be necessary.

If acute rupture of the forearm flexor mass is diagnosed, the patient is best treated nonoperatively. Surgical repair is tenuous, and the result is usually unsatisfactory. If medial instability is present exploration of the anterior oblique ligament should be performed.

Norwood et al. reported excellent results following primary repair of acute medial ruptures in recreational athletes who had sustained falls.[4] All patients regained full range of motion and returned to previous levels of performance. However, Barnes and Tullos reported poor results following repair of medial instability in professional and college level baseball pitchers.[7] These athletes had a prolonged rehabilitation and did not return to previous levels of performance. Acute rupture of the medial collateral ligament in high-performance pitchers is probably a nonexistent entity. Rather, there is a sudden failure of a ligament that has been attenuated as a result of chronic microtearing. Surgical repair or reconstruction should be performed in these athletes, but the prognosis must be guarded.

Surgical Technique. The elbow is approached medially through a curved longitudinal incision immediately anterior to the medial epicondyle (Fig. 25–4). Care should be taken to protect the posterior branch of the medial antebrachial nerve, which can cross the distal portion of the incision.

Hemorrhage within the ulnar nerve sheath is a usual finding. The nerve should be decompressed by extending the dissection proximally through the intermuscular septum and distally into the flexor carpi ulnaris muscle. Anterior transposition should be reserved for those instances in which there exists a great amount of medial injury or when a significant amount of dissection has been performed. In these cases the nerve can become compressed by abundant scar tissue formation.

Following decompression of the nerve, the forearm flexor mass is dissected off the medial epicondyle and reflected anteriorly to expose the medial collateral ligament (Fig. 25–5). A middle tear of the anterior oblique band should be repaired with nonabsorbable suture using a modified Bunnell or mattress stitch and reinforced with an antebrachial fascial graft (Fig. 25–6A). If the anterior oblique ligament is disrupted proximally, it should be reinserted by weaving a nonabsorbable suture through the substance of the ligament. The suture is then passed through drill holes in the medial epicondyle and tied with the elbow at 30 degrees from full extension (Fig. 25–6B). Avulsions of the ligament from its insertion on the coronoid process can be repaired using sutures passed through drill holes

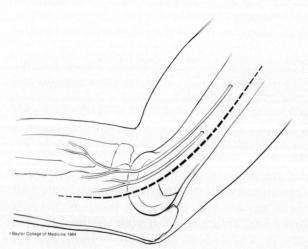

FIGURE 25–4. Skin incision for approach to the medial elbow. The incision is made anteriorly to avoid painful scarring over the epicondyle.

Baylor College of Medicine 1984

FIGURE 25–5. Approach to the medial aspect of the elbow with retraction of the flexor mass anteriorly exposing the medial collateral ligament.

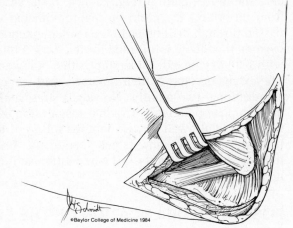

©Baylor College of Medicine 1984

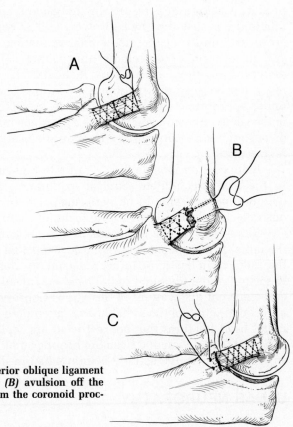

FIGURE 25–6. Repair of the anterior oblique ligament following *(A)* middle area tear, *(B)* avulsion off the epicondyle, and *(C)* avulsion from the coronoid process.

©Baylor College of Medicine 1983

or a staple for fixation (Fig. 25–6C). If the forearm flexor mass is avulsed from its origin, it should be reapproximated using nonabsorbable suture passed through drill holes in the medial epicondyle. Following routine skin closure, the elbow is splinted for ten days. Protected motion in a cast brace with a 30-degree extension stop is then allowed for a period of one month. The extension stop is then removed, and use of the brace is continued for an additional two months. No valgus stress activity is allowed before three months postoperatively. Gradual resumption of controlled noncompetitive throwing is allowed for two months followed by competitive activity on a limited basis at six months postoperatively. Reassessment of the elbow and the decision to return to full competitive activity is made at the end of six months.

POSTERIOR DISLOCATION OF THE ELBOW

The treatment of posterior dislocation of the elbow has traditionally been closed reduction followed by cast immobilization. This method has produced satisfactory results in the general population. However, when this injury is sustained by a throwing athlete special consideration must be given to stability of the elbow after reduction. Following hyperextension and dislocation of the elbow, the medial collateral ligament is always disrupted or attenuated. Frank instability is usually not apparent after reduction because of involuntary guarding. Therefore, a valgus stress test under appropriate anesthesia is usually necessary to evaluate the stability of the elbow. A significant incidence of valgus instablity following reduction of posterior dislocations and fracture dislocations of the elbow has been reported.[5, 8]

It appears reasonable that in order to prevent chronic valgus instability in the throwing athlete surgical exploration and repair of the anterior oblique ligament should be performed if radiographic stress testing demonstrates instability. The surgical technique and postoperative management are the same as for the management of acute valgus instability. Fractures of the radial head as a concomitant injury must be addressed separately, since the radiocapitellar joint forms a secondary defense against valgus stress. Resection of the fractured radial head may result in acute valgus instability and recurrent dislocations of the elbow. Conservation with the preservation or reconstruction of the radial head is attempted in the athlete. Comminuted radial head fractures that are restricted are replaced with a Silastic spacer as a stent to allow medial ligament healing and to give lateral radiocapitellar support. Competitive activity is terminated in these cases.

ULNAR NEUROPATHY

The location of the ulnar nerve medially within the cubital tunnel makes it highly susceptible to the valgus stresses encountered in throwing sports. Ulnar nerve symptoms are caused by compression or fixation of the nerve by adhesions and are aggravated by repetitive throwing. Subluxation of the nerve, although usually asymptomatic, can become painful if the nerve is tethered proximally or distally to the elbow or if the nerve receives a direct blow while it is subluxated on the condyle.

The diagnosis of ulnar neuropathy at the elbow is not always straightforward, since there are often few, if any, objective neurologic changes. Initially the electromyogram usually does not show signs of neurologic change, although it may indicate a delay in conduction across the cubital tunnel. The patient may have subtle changes in two-point discrimination over the ulnar nerve sensory distribution as well as loss of fine intrinsic muscle control. The patient with entrapment of the nerve has tenderness and a positive Tinel's sign behind the medial epicondyle, while a symptomatic subluxating ulnar nerve usually is tender and demonstrates a positive Tinel's sign proximal to the epicondyle, usually where the nerve is tethered by the intermuscular septum.

Ulnar neuropathy at the elbow must be differentiated from entrapment of the nerve at the wrist within Guyon's canal as well as cervical radiculopathy or compression of the nerve by extrinsic masses such as·lipoma or a ganglion arising from the medial elbow. Also, in any throwing athlete who complains of persistent medial elbow pain, consideration should be given to the diagnosis of a chronic compartment syndrome involving the forearm flexor mass. The diagnosis is confirmed by intracompartmental pressure measurements, and the patient is treated with appropriate fasciotomies.

Repositioning of the ulnar nerve deeper in the forearm musculature has been advocated by some surgeons who believe that the nerve is better protected in this position.[9] However, the authors have observed extensive scarring and compression of the ulnar nerve following this procedure. This is particularly true in the throwing athlete in whom the hypertrophied forearm flexor mass may compress the nerve during contraction.

Subcutaneous transposition of the ulnar nerve has been advocated as a means to avoid compression of the nerve by the forearm musculature.[10] However, the nerve is accompanied through the cubital tunnel by a posterior plexus of vessels, and fibrotic changes have been observed in the ulnar nerve, probably as the result of ischemia, following complete stripping of the nerve from this plexus in order to mobilize it anteriorly. The authors advocate anterior transposition of the nerve in cases involving extensive dissection on the medial side of the elbow such as occurs with a reconstruction of the medial collateral ligament. In these cases the extensive scarring that occurs can entrap the nerve if it is left in its anatomic position.

In the treatment of ulnar neuropathy, whether it be secondary to compression or subluxation of the nerve, the primary objective of surgical therapy is to release the nerve from all tethering or compressing structures with a minimal amount of trauma to the nerve itself. The authors utilize decompression and medial epicondylectomy similar to that described by

Neblett and Ehni as the usual procedure of choice to achieve these objectives.[11] It is recommended that an incision be made slightly anterior to the medial epicondyle, with care being taken to avoid the posterior branch of the medial antebrachial nerve, which can pass across the distal portion of the incision (Fig. 25–4). The nerve is then freed from surrounding fascial and soft tissue, but no extensive dissection should be made posterior to the nerve in order to preserve the vascular plexus that accompanies it. The nerve is then decompressed in situ by reflecting the flexor mass off the epicondyle and resecting the epicondyle medial to the insertion of the medial collateral ligament (Fig. 25–7). The flexor mass is then reapproximated to the remaining epicondyle and fascia (Fig. 25–8). This allows unobstructed excursion of the nerve anteriorly as the elbow is taken through a range of motion. Care must be taken not to resect too much of the epicondyle; otherwise instability of the elbow can result.

Simple external neurolysis should be performed when the epineurium is fibrotic. A more extensive neurolysis may lead to excessive intraneural fibrosis. The ulnar nerve should be freed proximally as it passes around the intermuscular septum as well as distally as it passes between the two heads of the flexor carpi ulnaris. The intermuscular septum is resected to prevent recurrence of any tethering proximal to the cubital tunnel (Fig. 25–7). Meticulous hemostasis should be achieved prior to skin closure, and a bulky compressive dressing should be applied. A splint is worn for five days postoperatively, and then active motion is initiated.

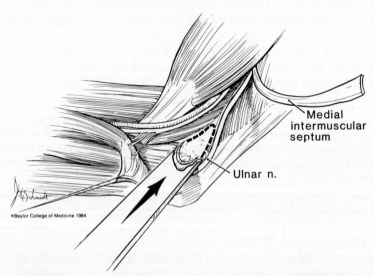

FIGURE 25–7. Ulnar nerve decompression demonstrating proximal resection of the intermuscular septum, elevation of the common flexor-pronator origin, and medial epicondylectomy.

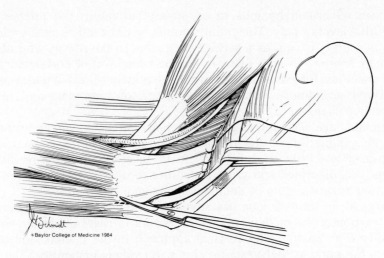

FIGURE 25–8. Resuture of the flexor-pronator origin to the periosteum and soft tissues and release of the flexor carpi ulnaris.

CHRONIC VALGUS INSTABILITY AND LOOSE BODY FORMATION

The arm of a throwing athlete can be expected to develop adaptive changes after years of use. General hypertrophy of the arm is usually seen in professional baseball pitchers. Fibrosis of the flexor-pronator group, enlargement of the trochlea, and increased cubitus valgus cause the loss of terminal extension usually present in these athletes. These changes do not appear to interfere with performance.[12]

The chronic valgus stresses generated during the acceleration phase of pitching as well as the forced extension during the follow-through motion lead to degenerative changes that compromise performance of the arm. Attenuation of the medial collateral ligament leads to valgus instability, which causes overload of other structures within the elbow. The radiocapitellar joint, which normally is not loaded during throwing, is subjected to compressive loading, which may lead to degenerative change and loose body formation. In the adolescent pitcher this mechanism may be the cause of osteochondritis dissecans of the capitellum. Medial collateral ligament attenuation also allows the olecranon to ride medially, impinging on the lateral trochlea and olecranon fossa and causing spur formation and eventual loose body formation at the tip of the olecranon, which also can become a source of loose bodies.

Valgus instability eventually compromises a competitive level of performance in the throwing athlete such as the baseball pitcher. Reconstructive procedures on the medial side of the elbow such as removal of the coronoid traction spur and reconstruction of the medial collateral ligament have been advocated by Jobe in an attempt to return the pitcher to a competitive level of play. The authors do not recommend reconstruction of valgus instability except as a salvage procedure in the player who desires "one more season" or who plans to decrease his level of performance—to pursue coaching, for example. A return to the previous level of performance, if achieved, eventually results in the return of symptoms and further degenerative changes.

Patients have been encountered who have iatrogenic valgus instability following exploration of the medial collateral ligament and removal of calcific masses within its substance. In these cases the anterior oblique ligament was disrupted and gross instability resulted. These patients benefited from reconstruction of the medial collateral ligament.

Surgical Technique. Jobe has advocated a tendon graft procedure for reconstruction of the medial collateral ligament in cases of chronic valgus instability (Fig. 25–9).* The surgical approach to the medial side of the elbow is the same as that described for acute valgus instability. The joint is inspected for loose bodies, and then one-eighth–inch to one-quarter–inch drill holes are placed in the medial epicondyle and in the olecranon-coronoid junction by passing from the anterior to the posterior side. A tendon graft using the palmaris longus, the fascia lata, or the long toe

*Jobe, F. W.: Personal communication.

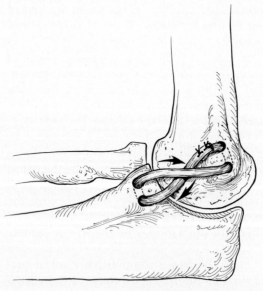

FIGURE 25–9. Reconstruction of the medial collateral ligament as described by Jobe (personal communication).

©Baylor College of Medicine 1983

extensor is then "harvested" and passed through the drill holes in a figure-eight or parallel fashion. The tension of the graft is adjusted with the arm in 30 degrees of flexion, and the tendon is then sutured to itself with nonabsorbable material. With proper tension and position of the graft, the elbow should demonstrate full passive range of motion prior to closure. Anterior transposition of the ulnar nerve is usually indicated. After splinting for ten days, protected motion is allowed in a cast brace with a 30-degree extension stop. After one month the extension stop is removed, and the brace is used for an additional two months.

When valgus instability is present with an intact but attenuated anterior oblique ligament, reconstruction can be performed by transferring the medial epicondyle with the medial collateral ligament proximally. The surgical exposure is the same as for acute valgus instability. The anterior oblique ligament is exposed and dissected from the posterior oblique fibers. An osteotome is then used to transect the base of the medial epicondyle laterally with the origin of the anterior oblique ligament attached. The epicondyle with the attached ligament is then reflected distally, and the joint is debrided as necessary. The epicondyle is then advanced proximally and anteriorly on the humerus and secured with a cortical screw and washer with the elbow in 30 degrees of flexion (Fig. 25–10). The ulnar nerve is then transposed anteriorly, and the wound is closed. Postoperative bracing and rehabilitation are the same as for acute valgus instability.

Removal of loose bodies almost always provides some symptomatic

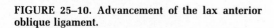
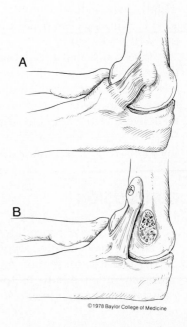

FIGURE 25–10. Advancement of the lax anterior oblique ligament.

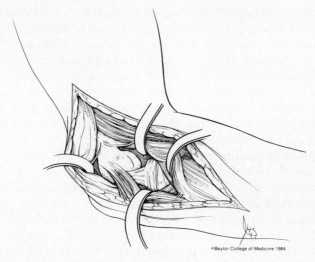

©Baylor College of Medicine 1984

FIGURE 25–11. Posterolateral approach to the elbow for retrieval of loose bodies from the posterior compartment or radiocapitellar joint.

relief to the elbow with valgus instability. However, the procedure is palliative, and symptoms may return with further throwing. The elbow is best approached posterolaterally by entering the point posterior to the anconeus in order to retrieve loose bodies. The incision can be extended distally when debridement of the radiocapitellar joint is indicated (Fig. 25–11). The success of arthroscopic removal of loose bodies depends on the skill of the surgeon.

Jobe states that the patient whose elbow has degenerative changes in the radiocapitellar joint has a poor prognosis for return to play.[13] He advocates inspection of the joint at the time of arthrotomy for loose body removal. However, this requires that the arthrotomy be extended distally to visualize a radiocapitellar joint that may not require debridement. Arthroscopic examination or arthrotomograms may be used to adequately evaluate the joint without the morbidity of additional dissection.

CONCLUSION

Reconstructive procedures on the elbow of the high-performance throwing athlete have limited applications. The involved pathologic processes are degenerative in nature, and surgery cannot be expected to increase the tolerance of an elbow to the repetitive traumatic stresses that it must withstand if the previous level of performance is resumed.

REFERENCES

1. Watson-Jones, R.: Fractures and Dislocations. Vol. II. Williams & Wilkins, 1962, p. 544.
2. Bebe: Can J Surg. 18:137, 1965.
3. Woods, G. W., and Tullos, H. S.: Elbow instability and medial epicondyle fractures. Am J Sports Med 5:23, 1977.
4. Norwood, L. A., Shook, J. A., and Andrews, J. R.: Acute medial elbow ruptures. Am J Sports Med 9:16, 1981.
5. Shepard, D. M., Bennett, J. B., and Tullo, H. S.: Acute Traumatic Elbow Instability in the Adult Patient: Diagnosis and Management. In press.
6. Waris, W.: Elbow injuries in javelin throwers. Acta Chir Scand 93:563, 1946.
7. Barnes, D. A., and Tullos, H. S.: An analysis of 100 symptomatic baseball players. Am J Sports Med 6:62, 1978.
8. Tullos, H. S., Bennett, J. B., and Woods, G. W.: Unpublished data.
9. Levy, D. M., and Apfelberg, D. B.: Results of anterior transposition for ulnar neuropathy at the elbow. Am J Surg 123:304, 1972.
10. Eaton, R. G., Crowe, J. F., and Parkes III, J. C.: Anterior transposition of the ulnar nerve using a non-compressing fasciodermal sling. J Bone Joint Surg 62A:820, 1980.
11. Neblett, C., and Ehni, G.: Medical epicondylectomy for ulnar palsy. J Neurosurg 32:55, 1970.
12. King, J. W., Brelsford, H. J., and Tullos, H. S.: Analysis of the pitching arm of the professional baseball pitcher. Clin Orthop 67:116, 1969.
13. Indelicato, P. A., Jobe, F. W., Kerlan, R. K., Carter, V. S., Shields, C. L., and Lombardo, S.: Correctible elbow lesions in professional baseball players. Am J Sports Med 7:72, 1979.

VALGUS EXTENSION OVERLOAD IN THE PITCHING ELBOW

JAMES R. ANDREWS, M.D. / FRANK WILSON, M.D.

INTRODUCTION

Pain in the pitching arm is a common problem for baseball players at all levels of participation. It is the purpose of this chapter to emphasize the location of osteophyte production on the medial aspect of the olecranon as it abuts against the medial aspect of the olecranon fossa. The significance of this lesion is underrated, since most emphasis in the past has been on the posterior olecranon osteophyte caused mainly by the extension overload syndrome. The true symptomatic lesion is caused by the posteromedial osteophyte as it abuts into the medial margin of the olecranon fossa (Fig. 26–1). This osteophyte can create a painful area of degenerative changes to the articular cartilage on the medial aspect of the olecranon fossa as well.

Although the lesion has been recognized previously, little attention has been directed to surgical treatment. This lesion may be an isolated phenomenon, or it may occur with more severe degenerative problems about the elbow. The authors believe that this isolated lesion occurs more frequently than is commonly recognized and emphasize early recognition and aggressive surgical intervention.

According to Tullos and King,[1] 50 per cent of all professional baseball pitchers experience sufficient elbow or shoulder joint symptoms to keep them from pitching at various times in their careers. George Bennett[2, 3] was the first to direct attention to problems that occur in the pitching elbow.

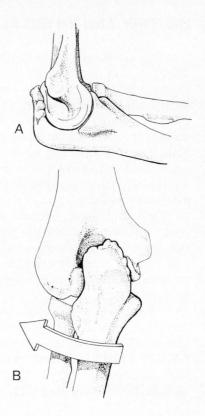

FIGURE 26–1. An illustration of *(A)* a side view of the elbow shows the medial extent of osteophytes around the olecranon. *(B)* The posterior aspect of the olecranon showing the extent of posterior and posteromedial osteophytes as the elbow impinges into the olecranon fossa. The arrow represents the direction of dynamic stress and resultant impingement of the olecranon process in the olecranon fossa.

Since then much has been written about baseball players' elbows, and many problems have been described. Slocum[4] has classified throwers' injuries as medial tension overload and lateral compression injuries. Barnes and Tullos[5] have added subclassifications of these categories according to various bony and muscular lesions.

It is known that a throwing athlete's arm undergoes general bony as well as muscular hypertrophy.[6] King[1] pointed out that 50 per cent of all pitchers have flexion contractures and that approximately 30 per cent of these players have cubitus valgus deformities. He was the first to recognize that the combination of hypertrophy of the olecranon fossa and the humerus, with cubitus valgus deformation, causes impingement on the medial aspect of the olecranon fossa. Indelicato and Jobe[7] recognized this area of pathology and thought that it was caused primarily by stress in the acceleration phase of the pitching mechanism. Some authors feel that players seldom return to competitive pitching when these bony changes occur.[8] However, symptomatic cases of the valgus extension overload syndrome that are recognized and treated surgically have predictable results that allow full return of function to the arm so that the athlete can pitch once again.

HISTORY AND PHYSICAL FINDINGS

The major complaint of pitchers with valgus extension overload syndrome is pain in the elbow. It may be difficult to determine exactly where the pain is in the elbow, and when taking a history from a pitcher it may be difficult to determine when the pain occurs in his pitching motion. Most pitchers complain that they notice a loss of control. After two or three innings the pain gradually increases and the pitches tend to rise and sail high. There is a painful inhibition of movement that gradually causes the pitchers to tire easily and to essentially become ineffective. The pitchers felt that the pain occurred when they were trying to whip the arm to gain maximal speed.

On examination, pitchers with valgus overload syndrome demonstrate pain with forced extension with a combination of valgus stress. Forced extension may not always produce pain without the valgus stretch maneuver. Thus, a combination of valgus stress and extension appears to cause the pain. In addition there may be local pain posteriorly over the olecranon in some cases.

Radiographic evaluation in most cases demonstrates the typical posterior osteophyte at the tip of the olecranon process (Fig. 26–2). However, identification of the posterior medial osteophyte that causes the painful inhibition can be difficult. Axial projections at various degrees of flexion were recorded to try to identify this posterior medial osteophyte. The authors have found that with the elbow flexed 100 degrees and the arm

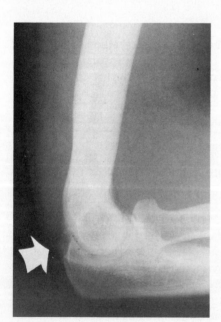

FIGURE 26–2. A routine lateral radiographic film shows the posterior osteophyte on the olecranon tip.

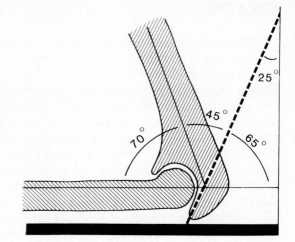

FIGURE 26–3. The technique of axial viewing that best demonstrates articulation of the olecranon with the trochlea and posteromedial osteophyte.

lying on the cassette, the beam should be angled 45 degrees to the ulna, as seen in Figure 26–3. This orientation gives the best view of the olecranon as it articulates with the olecranon fossa and puts the medial aspect of the olecranon in profile, as seen in Figure 26–4. Rarely, no bony osteophyte is seen, but at surgery there is always an exostosis medially that is sometimes purely cartilaginous.

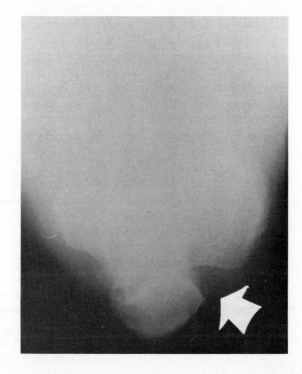

FIGURE 26–4. Radiographic film showing articulation of the olecranon with the trochlea and posteromedial osteophyte on profile.

TREATMENT

The authors' treatment protocol always begins with a physical therapy program and a period of observation. Physical therapy is beneficial to the overall conditioning of the athlete and for eventual postoperative return to athletic activity. The overall goal of physical therapy is to increase the functional strength of the elbow and to attempt to relieve the pain. Elaborate physical therapy protocols have been established but are too lengthy for this presentation. Basically, strengthening and flexibility are emphasized through high repetitions and low weight training. Therapy modalities such as heat, ultrasound, and phonophoresis along with friction massage have been employed. This period of observation, which includes the physical therapy portion, allows careful evaluation of the symptoms and cure of the minor sprains and results of strain. If conservative measures have not been sufficient and the diagnosis made by physical examination and radiography is consistent with the valgus extension overload syndrome, the authors recommend surgical intervention.

SURGICAL TECHNIQUE

The authors' surgical approach begins with a straight skin incision over the lateral epicondylar ridge of the humerus and extending 4 to 5 cm distally. The triceps tendon is identified and sharply elevated off the epicondylar ridge of the humerus. This exposes the posterior compartment of the elbow. The anconeous muscle fibers are elevated off the humerus and retracted out of view, thus allowing visualization of the synovium and posterior compartment. Once the synovium has been opened various degrees of flexion and extension, with varus stress, give good visualization of the entire olecranon process. A one-quarter–inch osteotome is used to make a straight osteotomy of approximately 1 cm of the olecranon process (see Fig. 26–5A). When the osteotomy is being done, the margin of error should be in the direction of overestimation of the cut into the normal olecranon process so as not to risk leaving any of the posterior osteophyte. Instability is not created with this small osteotomy.[9] The posterior osteophyte is thus removed, allowing exposure to the more important lesion on the posterior medial aspect of the olecranon.

A one-eighth–inch or one-quarter–inch curved osteotome can be used to make a curved cut into the posterior medial olecranon (Fig. 26–5B) to remove the posterior medial osteophyte. Unless care is taken in making the second cut, the posterior medial lesion can be missed. The medial wall of the olecranon fossa can be visualized once a second osteotomy has been done, and any other interfering osteophyte can be cut away with a rongeur. Often an area of chondromalacia on this wall can be seen, and enough of the posterior medial olecranon tip must be removed to clear this area and

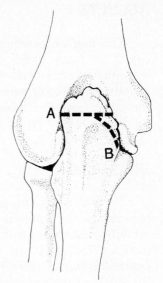

FIGURE 26–5. *(A)* Posterior view of the olecranon with the first cut made straight across. *(B)* The second cut is made with a curved osteotome.

prevent further impingement. Once decompression has been accomplished in this manner, no further treatment is needed in this area. The ulnar nerve lies more posterior and medial to the osteotomy incision and is therefore not encountered in this approach. Adequate irrigation of the wound is recommended to remove any debris or loose bodies. The triceps interval is then closed back to the epicondylar ridge with a heavy synthetic absorbable suture. Nonabsorbable sutures may produce suture irritation in the pitcher's elbow.

After seven to ten days of splinting, active and passive assist programs are instituted by the physical therapist. Pendulum exercises and gentle mobilization techniques are added as pain subsides. During the next four- to six-week interval as the range of motion returns and the pain subsides, a long toss, short toss program (see Chapter 3), similar to that recommended by Frank Jobe, is begun.* This program allows the athlete to begin in center field by throwing the ball in an easy overhand toss and trying to emphasize normal body mechanics and to allow the ball to roll to second base. He gradually increases the speed so that he can "one-hop" the ball to second base, and after a week or two he can throw it the entire distance.

Throwing time is usually limited to about 15 minutes per day during this interval. At the same time strengthening, flexibility, and ice therapy modalities are continued. The athlete then progresses to 30 feet and begins throwing at half speed for 15 minutes a day, then gradually advances to 60 feet at half speed, and finally to full speed over the six- to seven-week interval.

---

*Jobe, W., M.D., 1983: Personal communication.

RESULTS

Five baseball pitchers, three college and two professional, of an average age of 24 years, underwent surgical excision of a painful posteromedial osteophyte.[10] Preoperative symptoms averaged 2.6 years in duration and usually consisted of pain in the elbow between the acceleration and follow-through phases of pitching. With an average follow-up of 1 year, all of the pitchers returned for one full season at maximal pitching effectiveness.

DISCUSSION

Injuries about the pitching elbow occur in numerous ways. This is because of the unusual stresses applied to the elbow joint during the pitching maneuver. It is essential to understand the basic aspects of the pitching movement in order to recognize the different areas of stress concentration about the elbow. Slocum[4] has outlined the essential steps in the pitching mechanism in the basic overload syndromes. However, it is often hard to separate the medial tension, lateral compression, and extension overload syndromes as described by him.

King, Andrews, Tullos, and others[1, 11, 12] have analyzed and divided the throwing mechanism into various phases, which include the wind-up or cocking phase, the acceleration phase, and the follow-through. Andrews et al.[10] have emphasized these phases in trying to correlate the actual mechanics in the elbow joint to the stress syndromes. Bennett[2] was first to recognize that this kind of stress on the elbow could result in "exfoliation of cartilage, which could either form loose bodies or cartilaginous masses on the adjacent surfaces of the olecranon and the internal condyle of the humerus." Indelicato et al.[7] have also recognized this problem and relate it to the valgus overload acceleration phase of the pitching mechanism.

The authors believe that the mechanism of injury in the valgus extension overload syndrome occurs in the early acceleration phase of pitching. In this early phase of acceleration excessive valgus stresses are applied to the elbow and cause a wedging effect of the olecranon in the olecranon fossa, as shown in Figure 26–1. This impingement leads to osteophyte production at the posterior and posteromedial aspects of the olecranon tip and can cause a "kissing lesion" of chondromalacia on the adjacent area of the olecranon fossa.

SUMMARY

The authors believe that a major source of pain in the pitcher's elbow can be osteophyte production as a result of impingement of the olecranon process and the olecranon fossa during the acceleration phase of pitching.

A high index of suspicion and awareness of this entity are necessary when throwers have the typical pain on pitching that increases early in the game. They also frequently complain that they just cannot "let it go." Sometimes they notice a gradual loss of control that causes early release, resulting in pitches thrown too high. Careful analysis of the pitching mechanism should be performed by the coaches, trainers, and physicians. If errors are found, changes should be made early. However, in most cases the pain in the elbow is what causes the disturbance in the pitching movement, and the athlete is merely compensating for this problem. If the athlete cannot perform at his maximal potential because of the valgus extension overload, surgical correction should not be delayed.

In the attempt to relieve pain and correct deformity the words of Hugh Tullos should be remembered: "We do not fix baseball players, we only temporarily improve them. If they continue to pitch, they will continue to have their problems."*

---

*Tullos, H. S., 1983: Personal communication.

REFERENCES

1. King, J. W., Brelsford, H. J., and Tullos, H. S.: Analysis of the pitching arm of the professional baseball pitcher. Clin Orthop 67:116, 1969.
2. Bennett, G. E.: Elbow and shoulder lesions of baseball players. Am J Surg 98:484, 1959.
3. Bennett, G. E.: Shoulder and elbow lesions of the professional baseball pitcher. JAMA 117:510, 1941.
4. Slocum, D. B.: Classification of elbow injuries from baseball players. Am J Sports Med 6:62, 1978.
5. Barnes, D. A., and Tullos, H. S.: An analysis of 100 symptomatic baseball players. Am J Sports Med 6:62, 1978.
6. Jones, H. H., Priest, J. D., Hayes, W. C., Tichenor, C. C., and Nagel, D. A.: Humeral hypertrophy in response to exercise. J Bone Joint Surg 59A:204, 1977.
7. Indelicato, P. A., Jobe, F. W., Kerlan, R. K., Carter, V. S., Shields, C. L., and Lombardo, S. J.: Correctable elbow lesions in professional baseball players: A review of 25 cases. Am J Sports Med 7:72, 1979.
8. De Haven, K. E., and Evarts, C. M.: Throwing injuries of the elbow in athletes. Orthop Clin North Am 4:301, 1973.
9. Gartsman, G. M., Sculco, T. P., Otis, J. C.: Operative treatment of olecranon fractures. J Bone Joint Surg 63A:718, 1981.
10. Wilson, F. D., Andrews, J. R., Blackburn, T. A., and McCluskey, G.: Valgus extension overload in the pitching elbow. Am J Sports Med 11:83, 1983.
11. Andrews, J. R., McCluskey, G. M., and McLeod, W. D.: Musculo-tendinous injuries of the shoulder and elbow in athletes. Schering Symposium. The Journal of the National Athletic Trainers Association II, Summer 1976.
12. Tullos, H. S., King, J. W.: Throwing mechanism in sports. Orthop Clin North Am 4:709, 1973.

CONDITIONING
AND
REHABILITATION

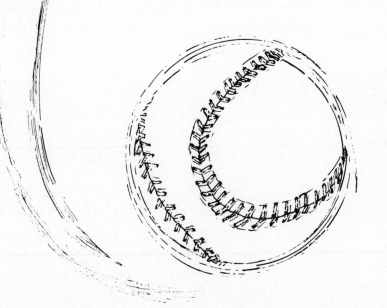

27

SPRING TRAINING CONDITIONING FOR THE THROWING SHOULDER*

CHARLES P. GREENE

The throwing motion imposes tremendous stress on the shoulder. A look at the history of a throwing injury usually shows that the cause may have involved throwing too often, working on new pitches, pitching batting practice frequently, poor conditioning (lack of strength and flexibility), and improper throwing technique.

The disabling shoulder injury is usually not the result of one forceful throw or one hard workout but rather the result of repetitive injury with accompanying soreness, lack of full relaxation, weakness, and limited motion. Irritation with resulting inflammation is the main enemy of the throwing arm.

Only after a proper warm-up should a pitcher pick up a baseball. The pitcher should always warm up to throw and not throw to warm up. An efficient warm-up promotes numerous positive benefits for the pitcher. The primary reasons for warming up are:

1. To promote a psychologic feeling of readiness to perform
2. To increase body temperature and blood flow

*Adapted from Greene, C., Pearl, A., and Whieldon, T., *Maximize Performance, Minimize Injury*, Miami, Suniland Press, 1980.

3. To increase range of motion
4. To increase speed of movement

WARM-UP EXERCISES

A three- to five-pound weight can be used to perform a series of exercises to warm up all of the connective tissue and musculature involved in throwing (Fig. 27–1). These exercises should not be performed for the development of strength but solely to increase tissue temperature and blood flow. When exercising the shoulder, special emphasis should be given to full range of motion.

Partner stretching exercises can be used to passively take the throwing arm through its most extreme range of motion before a baseball is thrown. The extreme positions encountered during throwing then feel familiar and comfortable, and tissue tearing can be minimized.

Guidelines for the Partner Stretching Program

1. Stretching with a partner is more beneficial than stretching alone.
2. Gradual stretching should have two phases of 30 seconds each in length. In the first phase the partner applies gentle pressure, which is gradually increased until an easy stretching sensation is experienced. This

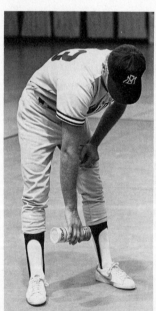

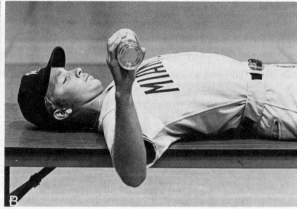

FIGURE 27–1. *A* and *B*. Weight exercises are performed to increase tissue temperature and blood flow, not to develop strength. The athlete in this illustration is using a tennis ball can full of sand.

position is held for 30 seconds. In the second phase the partner gradually increases the gentle pressure until the stretching sensation becomes more intense but not to the point of actual pain or discomfort. This position is maintained for 30 seconds. The athlete should stretch, not strain.

3.   The athlete should try to maintain continued relaxation as he is stretching and to breathe normally.

4.   Everyone is different in his range of flexibility, and stretching should never become a contest between athletes. The athlete should always strive for improvement in his individual range of motion.

SHOULDER TRAINING DRILLS

Throwing the full 60-foot distance every day is very taxing on the arm and therefore it is recommended that this type of practice be used only on alternate days. However, since repetition is the key to developing sound skills, daily drills of a less vigorous nature may be utilized. For this purpose a series of drills that allow for proper use of the shoulder are described:

1.   Each drill is designed to allow for daily repetition with a minimal amount of stress.

2.   The drills are performed at a much shorter pitching distance (30 to 40 feet is recommended).

Chair Drill. The purpose of this drill is to force the pitcher to throw over his stride leg, which is the base of support for the entire delivery. By raising the pivot foot and resting it on the seat of a chair the weight of the body is transferred to the opposite side (Fig. 27–2). This causes the entire pitching action to vault over the left leg if the pitcher is right-handed. This vaulting action allows the total force of the delivery to be transferred to the ball to produce a more effective pitch.

Of further benefit is the large number of repetitions that can be practiced with this drill, since the pitcher is not using the entire force of the body. The restriction caused by the chair does not allow a total effort, and therefore the drill does not cause the same fatigue experienced when pitching with a full delivery.

Stand-Up Drill. This drill is the next step in the progression from the chair drill to the full delivery. While it includes the same elements as in the chair drill it allows the pitcher to experience more forceful use of the lower body. By keeping the pivot foot back and rotating the heel over the toe while throwing, the athlete acquires the feeling of hip action (Fig. 27–3).

Form Drill. Pitchers can practice their "form" by throwing directly against a wall or a screen that provides a rebounding capability (Fig. 27–4). The pitcher stands about 20 to 25 feet away from the wall and experiences the feeling of throwing while getting the shoulder really loose.

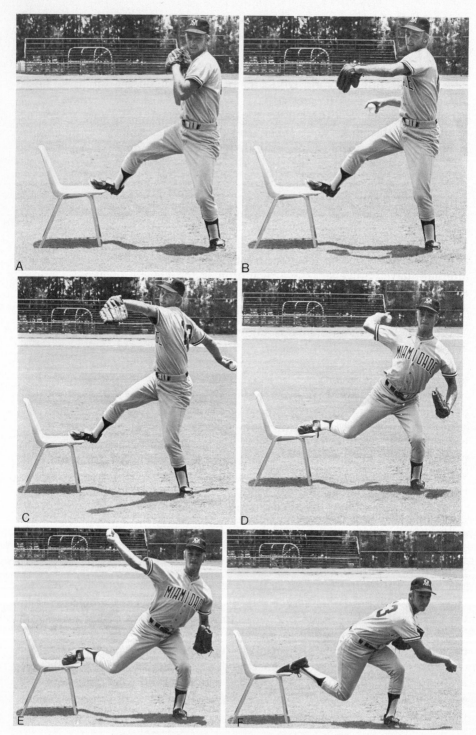

FIGURE 27–2. *A–F*, The chair drill is illustrated.

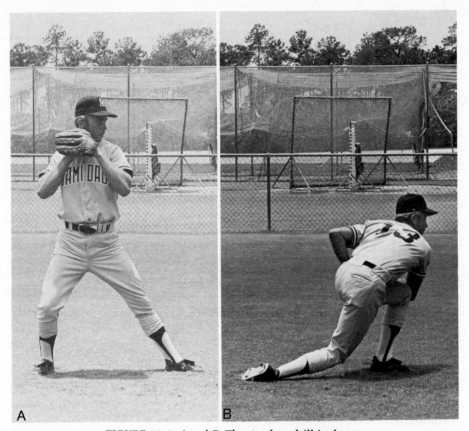

FIGURE 27–3. *A* and *B*. The stand-up drill is shown.

If these drills are incorporated with pitching the regulation distance, the shoulder can get the necessary repetition without undue fatigue.

Maximizing pitching performance while minimizing risk of injury to the throwing shoulder involves a team effort between the athlete, coach, trainer, and team physician.

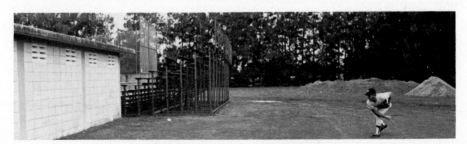

FIGURE 27–4. The form drill is shown.

GENERAL TRAINING TECHNIQUES TO WARM UP AND COOL DOWN THE THROWING ARM

DON FAULS, A.T.C.

I. THE WARM-UP

Introduction

Every individual has his or her method of performing a pregame warm-up. The trainer should not alter a player's warm-up routine unless the individual is having problems. Problems can be manifested as uncontrollable pitches, ineffective starts, stiffness, and so forth.

Most pitchers have developed their own techniques of warming up as they progress in their careers. Some want to warm up alone as they loosen up for a game. Some pitchers request a short rubdown before they start their pregame warm-up. Other pitchers want their arm stretched before they start throwing.

If the opinion is held that pitching is 70 per cent of the game of baseball, then the trainer should spend that percentage of his time with the pitchers.

Psychologic Considerations

Because of the relative importance placed on the pitcher by other members of the baseball team, coaching staff, and fans, many baseball pitchers develop unique personalities. Some are loners who wish to be left alone, while others interact quite readily. Both types of individuals need encouragement and support. If a certain pitcher appears to need help with his pitching the trainer should be available for consultation. The time during which most pitchers are receptive to suggestions is when they are pitching poorly and struggling. However, the trainer can provide suggestions and help not just on the playing field. The trainer should engage in conversation with the injured or troubled athlete and offer help at opportune times, such as when dining or while riding in a bus or car to an away game. Topics such as career goals, pitching style, and injury patterns, among others, can be discussed, and important ground work can be established that can be later "translated" to performance on the pitching mound.

Arm Stretching

If a pitcher is tight and has demonstrated trouble loosening up, an arm stretch may be beneficial. This routine is performed prior to the pitcher's individual warm-up. The author believes that this loosens up the pitcher's action more quickly and can save warm-up pitches. A good arm stretch performed before the warm-up can save the pitcher as many as 25 pitches. If this is so, those pitches can be in reserve, available for use late in the game. The pitching arm has only so many effective pitches on a given day. Anything that can be done to preserve those pitches until later in the game is obviously beneficial to the pitcher.

The arm stretch described here, which has been used by the author for the past 30 years, has enjoyed great success both at the collegiate and the professional baseball levels.[1] It has also been used by quarterbacks before practice or a game.

The general principals to be followed in all the stretches are:

1. The stretches should be performed *before* the practice session.

2. Within 15 minutes after the stretches have been done, the athlete should begin throwing as he would for a normal warm-up.

3. The athletic trainer does all the movement during the routine, while the athlete lies relaxed.

4. While doing the stretches, it may be necessary for the trainer to keep reminding the athlete to relax.

5. The muscles should be stretched to their limit. Pain, however, should be the determining factor.

6. It is important that (a) the stretches be performed by the trainer in their presented order and (b) the stretches be done one after another, since continuity must be a major goal. Continuity means that each stretch should overlap its predecessor so that stretch 1 flows into stretch 2, and so forth.

7. The number of stretches should be varied to fit the athlete. Some athletes need more stretches than others and some less. The trainer should use his professional judgment.

8. The arm stretch should be shown to the athletes. The trainer must not insist on its use. The athletes should be allowed to make up their own minds. However, if the trainer feels that someone needs this exercise and is hesitant or resistant, a little suggestive selling may get the athlete to try this exercise.

9. The stretches and their explanations are for right-handed throwers. Obvious alterations should be made when working with a left-handed thrower.

ORDER OF STRETCHES

I. **POSITION ONE**
   a. STRETCH 1—SHOULDER ROLL
   b. STRETCH 2—PECTORAL STRETCH
   c. STRETCH 3—SHOULDER HYPEREXTENSION
   d. STRETCH 4—SHOULDER HYPERFLEXION
   e. STRETCH 5—SHOULDER CIRCLES

II. **POSITION TWO**
   a. STRETCH 6—THE "PUMP" STRETCH
   b. STRETCH 7—ELBOW CIRCLES
   c. STRETCH 8—WRIST CIRCLES
   d. STRETCH 9—KNUCKLE POPS
   e. STRETCH 10—ARM WAVES

Position One. The athlete lies on his side, facing the athletic trainer. His throwing arm is held at the side, and his head rests flat on the nonthrowing arm.

STRETCH 1: SHOULDER ROLL. The pitcher's arm is placed on the athletic trainer's left forearm. The athletic trainer cups the pitcher's shoulder with both hands (Fig. 28–1) and rotates the shoulder girdle ten times clockwise and counterclockwise. The goal is to move the scapula and clavicle, not the humerus. Rotation is performed in a small circle.

FOR CONTINUITY (STRETCH 1 TO STRETCH 2). The pitcher's arm is flipped from the trainer's left forearm to the trainer's right forearm.

STRETCH 2: PECTORAL STRETCH. The athletic trainer places his right hand on the athlete's scapula. The athlete's arm is then bent at the elbow and laid along and across the trainer's right forearm so that the humerus is parallel to the table above the head. The trainer rests his left elbow against the athlete's hip and places his left hand on the scapula so that the fingers of his two hands touch (Fig. 28–2). The trainer then pulls the scapula toward him and pushes the arm with his right elbow while he makes sure that the athlete's arm remains parallel to the table. As the athlete's arm moves behind his head the trainer may need to lean over the athlete's body. The arm is held on stretch for two to three seconds and released, and stretch is reapplied three to five times.

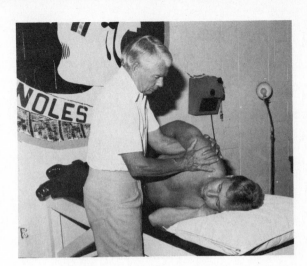

FIGURE 28–1. The shoulder roll.

FOR CONTINUITY (STRETCH 2 TO STRETCH 3). The athlete's arm is flipped from the trainer's right forearm to the trainer's left hand.

STRETCH 3: SHOULDER HYPEREXTENSION. The athletic trainer places his right hand on the athlete's scapula and grasps the athlete's right wrist or lower forearm with the left hand (Fig. 28–3). The athlete's arm is then pushed back as far as possible while keeping the elbow straight and the arm parallel to the table. As the arm is stretched back, firm pressure should be applied to the scapula. After two to three seconds the stretch should be released a little, then reapplied. This procedure is repeated three to five times.

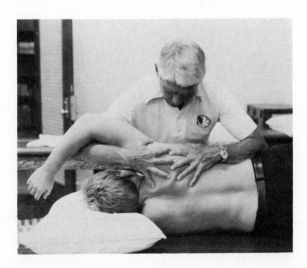

FIGURE 28–2. The pectoral stretch.

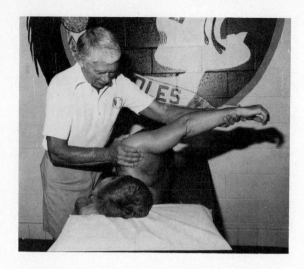

FIGURE 28–3. Shoulder hyperextension.

FOR CONTINUITY (STRETCH 3 TO STRETCH 4). The athlete's arm is transferred from the trainer's left hand to the right hand and brought over the athlete's ear.

STRETCH 4: SHOULDER HYPERFLEXION. The trainer's right hand is slid from the athlete's wrist to the palm and the trainer's left hand from the elbow to just above the wrist.

The trainer cups his left hand over the top of the athlete's shoulder (Fig. 28–4). The athlete's right wrist is then grasped with the trainer's right hand. The athlete's arm is extended over his ear but parallel to the table. The athlete's arm is then pushed down toward the table as far as possible, with the elbow kept straight and the arm parallel to the table. As the arm is stretched down, firm pressure should be applied to the tip of the shoulder.

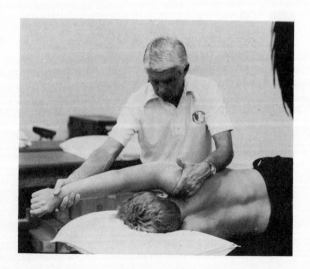

FIGURE 28–4. Shoulder hyperflexion

(The trainer's left hand is used as a fulcrum.) After two to three seconds the stretch is released a little, then reapplied. The procedure is repeated three to five times with the arm stretched a little more each time.

FOR CONTINUITY (STRETCH 4 TO STRETCH 5). The athlete's arm comes from over his ear toward his hip and bends at the elbow. The trainer's left hand then cups the athlete's elbow. The trainer's right hand is placed on the top of the athlete's wrist, and the rotation motion begins with the trainer's left hand pushing the athlete's elbow.

STRETCH 5: SHOULDER CIRCLES. With the elbow bent to 90 degrees the trainer grasps the athlete's wrist with his right hand, and the elbow is cupped with the left hand (Fig. 28–5). With the forearm kept parallel to the table, the upper arm is rotated in as big a circle as possible, both clockwise and counterclockwise, five to eight times.

It is important to exaggerate the circle at the top of the arc. Also, a patterned slow speed of movement should be used.

Position Two. The athlete rolls over onto his back so that the throwing side of his body is at the opposite edge of the table, and the shoulder and arm are just barely off the table's edge.

STRETCH 6: "THE PUMP" STRETCH. The athletic trainer, in a crouched position, grasps the athlete's arm just above the wrist with his right hand and lifts it into the air. He slides his left hand up under the athlete's arm, through the armpit, and places it on the athlete's chest (Fig. 28–6). The athlete's arm is then cradled (supported) by the trainer's anterior elbow joint. With the trainer's left arm used as a fulcrum, the athlete's arm is moved back perpendicular to the body, and the trainer pushes the athlete's arm back. The elbow during this stretch is in full extension. The stretch is held for three to four seconds, relaxed, and repeated three to five times.

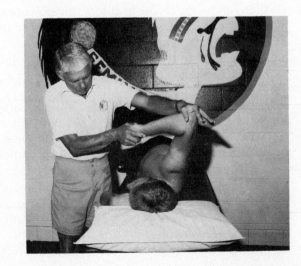

FIGURE 28–5. Shoulder circles.

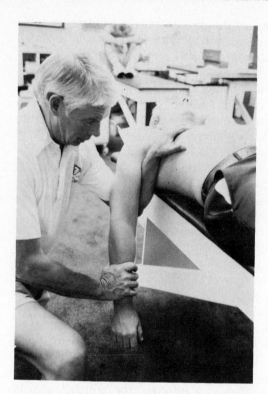

FIGURE 28–6. The "pump" stretch.

FOR CONTINUITY (STRETCH 6 TO STRETCH 7). The trainer stands up, slides his right hand to the athlete's palm and his left hand from the athlete's chest to the athlete's elbow, and cups it.

STRETCH 7: ELBOW CIRCLES. The athletic trainer grasps the athlete's arm just above the elbow with his left hand and the wrist with his right hand. He then rotates the elbow in as large an arc as possible. Rotation is performed clockwise and counterclockwise, four to five times in each direction (Fig. 28–7).

FOR CONTINUITY (STRETCH 7 TO STRETCH 8). The trainer's right hand is slid from the athlete's wrist to the palm and the trainer's left hand from the elbow to just above the wrist.

The athletic trainer grasps the athlete's arm just above the wrist with his left hand and the athlete's palm with his right hand. He then rotates the wrist clockwise and counterclockwise three to five times. (Fig. 28–8).

STRETCH 9: KNUCKLE POP. The athletic trainer grasps the athlete's hand with his left hand and each finger, one at a time, with his right hand. The trainer then pulls on each finger with moderate pressure. Each finger is pulled only once. It is not necessary to hear a pop.

STRETCH 10: ARM WAVES. The athletic trainer grasps the athlete's hand with both of his hands and lifts up and down, causing the athlete's arm to wave (Fig. 28–9). The athlete should be very relaxed and the arm very limp.

FIGURE 28–7. Elbow circles.

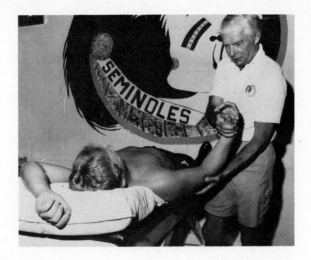

After three to five waves the athletic trainer throws the arm and hand to the athlete's chest. The arm should flop onto the athlete's chest if he is relaxed.

The pitcher is now ready to begin his individual warm-up routine and actually to begin throwing the baseball.

Pitching Tips

A pitcher should always have at least two sweat shirts. A soaked sweat shirt can get quite heavy, and the pitcher does not need this extra weight, especially late in the game.

FIGURE 28–8. Wrist circles.

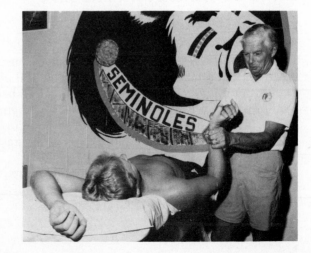

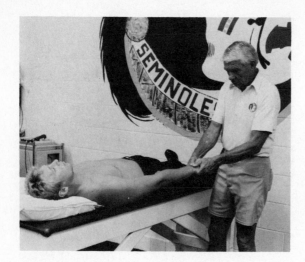

FIGURE 28–9. Arm waves.

In addition to plenty of fluids, on hot and humid days a mixture of ice water and aromatic spirits of ammonia is quite effective in reviving a tiring player. The author uses two ounces of ammonia in an 11-quart pail of ice water. A towel is placed in this mixture, wrung out, and the player's face and neck are wiped off with the towel. While the towel is over the player's face, he should take a deep breath. This can heighten the pitcher's senses and give him a "second wind." This is rarely recommended before the fifth inning because a player can only be revived so many times.

II. THE COOLING DOWN PROCESS

Introduction

Nearly all trainers at the present time recommend the postgame "icing down" of the pitcher's arm. This is a good and effective process to control swelling or injury, or both. However, the author believes that not all pitchers require postplay "icing down" and that this regimen should not be started unless the player wants it or has a specific injury. If a pitcher is throwing well and not having any problems, chances are that he does not need to "ice down" his arm.

Some pitchers always ask to have their arms "iced down" and feel that they have to have something wrong with their arms all the time. Some of these players are malingerers and may only be looking for an excuse in case they do not perform well.

Technique

There are several different methods available to cool the throwing athlete's arm. One technique is to apply several ice bags from the shoulder to the wrist, which are held in place with elastic bandages. It seems to be advisable to elevate the arm while doing this. Elevation of the arm is facilitated by the use of a handle attached to a rope connected to the ceiling. While the pitcher is lying down with the arm covered with ice bags, the arm is raised and the handle is grasped and held in this position for 15 to 20 minutes. The amount of time that the ice is applied depends on the severity of the injury, the tolerance of the player, and the experience of the trainer.

Another method of cooling the arm is by using ice water. With the aid of some form of container into which the pitcher can get most of his arm, the entire arm is submerged in the water. Ice bags can be placed on those areas not covered by the water. Usually the arm is wrapped with a towel when this method is used. This method can cause extreme pain in the elbow area and may even cause irritation of the ulnar nerve. Because many players cannot tolerate such pain for very long, having the pitcher dip the elbow in and out of the water until he gets used to the water may help in administering this technique.

An alternative to the use of ice or cryotherapy is the postgame arm massage. The arm is elevated above the head, and a rope with a handle attached is grasped by the player. The arm is massaged with alcohol or some lubricant. The massage should be started in the area of the shoulder and progress to the elbow and forearm. The actual massage stroke is always toward the heart. This method should not be used too long, since the pitcher's arm is already tired from pitching and massaging is a tiring process. Four or five minutes usually suffices. This method is called "milking the arm," and the goal is to eliminate some of the swelling that occurs during pitching. After this "milking" process the arm, back, and neck are rubbed with alcohol.

THE POSTPITCHING DAY

After having pitched a complete game of seven innings or after having thrown a certain number of pitches, a player is usually fairly stiff or sore on the next day. Some pitchers can pitch a couple of innings the next day; others cannot. On the first postpitching day one way to eliminate some of the stiffness and to exercise generally is to have the pitcher back up one of his fellow teammate pitchers during batting practice. The bending and extra movements that are required and the fielding of balls and bending down and picking up provide a good workout, with sufficient bending and stretching, and loosen up a player's tight muscles.

SUMMARY

The techniques of warming up and cooling down of the throwing arm as described here have been used successfully by the author for over 30 years. Although each trainer and each player develop a specific routine, the techniques described here may serve to broaden the trainer's approach to the care of the throwing arm.

REFERENCES

1. Madaleno, J. A.: The Fauls shoulder stretch. Journal of the National Athletic Trainers' Association. 16:187, 1981.

THE OFF-SEASON PROGRAM FOR THE THROWING ARM

TURNER A. BLACKBURN, A.T.C., R.P.T.

INTRODUCTION

The purpose of this chapter is to present a practical program for the conditioning of the entire throwing arm that can be used at all levels of achievement, including high school, college, and professional levels. It is applicable to the in-season rehabilitation of the throwing arm as well. This program can be utilized by each individual player at his own discretion and often can be performed without supervision. One of the most common mistakes that baseball players make with regard to conditioning and rehabilitation of the throwing arm is that they appear at spring training camp with expectations of getting the arm into condition at that time, rather than coming to spring training camp already conditioned. The baseball player should come to spring training in excellent condition and not expect to get the throwing arm in this excellent condition once he gets to camp. Therefore, an exercise program to be performed during the off-season for the throwing arm is of utmost importance.

An important consideration in the planning of an off-season program is whether the athlete's arm is healthy or injured. This determines the type of program to prescribe for the throwing athlete and how frequently it should be performed. The three most important aspects to which the off-season program should be directed are (1) strength and weight training, (2) conditioning, and (3) flexibility.

The strength training program is designed to provide endurance strength to the throwing athlete's arm and not just pure physical strength. This endurance strength is best achieved by utilizing a program of numerous repetitions and low weight. Endurance is of utmost importance because pitchers are sometimes required to throw 100 to 150 pitches during a single game. The high repetition and low weight program develops not only strength but the endurance the player needs to throw during these long periods of time. The program should be customized and very specific to each individual thrower and to his injury pattern, if he has one. Numerous repetitions usually consist of five sets of ten repetitions. In dealing with the injured throwing arm, possibly no weight should be used at first. The athlete gradually works up to at least five pounds. The weight is progressively increased as he becomes stronger. These endurance exercises should be performed three times a day; however, the noninjured athletes who want to maintain strength during the off-season can work just once a day on these exercises.

Increasing the strength of the thrower should make him a more accurate and stronger pitcher. There is controversy concerning the role that weight machines play in this strengthening program. Many expensive strength machines are presently being utilized by various Major League baseball organizations. It is important that the players using these machines know how to utilize them in a safe fashion and work on specific exercises required to strengthen the muscles utilized in throwing a baseball. It is important that too much bulk not be developed and that proper attention be given to flexibility. Lack of emphasis on flexibility is the most common error in most conditioning programs. The injured throwing arm should have obtained a normal range of motion and flexibility, and the player should have returned to full throwing capabilities before any weight machines are utilized. These weight training machines are excellent for making the normal shoulder even stronger. However, they do not work very well in returning the abnormal or injured shoulder to normal condition.

WEIGHT TRAINING FOR THE THROWING ARM

The following weight training program is designed to correspond with the various phases of throwing: wind-up, cocking, acceleration, follow-through, and deceleration.

In the wind-up phase, which can vary substantially from player to player, there are no specific exercises. In the cocking phase the external rotators, the muscles concerned with shoulder suspension, the horizontal abductors, and the scapular stabilizers are important and need to be strengthened appropriately. The shoulder girdle is a suspension system, and proximal stabilization of the scapula on the chest wall is very important. The shoulder shrug with scapular abduction is an excellent exercise for strengthening the entire shoulder girdle and scapular stabilizers as well as

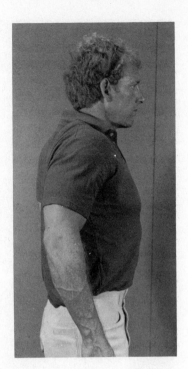

FIGURE 29–1. Shoulder shrug with scapular abduction.

the trapezius muscle (Fig. 29–1). Strengthening of the anterior and middle portions of the deltoid muscle should be performed because these muscles help the individual to bring the arm into the cocked position. The athlete utilizes flexion and abduction, working through the range of motion slowly and deliberately. There is a pause of a count of two at the end of the range of motion (Figs. 29–2A, B).

The supraspinatus portion of the rotator cuff is exercised by lifting the arm up to the horizontal level with the arm in the "empty can" position, which places the arm at full internal rotation with the thumbs pointing toward the ground and the arm pulled into 30-degree horizontal abduction. This position isolates the supraspinatus portion of the rotator cuff (Fig. 29–3). The other rotator cuff muscles (infraspinatus and teres minor) are best exercised with the individual prone and the humerus supported on the table at 90-degree abduction with the elbow off the table and flexed 90 degrees. The athlete rotates the humerus into the fullest amount of external rotation possible, pauses, and relaxes (Fig. 29–4).

The posterior portion of the deltoid muscle and the other horizontal abductors can be exercised with the athlete in the prone position and the arm hanging completely off the table. The arm is lifted from the body until the hand is at eye level. This exercise puts major emphasis on the teres minor and other portions of the rotator cuff as well as the scapular stabilizers (Fig. 29–5).

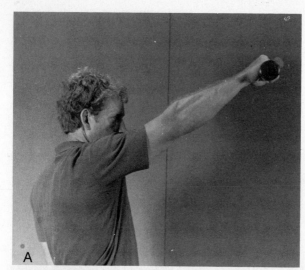

FIGURE 29–2A. The anterior portion of the deltoid muscle is strengthened by forward flexion exercises.

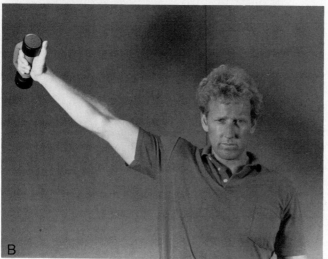

FIGURE 29–2B. The middle portion of the deltoid muscle is strengthened by abduction exercises.

The horizontal adductors, shoulder depressors, and internal rotators are important during the acceleration phase of throwing and are strengthened by the sitting pushup or the dip. The athlete works up to five sets of ten repetitions (Fig. 29–6). Another satisfactory exercise for strengthening the internal rotators and shoulder depressors is the pushup. This should be used cautiously by athletes who have either bicipital tendinitis or anterior subluxation of the shoulder. As with most of the other shoulder exercises the pushup is performed by utilizing numerous repetitions to develop endurance and strength. The pushups can be modified and performed

FIGURE 29–3. The supraspinatus tendon of the rotator cuff can be isolated for testing by internally rotating and abducting the humerus.

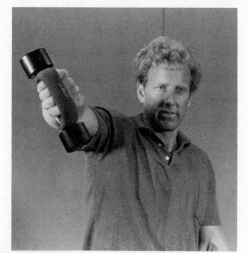

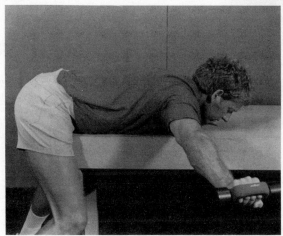

FIGURE 29–4. Shoulder position for strengthening the external rotators.

FIGURE 29–5. Strengthening exercise for the posterior portion of the deltoid muscle and the rotator cuff.

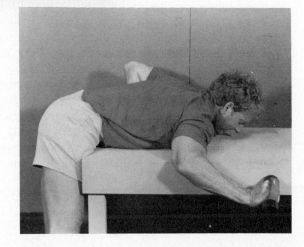

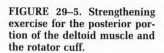

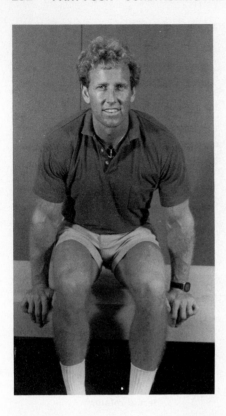

FIGURE 29–6. The sitting pushup or dip for strengthening the shoulder depressor, horizontal adductor, and internal rotator muscles.

against a wall or table so that the forces can be lessened across the anterior portion of the shoulder (Fig. 29–7).

The bench press is another commonly performed exercise to strengthen the shoulder and upper arm musculature. As the weight is lowered against the chest, the anterior portion of the shoulder is stressed and may exacerbate bicipital tendinitis or anterior subluxation of the shoulder. If the player has one of these problems he should do the bench press by bringing the humerus just parallel to the body and should not allow the bar to touch the chest. This lessens the stress on the anterior structures of the shoulder. It is important not to bounce when performing the bench press. Often the younger athletes attempt to lift heavier weights by bouncing the bar off the chest. This can only lead to injury, and these abnormal forces are transmitted to the shoulder and stretch the anterior capsule. The condition of a posteriorly subluxating shoulder occasionally is worsened by the bench press, particularly if a closed hand grip is used. If a posterior shoulder subluxation becomes a problem during the bench press a wider grip should be used so that the forces are transmitted more toward the center of the joint, rather than to the posterior structures of the joint. Another exercise that may be irritating to an athlete with biceps tendinitis or anterior subluxation of the shoulder is a full bar dip.

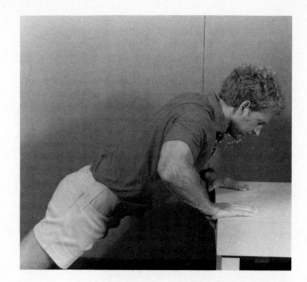

FIGURE 29–7. Modified pushup.

The biceps and triceps muscles are important to the throwing arm and are strengthened by utilizing the french curl for the triceps and the biceps or the elbow curl for the biceps (Figs. 29–8, 29–9).

ISOMETRIC EXERCISES

The throwing shoulder may also be strengthened by isometric exercises. These exercises should be performed in several different positions through the full range of motion and held for at least six counts. The athlete should perform 25 to 30 contractions at least three times a day. These can be done in a variety of positions and can be administered by the athlete himself, by using one of his teammates, or by utilizing a wall or strap apparatus to give resistance. These isometric exercises can be performed at home or on the road, since there is no need for special equipment.

FLEXIBILITY EXERCISES

Flexibility is of paramount importance in the prevention of throwing injuries. The throwing motion requires the shoulder to be placed in extremes of abduction and external rotation, and thus particular flexibility is needed in these range-of-motion areas. External rotation flexibility exercises are performed in three positions: 90-degree, 135-degree, and full abduction (Fig. 29–10). These should be performed by doing at least 25 repetitions, holding each for a count of five. The player should stretch at least once per day before throwing and more frequently if there has been a shoulder

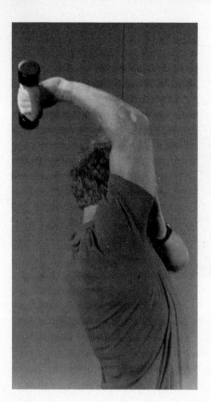

FIGURE 29–8. French curl exercise for strengthening the triceps muscle.

FIGURE 29–9. Biceps or elbow curl for strengthening the biceps muscle.

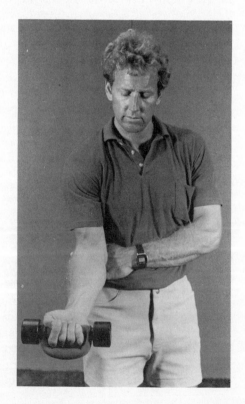

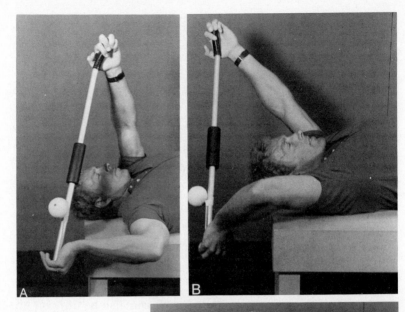

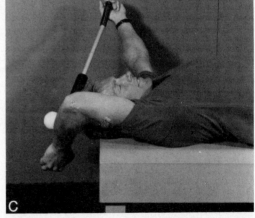

FIGURE 29–10. External rotation flexibility exercises performed with the shoulder abducted *(A)* 90 degrees, *(B)* 135 degrees, and *(C)* in full abduction.

injury. Abduction flexibility exercises are performed by sliding the arm up along the treatment table and trying to keep the arm down on the table as the athlete pulls with his other hand. A hammer is very helpful with this pull-through, as is a baseball bat, a baton, a broomstick, or a cane.

Although extremes of internal rotation are not utilized as much as the extremes of external rotation during the throwing act, the external rotators still need to be stretched so that the athlete can obtain proper internal rotation. This is performed by having the athlete lie supine with the arm at 90 degrees. A wand is used to perform an active assist type of stretching of the external rotators as the arm is moved into internal rotation (Fig. 29–11).

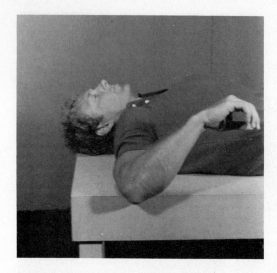

FIGURE 29–11. Internally rotating the shoulder stretches the external rotator muscles.

An overhead rope and pulley system can also be utilized effectively to stress the capsule and to warm up the throwing arm. It is important that this exercise be performed with the arm in full abduction and external rotation and raised up toward the head as far as possible.

Because horizontal adduction is important during the follow-through phase of throwing, the posterior structures of the shoulder need to be flexible and properly stretched (Fig. 29–12). This stretching is performed 25 times and held for a count of five. Hanging from an overhead bar is also a good way to stretch the capsule, provided that there are no subluxation problems.

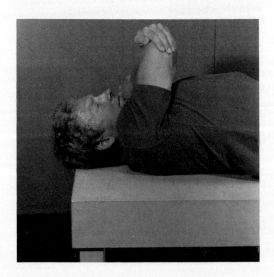

FIGURE 29–12. Stretching exercise for the posterior shoulder structures.

The Codman's or pendulum exercises are also a satisfactory method of loosening up the throwing arm. These exercises are most commonly used in postinjury and postsurgical situations. However, they may also be performed to loosen up the arm before throwing. These exercises should be done in a clockwise and counterclockwise fashion from front to back and side to side as well. The chest should be parallel with the floor while they are being performed (Fig. 29–13).

In addition to the flexibility and warm-up techniques described earlier, there are various mobilization techniques that are instrumental in loosening up the throwing shoulder, particularly the capsule of the shoulder prior to throwing. These techniques are described in other chapters and are not described further here.

Not only the shoulder and upper arm need to be flexible and have proper endurance strength for the throwing mechanism, but the forearm, hand, and wrist all need to be properly conditioned to prevent injury. Flexibility of the forearm is very important, since many of the muscles in the forearm cross both the elbow and the wrist joints. The extensors are stretched with the elbow in full extension and the hand and wrist pulled down into full flexion (Fig. 29–14). This position is held for a count of ten or longer and repeated at least 25 times. The flexors are also stretched with the elbow in full extension. It is important when the wrist is pulled into full extension that the forearm be held in full supination so that the pronator teres muscle may also be stretched (Fig. 29–15).

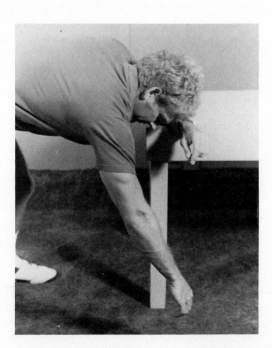

FIGURE 29–13. Pendulum exercises.

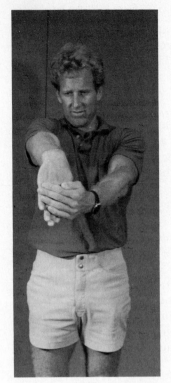

FIGURE 29–14. Stretching exercise for wrist extensor muscles.

FIGURE 29–15. Stretching exercise for wrist flexor muscles.

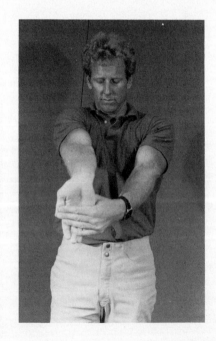

STRENGTHENING EXERCISES

Strengthening exercises for the forearm consist of five sets of ten repetitions with one to five pounds of resistance for the forearm flexors, extensors, pronators, and supinators (Fig. 29–16 to 29–19). These exercises are performed by pulling the wrist through the full movement in both directions at a slow pace and avoiding a fast "fanning" motion as the exercises are performed. The athlete is positioned with the forearm on the table, on the thigh, or on the arm of the chair so as to stabilize the upper arm and forearm. The wrist can then move through uninhibited full range of motion.

Grip strength is also important to the throwing athlete. Grip strength can be increased by performing exercises with therapeutic putty or some type of commercially available grip apparatus. Such exercises can be performed by the athlete throughout the day at his leisure.

Because the entire body is involved in the throwing act, flexibility and strengthening of the trunk are also important. Flexibility exercises for trunk rotation and strengthening curls, abdominal rotational curls, and back extension strengthening exercises should be included in the throwing athlete's conditioning program.

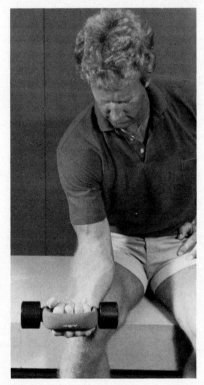

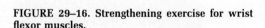

FIGURE 29–16. Strengthening exercise for wrist flexor muscles.

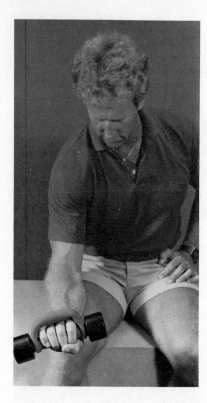

FIGURE 29–17. Strengthening exercise for wrist extensor muscles.

FIGURE 29–18. Strengthening exercise for the forearm pronator muscles.

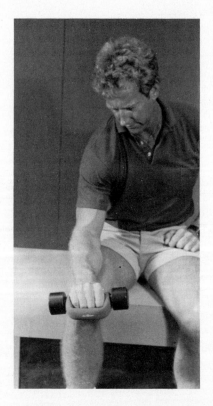

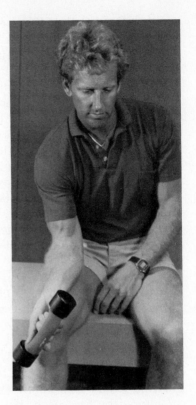

FIGURE 29–19. Strengthening exercise for the fore-arm supinator muscles.

Cardiovascular conditioning, especially during the winter, is also important. Running and bicycling are excellent conditioning exercises. Many athletes lose aerobic conditioning during the season because they are not running as much as during the spring. The lower extremities can be strengthened by running and cycling as well as by stair climbing and by exercises performed on various types of weight machines.

CONDITIONING AND RETURN TO THROWING AFTER INJURY

During the off-season the athlete should be throwing for at least 10 to 15 minutes three times a week to maintain proper strength and conditioning for the throwing arm. As spring training approaches, the athlete is able to increase his throwing so that he can arrive at training camp with his arm in condition and not produce an injury during the early phases of spring training.

The individual who is recovering from an injury should return to throwing with a long toss, short toss program. The arm should be warmed up with both the strengthening and the stretching exercises outlined previously as well as the use of heat and a few tosses at 10 to 15 feet to loosen up the throwing arm.

The long toss portion of the program for return to throwing is performed by having the player throw from center field to second base (a distance of 80 to 150 feet). If the individual is just beginning to throw again after an injury he throws just hard enough to allow the ball to roll into second base. This throwing is performed for four minutes. Following this throwing, a short toss program is performed for four minutes in which the athlete throws over a distance of 30 feet and works up to half speed. Initially these eight minutes of throwing can be done twice a day. As the athlete becomes stronger he increases the amount of throwing, the distance thrown, and the intensity with which each ball is thrown. The long toss portion of this program is increased by having the athlete throw just hard enough so that the ball reaches second base from the outfield on one bounce. He then eventually works to the level at which he can throw it this distance on the fly.

In the short toss program the athlete works 30 feet at half speed, to 60 feet at half speed, then to 60 feet at three-quarter speed, and finally to throwing off the mound. Following this sequence he begins to throw breaking pitches and works up to full speed. The long toss, short toss program can be performed as much as four times a day. The key to this program is to allow the individual to throw but never to let him become really fatigued. By following this program the athlete can throw more often than he would if he threw at just one session. This program needs to be monitored by the coach, the trainer, and the individual athlete to avoid throwing too hard. At times a rest day is needed, and in some instances throwing for two days and resting on the third day works very well.

It has been the purpose of this chapter to outline an exercise program for the throwing arm. This program may be used in the off-season as well as in the rehabilitation of the injured throwing arm. The key to these programs is the high repetition and low weight regimens with emphasis on flexibility, especially external rotation. The entire arm and body need to be flexible, to be conditioned, and to have adequate endurance strength. The conditioning of the throwing arm after injury should be done in a supervised and controlled fashion with daily goals set for the athlete. Progress is very unpredictable and varies from individual to individual. The ultimate goal of these training and rehabilitative programs is to return the athlete to full throwing potential.

STRENGTH/POWER TRAINING FOR BASEBALL PITCHERS*

THOMAS M. McLAUGHLIN, Ph.D.

INTRODUCTION

Throwing a baseball is one of the most complex and dramatic human sport motions that exists. The upper extremity and ball must be accelerated from rest to a linear release velocity that can be in excess of 100 miles per hour. Along with neuromuscular considerations, significant levels of muscle strength and power are required for optimal throwing performance. As demonstrated in research investigations,[1] resistive training has been found to produce development of strength and power as well as concomitant improvements in sports performance. In recent years the importance of resistive training in baseball has become increasingly apparent, with players and coaches alike seeking information on strength/power training methods.

As might be expected from such a forceful activity, the throwing mechanism has been shown to cause a significant number of injuries, especially in baseball pitchers. The frequency and severity of such throwing injuries have led to considerable interest within the baseball and sports medicine communities (as evidenced by this text) regarding strategies for

*The photographs used in this chapter were taken using a process developed by Mr. Austin Mitchell, scientific photographer, of Auburn, Alabama, who worked with the author. Information on this technique can be obtained from Mr. Mitchell.

the prevention and rehabilitation of such injuries. The beneficial effects of resistive exercise in both rehabilitation and prevention have strong experiential support and have also begun to be demonstrated in the research literature. In this regard resistive training appears to be of significant value to baseball, as has been the case for other sports.

The two major roles of strength/power training for baseball pitchers thus appear to be to maximize performance and to minimize injury. However, it is important to realize initially that it is by no means a simple task to design a strength/power program for baseball pitchers that is effective in achieving these two goals. Any such program must incorporate both research and empirical evidence from a variety of sources such as sport science researchers, sport orthopaedists, baseball coaches or pitchers, elite strength/power athletes involved in other sports, and so forth. When reviewing evidence from such varied sources, it is important to recognize that almost any strength/power program, no matter how ill-conceived, may produce some positive short-term results. This can often mask the superior long-term results produced by better designed programs, which adds to the confusion, misinformation, and conflicting claims that can confound all those seeking the optimal strength/power program for baseball pitchers. To help in this effort, this paper presents a strength/power training program based on research and experience and designed to maximize performance and minimize injury in baseball pitchers.

The rational design of a strength/power training program for baseball pitchers is based on three major steps (see Fig. 30–1). (1) First, through

Step 1: Determine the Biomechanical Needs of a Baseball Pitcher

MUSCLES INVOLVED AND RANGES OF MOTION

FUNCTIONS OF MUSCLES IN THROWING

Step 2: Select Best Strength/Power Exercises

CHOICE OF RESISTANCE (MACHINES, FREE WEIGHTS)

BIOMECHANICS OF STRENGTH/POWER EXERCISES

FIGURE 30–1. Steps in the design of a strength/power program.

Step 3: Incorporate into Theory of Training

CONCEPT OF PERIODIZATION

ADJUSTMENT OF PROGRAM TO SEASON

either biomechanical research or empirical evidence, the nature, magnitudes, and patterns of muscular involvement during throwing must be understood. This information must be determined in order to identify the key muscles and ranges of force application important in the throwing mechanism. It is also of additional value to ascertain the nature and frequency of any musculoskeletal injuries typical in baseball pitchers. (2) The second step entails selection of the strength/power exercises that best work the muscles of importance to throwing. Involved here is determination of the type and level of muscular involvement occurring during performance of various strength/power exercises. The objective is also to discover the proper techniques for performing a given strength/power exercise in order to best work (both effectively and safely) the key muscles of importance to throwing. (3) The third step involves consideration of an overall theory of strength/power training that is scientifically valid and within which can be blended the previous two steps in the design and implementation of a strength/power program for baseball pitchers. The baseball season's overall training plan and strength/power workouts can then be structured accordingly.

STEP ONE: THE BIOMECHANICAL DEMANDS OF PITCHING

Biomechanical research that determines the exact nature of muscular involvement in baseball pitching does not yet exist. This is not entirely unexpected, though, owing to the complexity of the research protocol needed to effectively determine this information. To date, however, the three-dimensional kinematics (displacements, velocities, and accelerations), as well as kinetics (resultant forces and moments), have been determined for three types of pitches (see Chapter 2). Additionally, in a more recent study more advanced three-dimensional modeling techniques were used to calculate spatial forces and moments for a fastball pitch.[2] Such work is continuing and with time should provide better information about the musculoskeletal demands of throwing. Electromyographic data on muscle activity in pitching[3] are of additional value in determining which individual muscles are active and when, but prediction of force levels in these muscles is not possible from electromyography alone for such dynamic events as baseball pitching.

On the basis of the biomechanical data that exist to date on pitching as well as on kinesiological and coaching insights regarding muscles important to throwing, the three areas that were considered most important to develop in the pitcher were (1) general total body strength/power, (2) acceleration capacity of the arms and shoulder girdle, and (3) deceleration capacity of the arms and shoulder girdle.

STEP TWO: SELECTION OF THE BEST STRENGTH/POWER EXERCISES

The first consideration here is the method used to apply resistance during exercise, or basically whether free weights or machines of different types should be used in the strength/power training program. At present, on the basis of available research and empirical evidence, the use of free weights as the major form of resistance in strength/power programs offers significant advantages over the use of machines.[4-8] Among the benefits of free weight resistance over machines are nonconstrained acceleration and deceleration, specificity of training, loaded counter movements, more complete joint development, body size and geometric adaptability, and so forth. Particularly for a sport motion as complex and dynamic as a baseball pitch, the advantages of free weights over available exercise machinery as the choice for resistance are significant.

Recent biomechanical research indicates that small changes in technique during a weight training exercise can have significant consequences in performance, muscle involvement, and even potential injury.[9-14] Therefore, to effectively and safely develop key muscles important to throwing, a considerable amount of attention should be given to weight training exercise techniques. Biomechanics research on the techniques of free weight exercises is far from complete, since only recently has work been initiated to investigate muscular involvement during strength/power exercises. Based typically on the performances of elite Olympic lifters or power lifters, the preferred competitive techniques of the major lifts such as squat, bench press, clean and jerk, and snatch have been reasonably investigated to date.[9, 10, 11-14] Considerable work remains, however, regarding biomechanical research on the great number of remaining noncompetitive free weight exercises involved in strength/power training programs. Until such research is completed, kinesiological intuition and empirical evidence must be used to help select the exercises and related techniques that appear to best involve key muscles important to throwing.

STEP THREE: INCORPORATION OF OVERALL THEORY OF TRAINING

Although it is entirely conceivable that any number of theories of strength/power training may someday be found to be viable, the one discussed here is presently probably the most widely supported by research and empirical evidence.[5, 15-17] The concept of "periodization" that coaches have adopted nowadays in the sport training of athletes in track, swimming, and other events is equally important in the design and implementation of strength/power training. The periodization concepts of Selye and the Russian researcher Matveyev are important to follow in the design of a strength/power program for throwing.[3, 15] The basic idea of periodization is to gradually shift from high-volume and low-intensity training in the early period (or preparation phase) of the year to an emphasis on high intensity but low volume later in the season (or competition phase). Throughout the year the amount of training in technique increases parallel with the rise in intensity. After the competition phase there is finally a period of active rest in which volume and intensity are both low and the athlete engages in recreational sports.

The major purpose of the periodization of training is to prepare the athlete for optimal levels of performance at the end of the year's competitive season. In aiming for a peak in the athlete's performance in this way, overtraining is also avoided. In the strength/power programs typically used by United States coaches the emphasis, unfortunately, is on constantly getting athletes to push themselves more at every workout throughout the year. This type of training more quickly leads to chronic fatigue or over-training. Indeed, most strength/power programs in the United States typically involve a high probability of producing negative effects from over-training.

In recent years Stone et al.[16] have worked to apply the concepts of periodization to the strength/power training of athletes. Their study series has indicated that strength/power training programs based on periodization produce superior results to programs using other set and repetition combinations. The work by Stone et al.[16] is especially indicative of how significant the improvements in strength, power, and body composition can be when the concepts of periodization are properly applied.

SYNTHESIS: STRENGTH/POWER PROGRAM FOR BASEBALL PITCHERS

Taking into account the body of knowledge gleaned from both research and empirical evidence, a strength/power training program was generated for baseball pitchers. Figure 30–2 shows the resulting year-long overview of this program, which can be seen to be broken into four distinct phases. In the first phase a base cycle of ten weeks' duration is used to develop muscle strength and hypertrophy. After this preparatory base cycle has been completed the pitcher works for nine weeks in a power cycle, in which the intensity increases to the point at which the athlete performs only two repetitions per set. This results in a peaking of the athlete's performance in terms of power production just as the season begins. During the long (approximately 30-week) season, the pitcher follows a maintenance program in the attempt to prevent significant losses in the strength and power developed in the two off-season cycles. When the season is over it is important for the pitcher to take three weeks of active rest, in which recreational activities other than baseball or weight training are engaged in.

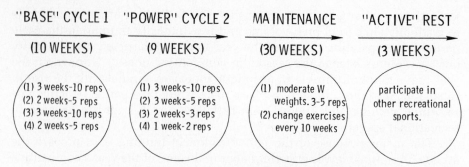

FIGURE 30–2. Year plan for baseball. Reps = repetitions.

In terms of specific training methods, Tables 30–1 to 30–3 give sample exercises for the base cycle, the power cycle, and the maintenance phases of the year. When reviewing these tables, it is important to also note Figure 30–2, which gives the repetitions to be used at different times during a cycle. For example, the first three weeks of the base cycle have the pitcher doing three sets of ten repetitions in all of the exercises shown in Table 30–2. If he could do wide grip bench presses on Monday with 200 pounds, he would use 170 pounds on Friday. As the athlete increases his 100 per cent poundages each week, the lighter percentages are increased appropriately.

In order to fully benefit from this program, a number of specific points need to be made. (1) The exercises in Tables 30–1 to 30–3 should be followed in the order given, with the compound, larger muscle mass exercises coming earlier in the workout. (2) Only free weights are used, and whenever possible dumbbells are preferred because of associated greater degrees of freedom. (3) A preworkout warm-up should be used before all workouts, and this should include flexibility work followed by light total body exercises for three sets of ten repetitions using only the bar for light clean and jerks. (4) Each exercise in Tables 30–1 to 30–3 should begin with one light to moderate specific warm-up set using the same repetitions as called for in that day's exercise. (5) All exercises in these tables should be done for three sets. (6) Poundage used on the 100 per cent intensity days should be increased whenever possible (as long as good technique is not sacrificed), and that used on the lighter-percentage days should be scaled upward proportionately. (7) In all exercises, emphasis should be placed on being as "explosive" as possible (to work as closely as possible to the force/velocity curve). (8) All sets of a given exercise should be completed before the next exercise is begun, with approximately two minutes' rest between sets. (9) Each workout should also be ended with flexibility work as time permits.

Regarding the techniques used in performing these exercises every effort should be made to perform the movements properly. If the techniques of these strength/power exercises are not understood, then reference should be made to such sources as the referenced articles, the *National Strength*

TABLE 30–1. SAMPLE PROGRAM FOR BASE CYCLE 1

	MONDAY		WEDNESDAY		FRIDAY
	Exercises	*Intensity**	*Exercises*	*Intensity*	FRIDAY
(1)	Wide grip bench press	(100%)	(1) Medium stance squats	(100%)	(1) Same exercises as in Monday workout, except that no squats are performed
(2)	Wide grip bent rowing	(100%)	(2) Wide grip high pulls	(100%)	
(3)	Lying triceps press	(100%)	(3) Wide grip shrugs	(100%)	
(4)	Concentration curl	(100%)	(4) Back extensions	(100%)	(2) Intensity is 85% for all exercises.
(5)	Dumbbell press	(100%)	(5) Abdominal curl-ups	(100%)	
(6)	Shoulder laterals	(100%)	(6) Dumbbell chest flies	(70%)	
(7)	Barbell T-bench press	(100%)	(7) Wide grip lateral pulls to chest	(70%)	
(8)	Medium stance squats*	(50%)	(8) Shoulder laterals	(70%)	
(9)	Abdominal curl-ups*	(50%)	(9) Forearms (optional)	(70%)	
(10)	Forearms (optional)	(100%)			

*Intensity is based on the amount of weight the athlete can lift for a required set and repetition combination. For example, 100 per cent means that the maximal weight used is that which permits performance of all three sets of whatever repetitions are used (as indicated in Fig. 30–2).

TABLE 30–2. SAMPLE PROGRAM FOR POWER CYCLE 2

	MONDAY		WEDNESDAY		FRIDAY
	Exercises	*Intensity**	*Exercises*	*Intensity*	FRIDAY
(1)	Dumbbell bench press	(100%)	(1) Wide stance (outside shoulder width squats)	(100%)	(1) Same exercises as in Monday workout, except that no squats are performed
(2)	Dumbbell bent rowing	(100%)			
(3)	Close grip (approximately 6") bench press	(100%)	(2) Medium grip high pulls	(100%)	
			(3) Medium grip shrugs	(100%)	(2) Intensity is 85% for all exercises.
(4)	Supinating dumbbell curl	(100%)	(4) Back extensions	(100%)	
(5)	Dumbbell press	(100%)	(5) Abdominal curl-ups	(100%)	
(6)	Shoulder laterals	(100%)	(6) Dumbbell chest flies	(70%)	
(7)	Dumbbell T-bench press	(100%)	(7) Medium grip lateral pulls to chest	(70%)	
(8)	Wide stance outside (shoulder-width) squats	(100%)	(8) Shoulder laterals	(70%)	
(9)	Abdominal curl-ups	(50%)	(9) Forearms (optional)	(70%)	
(10)	Forearms (optional)	(100%)			

*Intensity is based on the amount of weight the athlete can lift for a required set and repetition combination. For example, 100 per cent means that the maximal weight used is that which permits performance of all three sets of whatever repetitions are used (as indicated in Fig. 30–2).

TABLE 30–3. SAMPLE PROGRAMS FOR MAINTENANCE (IN SEASON)

(1) First 10 Weeks		(2) Second 10 Weeks	
Day One	Day Two	Day One	Day Two
(1) Squats (¼ only) medium stance*	(1) Squats, medium stance	(1) Outside shoulder stance squats	(1) Outside shoulder stance squats
(2) Wide grip bench press	(2) Wide grip high pulls	(2) Dumbbell bench press	(2) Medium grip shrugs
(3) Wide grip bent rowing	(3) Concentration curls	(3) Dumbbell bent rowing	(3) Dumbbell press
(4) Dumbbell press	(4) Lying triceps press	(4) Shoulder laterals	(4) Twist curls
(5) Back extensions	(5) Shoulder laterals	(5) Back extensions	(5) Close grip bench press
(6) Abdominal curl-ups	(6) Barbell T-bench press	(6) Abdominal curl-ups	(6) Dumbbell T-bench
(7) Forearms (optional)	(7) Abdominal curl-ups	(7) Forearms (optional)	(7) Abdominal curl-ups
	(8) Forearms (optional)		(8) Forearms (optional)

*Intensity for the entire maintenance program is approximately 70 to 85 per cent for all exercises. As shown in Fig. 30–2, three sets of three to five repetitions are used for all exercises.

and Conditioning Association Journal, strength/power athletes, the author, or other sources. The first few weeks of each cycle in particular should be spent in demonstrating and emphasizing the proper techniques of new exercises to the pitchers. Technique in all exercises should be monitored continuously throughout the year, especially at the end of the power cycle, when the heaviest weights are used.

Tables 30–1 to 30–3 show that much mechanical variation is used in the program. In other words, different exercises are used in workouts during the week, and exercises are either modified or replaced by similar movements every cycle or ten weeks. This process is important to continued improvement and follows the periodization concept. Regarding individual exercise techniques, it is not possible to discuss all the techniques here. The reader is again referred to the sources listed previously. Most of the exercises are named according to the typical jargon used by strength/power athletes and coaches. However, Figures 30–3 to 30–6 show some of the movements that need some technical clarification. Figure 30–3 shows the technique used in the dumbbell T-bench exercise, in which an elbow flexion angle of about 90 degrees is maintained throughout, and the upper arm stays in contact with the second bench. Figure 30–4 shows that the dumbbell press exercise is performed with the palms facing the head, not forward. The shoulder laterals shown in Figure 30–5 should be done with lighter dumbbells and with emphasis on acceleration and deceleration, especially at the end points of the exercise. As an excellent warm-up for pitchers before throwing, this exercise, as well as laterals in other planes, should be done with little or no weights over a smaller range near the shoulder level to emphasize short acceleration and deceleration motions. The back extension shown in Figure 30–6 illustrates the preferential body positioning, with bent knees, a flat back, and a raised support under the lumbar spine.

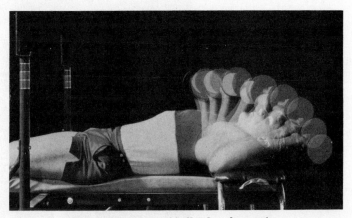

FIGURE 30–3. Dumbbell T-bench exercise.

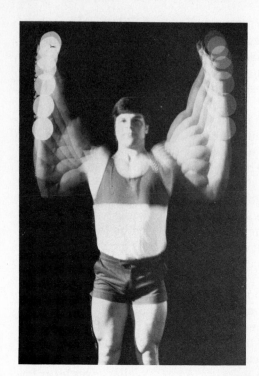

FIGURE 30–4. Dumbbell press.

FIGURE 30–5. Shoulder lateral.

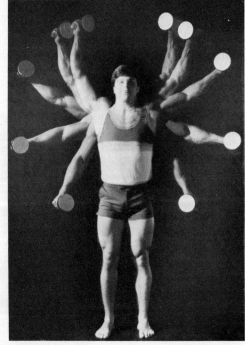

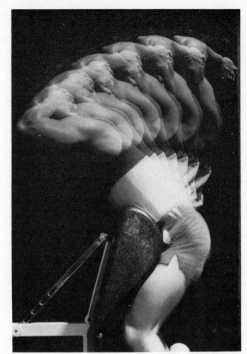

FIGURE 30–6. Back extensions.

REFERENCES

1. Atha, J.: Strengthening muscle. *In* D. I. Miller (ed.): Exercise and Sport Sciences Reviews. Vol. 9. Philadelphia, The Franklin Institute, 1981, pp. 1–74.
2. Horn, T.: An analytical solution to the determination of the resultant forces and torques occurring at the shoulder joint during baseball pitching. MS thesis. Atlanta, Auburn University, 1984.
3. Jobe, F. W., Tibone, J. E., Perry, J., and Moynes, D.: An EMG analysis of the shoulder in throwing and pitching. Am J Sports Med 11:3–5, 1983.
4. Garhammer, J.: Equipment for the development of athletic strength and power. National Strength and Conditioning Association Journal 3:6, 1981.
5. McLaughlin, T. M.: Strength building with free weights. *In* World Swimming Clinic Yearbook. American Swim Coaches Association, New Orleans, LA, 1980, pp. 157–168.
6. McLaughlin, T. M.: A consumer guide for selecting free weight or machine exercises. Part I. Powerlifting, USA 31–32, May, 1984.
7. Stone, M. H., and Garhammer, J.: Some thoughts on strength and power. National Strength and Conditioning Association Journal 3:5, 1981.
8. Stone, M. H.: Considerations in gaining strength-power training effect (machines vs. free weights). National Strength and Conditioning Association Journal 4:1, 1982.
9. Enoka, R. M.: The pull in Olympic weightlifting. Med Sci Sports 11:131–137, 1979.
10. Garhammer, J.: Biochemical characteristics of the 1978 world weightlifting champions. *In* Biomechanics VII-B. Baltimore, University Park Press, 1981, pp. 300–304.
11. Madsen, N., and McLaughlin, T. M.: Kinematic factors affecting performance and injury risk in the bench press exercise. Med Sci Sports Exerc 15:376–381, 1984.
12. McLaughlin, T. M., Dillman, C. J., and Lardner, T. J.: A kinematic model of performance in the parallel squat. Med Sci Sports 9:128–133, 1977.

13. McLaughlin, T. M., Lardner, T. J., and Dillman, C. J.: Kinetics of the parallel squat. Res Q 49:175–189, 1978.
14. McLaughlin, T. M., and Madsen, N.: Bench press techniques of elite heavyweight powerlifters. National Strength and Conditioning Association Journal (in press).
15. Garhammer, J.: Periodization of strength training for athletes. Track Technique 73:2398–2399, 1979.
16. Stone, M., O'Brien, H., Garhammer, J., McMillan, J., and Rozenek, R.: A theoretical model of strength training. National Strength and Conditioning Association Journal Aug/Sept, 36–39, 1982.
17. Tschiene, P.: Power training principles for top-class throwers. Track Technique 52:1642–1654, 1973.

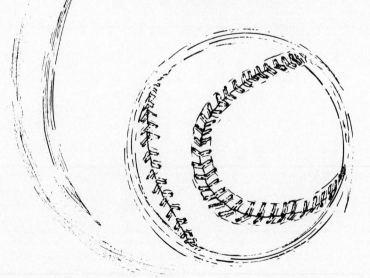

PART FIVE

THE THROWING MOTION IN OTHER SPORTS

TENNIS SERVING COMPARED WITH BASEBALL PITCHING

ROBERT LEACH, M.D.

The act of pitching a baseball and that of hitting a tennis serve are often compared in discussions of chronic shoulder rotator cuff problems. Baseball pitchers and tennis players have similar acute and chronic shoulder symptoms. However, there are major differences between the two actions despite the similarity of resulting shoulder disorders.

In tennis the player uses a racquet, which can be regarded as an extension of his arm, to strike the tennis ball. Much of the impact force of the racquet hitting the ball is dissipated at the racquet-ball interface by the strings and the racquet frame and even by the wrist and forearm so that less force is transmitted to the shoulder. The energy applied to the ball is provided by the speed of the arm and racquet and by the force applied to the ball. Both are a function of strength and leverage supplied by the arm's length and its extension, the racquet length. This energy causes a served tennis ball to go considerably faster than a pitched baseball. Many leading tennis players have had their serves consistently timed at over 120 miles per hour; the record timed by a radar gun is over 140 miles per hour. In contrast, the fastest Major League baseball pitchers throw the ball in the range of 93 to 97 miles per hour, with many not making 90 miles per hour.

The force generated to cause a tennis ball to go so fast apparently does not have a severe impact on the shoulder rotator cuff. A hard-fought three-set tennis match with scores of 6–4, 4–6, 6–4 would mean that each player would serve 15 games in the match. If nine serves per game is taken as an average, there would be 135 serves in the match. Obviously many matches are longer and others shorter. Under many circumstances a tennis player would serve this amount on a daily basis virtually throughout the year. In many instances players in college or on the professional tour or amateur circuit play doubles on the same day, which would increase the number of serves hit per day. A Major League baseball pitcher generally pitches every fourth day. In the course of a nine-inning game he usually throws between 110 and 130 pitches. On the day after such a game his arm is so sore that it is literally difficult to raise it. The second day following his pitching performance he feels better and can throw easily. By the third day after pitching he is working out normally and is ready to start either the fourth or fifth day after the previous game. Also, the baseball season is shorter than the tennis season, which is now year-round. Thus, there appears to be less force exerted on the shoulder structures in the tennis playing than in baseball pitching, if muscle soreness can be taken as a reflection of strain applied. In all probability the use of the racquet and the leverage imparted by this provides the increased force for delivering the ball and may decrease strain on the shoulder.

There are differences in the pitching motion compared with the usual tennis serve. The pitcher generally starts with a wind-up in which there is some internal rotation at the shoulder, and as the player cocks his arm the shoulder goes into extreme external rotation. There is a period of acceleration backward and then a major deceleration with a subsequent forward acceleration. There is great stress on the shoulder muscles at the deceleration point, and then the body comes forward and the arm uncocks and goes into the acceleration phase. The arm is then brought forcibly into internal rotation and adduction in this final phase as the ball is released (Fig. 31–1). The pitcher attempts to almost literally throw the arm away from the body and is prevented from doing this by the muscle tendon units around the shoulder, including the triceps and the rotator cuff. The specific pitch being thrown may determine how much internal rotation is actually occurring at the shoulder as well as the stresses put on the elbow and wrist as the pitcher follows through to deliver the final twist that determines how the ball performs.

In tennis most players start with the shoulder in neutral or slight internal rotation. As the racquet is raised and the racquet head is allowed to drop down behind the back there may be slight external rotation but much less than the amount of external rotation that the baseball pitcher has in his cocking phase (Fig. 31–2). The arm is then elevated, and as the racquet head goes up and forward there is some internal rotation of the arm but again less internal rotation and less adduction at the shoulder, even with the follow-through, than in the baseball pitcher. Also, the tennis player is not throwing the shoulder directly forward away from the body but is controlling the racquet as it hits the ball. This element of control seems to render less strain at muscle tendon units controlling the shoulder. Stress is

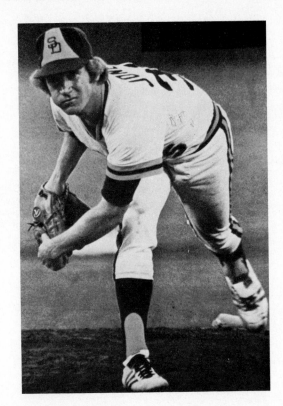

FIGURE 31–1. The follow-through demonstrates marked internal rotation in this baseball pitcher.

delivered to the elbow and the wrist, but there is less deceleration force around the shoulder in the tennis serve than in the baseball pitch.

The majority of rotator cuff problems occur in tennis players at age 40 or 50 who have played for a long period of time. Few young tennis players have major shoulder problems from which they are unable to recover. In contrast, in baseball pitching each year a certain number of baseball pitchers in high school, college, and the professional leagues have acute or chronic rotator cuff problems that end their baseball pitching careers.

Tennis players frequently play all of their lives. As they continue to play, the repetitive nature of serving and hitting overheads and high forehand and backhand volleys does seem to cause wear and tear on the rotator cuff. Many people in the Junior Veterans and Senior categories have chronic shoulder problems culminating with small attritional tears of the rotator cuff or chronic tendinitis. There are far fewer people who continue to pitch baseballs at age 45 or 55. However, in another throwing sport, softball, in which the pitching is underhand with a completely different stress on the shoulder, it is unusual to have shoulder problems. Many softball pitchers play well into their 40s.

Thus, there are major differences between the physical acts of pitching

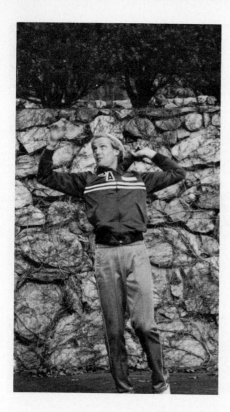

FIGURE 31–2. The early phase of a tennis serve shows only slight external rotation. The appearance of more shoulder external rotation is caused by laying back the wrist.

a baseball and hitting a tennis serve. In tennis the serving motion appears to be less violent with regard to the rotator cuff but if repeated over many years can cause gradual shoulder disability because of impingement of the rotator cuff against the coracoacromial arch. In baseball, pitching appears to be a more forceful motion with more marked internal rotation and adduction produced at the shoulder to force the anterior part of the rotator cuff against the coracoacromial arch.

WATER POLO INJURIES TO THE UPPER EXTREMITY

JOHN ROLLINS, M.D. / JAMES C. PUFFER, M.D. /
WILLIAM C. WHITING, Ph.D. / ROBERT J. GREGOR, Ph.D. /
GERALD A. M. FINERMAN, M.D.

Injuries to the upper extremity caused by the throwing motion in sports have generated extensive research and analysis. However, the inherent difficulties of the water environment have minimized examination of the throwing motion in water polo. Previous studies of throwing in water polo have been limited to a qualitative evaluation of wrist and shoulder movements and a two-dimensional cinematographic analysis of the overhand throw.[1,2]

Recently the authors have used three-dimensional techniques to analyze the mechanism of throwing in members of the United States Men's Water Polo Team. For these studies each player was filmed using two high-speed 16-mm motor-driven cameras with a phase-lock system that insured synchronous recordings from the cameras. Subjects were encouraged to throw with maximal velocity at a standard water polo goal. Appropriate locations of the shoulder, elbow, and wrist joint centers were marked so that they could be identified and analyzed digitally by a minicomputer. A direct linear transformation algorithm was used to provide three-dimensional coordinate locations of the shoulder, elbow, wrist, and ball. By utilizing computer techniques it was possible to calculate coordinates of the joint centers and the ball in three dimensions. Such analysis permits both descriptive and numerical analysis of the throwing motion in water polo.[3]

KINEMATIC ANALYSIS

The patterns of the throwing motion in the upper extremity in water polo are similar to those in other throwing sports such as baseball. There is an initial stance or positioning phase, the wind-up, the throw by forward motion of the arm, and the follow-through (Fig. 32–1 to 32–4). The actual throwing motion involves spinal rotation, humeral medial rotation, forward arm extension and pronation, and hand flexion with hip and lateral spine flexion at release. However, although the basic throwing mechanism is similar, there are certain important modifications in water polo. The initial stance includes holding the ball out of the water, positioning the opposite arm in front for balance, and an egg-beater motion of the legs to maintain position. The wind-up includes cocking of the throwing arm, vertical upward push with the leg kick, ball push-off, and a pull with the opposite or steadying arm. During the moment before throwing, the ipsilateral hip is abducted and the contralateral hip is flexed. The humerus is universally held oriented nearly perpendicular to the spinal axis (abducted 90 degrees through flexion of 90 degrees). Greater elbow flexion and external humeral

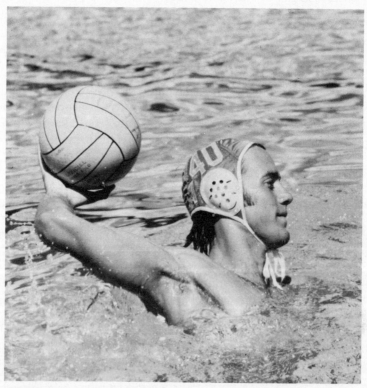

FIGURE 32–1. Initial positioning phase of water polo throwing motion.

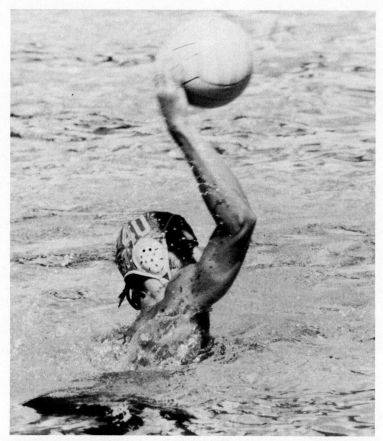

FIGURE 32–2. Throwing or acceleration phase of water polo throwing motion.

rotation are related to increased ball velocity. Forceful wrist flexion at the end of the throwing motion is minimal. Simultaneous with the arm motion there is lateral spine flexion and extension of the contralateral hip and knee. The follow-through involves hip and spine flexion while the arm is extended and internally rotated.

The authors' studies based on three-dimensional analysis have provided kinematic parameters of throwing in healthy members of the United States Water Polo Team. These data indicate that there is elbow peak angular velocity of approximately 1200 degrees per second. In comparison, high-velocity baseball throwers have been shown to extend their elbows at a rate in excess of 2200 degrees per second. This difference can be explained by the lack of ground support for water polo throwers and the necessity to propel a much larger ball. It is obvious that the task of accelerating a ball to an average release velocity of nearly 20 meters per second during 226

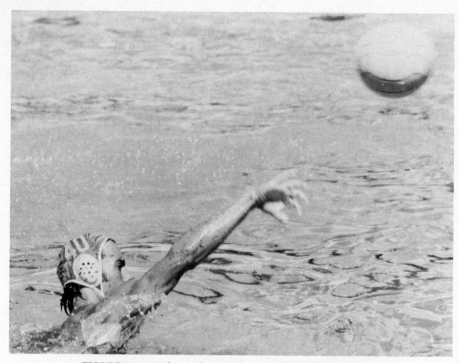

FIGURE 32–3. Release phase of water polo throwing motion.

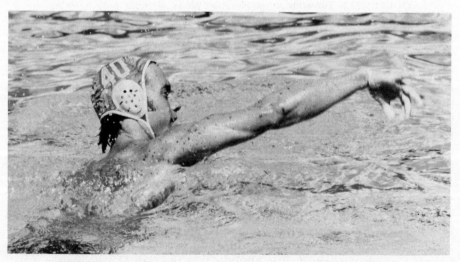

FIGURE 32–4. Follow-through phase of water polo throwing motion.

milliseconds involves considerable stress to the shoulder and upper extremity. It is hoped that further study and computer modeling will allow computation of the forces applied to the upper extremity in throwing motions. Representative kinematic parameters are presented in Table 32–1.[3]

INJURIES

Injuries to the upper extremity in water polo are quite similar to those in other throwing sports. Data for all injuries during 1982 for members of the United States National Water Polo Team revealed a 36 per cent incidence of rotator cuff tendinitis and a 2 per cent incidence of acromioclavicular joint degeneration. Kennedy[4] and Richardson[5] previously called attention to the incidence of acromial impingement syndrome in swimmers. Therefore, the water polo competitor is potentially at high risk, since he must condition himself both for swimming and for throwing.

The predominant injury pattern seen in water polo is subacromial impingement. Neer's anatomic dissections and explanation of the pathophysiology demonstrate that impingement occurs anteriorly under the acromion and coracoacromial ligament.[6] This injury occurs with the humerus flexed and internally rotated, in a position obtained during termination of the throwing motion. Usually the subacromial impingement syndrome is not severe enough to result in loss of competitive time. The data confirm that in 1982 no National Team player missed a game because of this complaint. The impingement syndrome is more frequently seen in international class competitors than in members of collegiate teams. This fact may be explained by the years of participation and increased demands of competition in international events. Occasionally more advanced stages of the subacromial impingement syndrome are evidenced by continued and

TABLE 32–1. KINEMATIC PARAMETERS OF AVERAGED THROW CYCLES[*3]

	MEAN	STANDARD ERROR
Duration of throw (millisecond)	226.6	9.1
Peak angular velocity (elbow) (degree/second)	1181.8	44.6
Angular velocity at release (elbow) (degree/second)	738.1	41.4
Time from peak angular velocity to release (milliseconds)	28.2	2.0
Elbow angle at peak angular velocity (degree)	126.6	2.1
Elbow angle at release (degree)	155.5	1.9
Ball velocity at release (meter/second)	19.3	0.5

*n = 14.

multiple episodes of injury. This syndrome responds to conservative treatment, including the application of ice after exercise and the judicious use of nonsteroidal anti-inflammatory agents. Long-term rest and even occasional local steroid injections may be required to treat this advanced injury. Severe degeneration and rotator cuff tear are common in water polo players.

The subacromial impingement syndrome must be differentiated from inflammation of the acromioclavicular joint. Water polo players with impingement syndrome complain of pain occurring throughout the throwing motion or at terminal release. Tenderness over the supraspinatus tendon and coracoacromial ligament are noted. Pain can be elicited by the combined flexion, adduction, internal rotation, or impingement test. The water polo player with acromioclavicular joint problems complains of severe pain with cocking of the arm, and examination reveals point tenderness over the acromioclavicular joint area.

Shoulder dislocation is frequently seen in the international competitor but also has been seen in the collegiate athlete. The mechanism of injury is striking of the arm by an opposing player, with forced abduction and external rotation causing a typical anterior dislocation of the shoulder. The incidence of shoulder dislocation occurring during water polo is approximately 1 to 2 per cent. Since water polo requires extensive swimming conditioning, selected paralysis related to traction of neural elements or compression by muscle hypertrophy has been noted. The most frequent of these neurologic complications is paralysis of the suprascapular nerve. The athlete frequently complains of weakness of the shoulder. Careful observations shows specific atrophy of the supraspinatus and infraspinatus muscles.

Elbow injuries are less frequent in water polo than in other throwing sports. This decreased frequency is probably due to the large ball size and reduced forceful flexion of the wrist in the terminal phase of throwing. Players who do have elbow pain almost always demonstrate evidence of medial epicondylitis on physical examination. Qualitative analysis of their shooting technique usually reveals that the ball is thrown in a side-arm fashion with forceful terminal wrist flexion rather than the more conventional overhead throw.

SUMMARY

Analysis of the throwing motion in water polo has shown numerous similarities to the basic throwing mechanism of other sports. However, the large ball and the inability to plant the feet creates specific differences that may increase the stress to the shoulder. The water polo player faces increased risk, since he must condition himself by an extensive swimming program and carry out a forceful throwing motion. The injury most frequently observed is the subacromial impingement syndrome. Fortunately this injury rarely leads to degeneration or rupture of the rotator cuff in this group of athletes.

REFERENCES

1. Clarys, J. P., and Lewillie, L.: The description of wrist and shoulder motion of different water polo shots using a simple light-trace technique. In First International Symposium on Biomechanics in Swimming, Water Polo and Diving, Proceedings. Bruxelles, University Libre de Bruxelles, 1971, pp. 249–256.
2. Davis, T., and Blanksby, B. A.: A cinematographic analysis of the overhand water polo throw. J Sports Med Phys Fitness 17:5–16, 1977.
3. Whiting, W.C., Puffer, J. C., Finerman, G. A. M., Gregor, R. J., and Maletis, G. B.: Three dimensional cinematographic analysis of water polo throwing in elite performers. Am J Sports Med (in press).
4. Kennedy, J. C., and Hawkins, R. J.: Swimmer's shoulder. Phys Sportsmed 2:34–38, 1974.
5. Richardson, A. B., Jobe, F. W., and Collins, H. B.: The shoulder in competitive swimming. Am J Sports Med 8:159–163, 1980.
6. Neer, C. S.: Anterior acromioplasty for the chronic impingement syndrome in the shoulder. J Bone Joint Surg 54A:41–50, 1972.

SHOULDER PROBLEMS IN SWIMMERS

FRANK A. PETTRONE, M.D.

INTRODUCTION

The purpose of this chapter is to analyze the effects of competitive swimming on the shoulder. Proper stroke technique is reviewed. The pathology of and recommendations for treatment of swimmer's shoulder are discussed. Suggestions for stroke correction are made.

Competitive swimming has long been a popular sport in the United States. With every Olympic games interest grows. There are probably now over 200,000 competitive year-round swimmers under 25 years of age in the United States and over one-half million part-time competitive swimmers, including swimmers in country clubs, recreational swimmers, and high school seniors who are training regularly. In addition, over one million people swim recreationally.

Training techniques in the United States currently range from 10,000 to 25,000 meters or 8 to 12 miles of swimming a day, six days a week. In a typical training regimen of swimming 10,000 meters a day for six days a week in a 12-month period each shoulder goes through 660,000 strokes. The Soviets, preparing their athletes for the 1980 Olympics, trained their swimmers at 30 miles a day. The consequence of arduous training schedules, in relation to early burnout, premature wearing out of the rotator cuff, and other overuse syndromes should be considered.

SWIMMING STROKES

Freestyle

In the freestyle stroke, the stroke motion consists of pulling down forcibly into adduction and internal rotation. Aproximately 90 per cent of the stroke propulsion comes from the upper extremities. During the pull-through phase, the latissimus dorsi, teres major, and triceps brachii muscles are active. In the recovery phase, the deltoid and trapezius muscles become dominant. The direction in which the hand travels during pull-through in freestyle swimming has been described as the inverted question mark by Councilman.[1] The hand is moving against still water, and the swimmer essentially pulls forward by utilizing water inertia. Coaches emphasize the longest arm pull possible in order to maximize forward propulsion from each stroke. This results in a longer smoother stroke with fewer strokes per distance.

Breast Stroke

In the breast stroke, butterfly, and backstroke the hands are also pulled through in an elliptical pattern, not a straight line. In the breast stroke the arms must move in a simultaneous and similar manner, and no out-of-water recovery of the arms is permitted. The legs must move in a simultaneous and similar manner. The frog kick must be used. The head must break the surface of the water at all times. The pull pattern of the arms is described as an inverted heart-shaped path.[1] The stroke begins with the palms facing diagonally outward. The arms are then pulled outward, downward, and back (but without crossing the midline).

Backstroke

In the backstroke the mechanism of force is similar to that in the breast stroke, the butterfly, and the backstroke, is replicable, but adds another problem. Starting in a position of maximal abduction, the arm goes into external rotation at the start of pull-through. This motion forces the humeral head forward and stretches the anterior capsule. The arm then progresses into adduction and internal rotation. During arm pull the elbow is bent 90 degrees. The hand should enter the water in a knifelike manner with the little finger first, and at recovery the thumb should leave the water first. The arm pull from the side describes an S-shaped pattern.[1]

Butterfly

In the butterfly both arms are recovered over the water while the legs kick upward and downward in a dolphin or fishtail kick. Two kicks of the legs are completed with each arm cycle. The arms' cycles must be similar and simultaneous. The arm pull-through pattern is described as an hourglass shape.[1]

SWIMMER'S SHOULDER

Swimmer's shoulder refers to the typical pain pattern of the subacromial impingement syndrome. The supraspinatus tendon, as the most superior component of the rotator cuff, passes beneath the coracoacromial arch (bone and ligament). The supraspinatus tendon is then most susceptible to abrasive wear with repetitive use.

The impingement phenomenon in swimmers is described as a "wringing out" of the rotator cuff as the arm adducts and internally rotates. MacNab[2] has demonstrated vessels filled at abduction that are "wrung out" as the arm is brought down and inward (Fig. 33–1). The mechanism of impingement is similar in the freestyle stroke, the butterfly, and the backstroke (Figs. 33–2 to 33–5). In each stroke there is internal rotation and adduction with the pull-through phase and external rotation with abduction in the recovery phase. The consequences of these training regimens on the shoulder are adaptation and hypertrophy; however, overuse syndromes also can occur. The rotator cuff can fray and develop an inflammatory response and edema. The result can be impingement. Past beliefs that childhood rotator cuff tears never occur may soon be questioned when children are observed who start competitive swimming with intense training at 6 years of age and continue until age 18. This overuse progresses to impingement syndromes. A number of studies[3, 4] that have looked at various elite world-class swimmers show that at least one half, probably even two thirds, of these athletes have developed impingement and shoulder problems severe enough to stop training for a significant period of time.

These problems are seen more often in the sprinter and the middle-distance swimmer than in the distance swimmer. Rotator cuff tendinitis is exacerbated by the use of hand paddles and foot-weight devices that are used to augment the work load and to increase the intensity of training. It is seen more commonly in early and midseason than in the highly competitive year-end season.

PATHOLOGY RELATED TO STROKE MECHANICS AND THEIR MODIFICATION

With adduction in these strokes (coming across the midline), impingement results in the anterior aspect of the cuff. Stroke modification can be

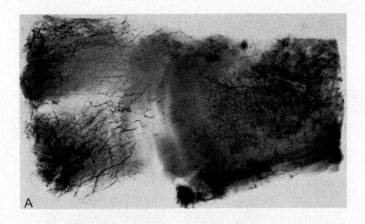

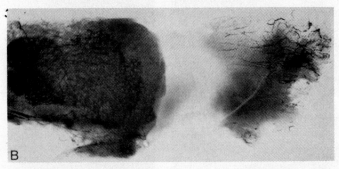

FIGURE 33–1. Injection study demonstrating vascularity of the rotator cuff: *A.* Injection with arm abducted. *B.* Injection with arm by the side in neutral rotation. It is to be noted that with the arm abducted there is almost full filling of the vessels to the point of insertion of the tendon, whereas with the arm by the side there is a large area of apparent avascularity. (Reprinted, with permission, from Rathbun, J. B., and MacNab, I., "The microvascular pattern of the rotator cuff," *Journal of Bone Joint Surgery* 52B:540, 1970.)

quite helpful at this point. Ideally the middle fingers in freestyle swimming should enter the water first. If the thumb and index fingers are first, this suggests too much internal rotation of the arm, and correction is needed. Increased elbow height at recovery and increased body roll can relieve shoulder impingement, especially in freestyle swimming. These modifications are used to correct the frequent error of straight arm recovery. In the freestyle stroke the impingement syndrome usually occurs on the dominant arm side, which is also the side on which a breath is taken.

The consequence of prolonged adduction of the shoulder, however, is prolonged hypovascularity of the supraspinatus muscle.[2] A possible correc-

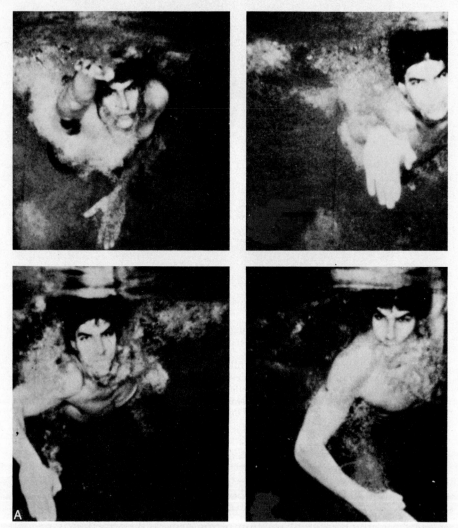

FIGURE 33–2. Freestyle swimming. (Reprinted, with permission, from Councilman, J., *The Science of Swimming*, New Jersey, Prentice Hall, 1968.)

Illustration continued on opposite page

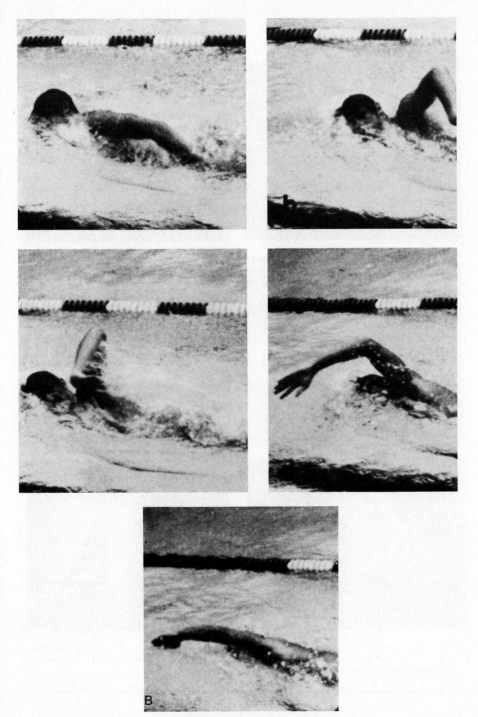

FIGURE 33–2. *Continued.*

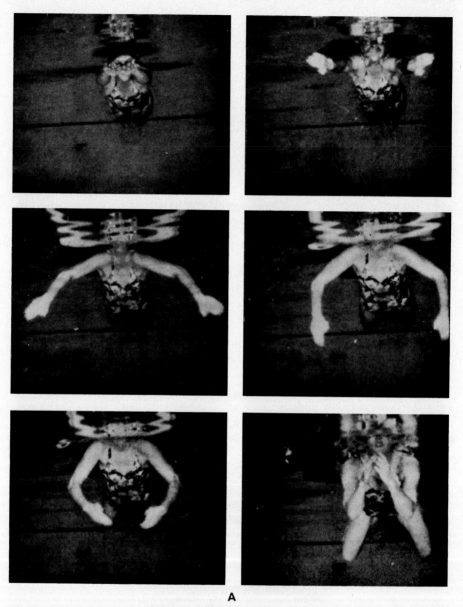

A

FIGURE 33–3. Breast stroke. (Reprinted, with permission, from Councilman, J., *The Science of Swimming*, New Jersey, Prentice Hall, 1968.)

Illustration continued on opposite page

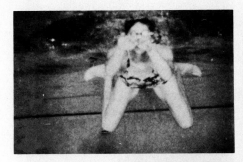
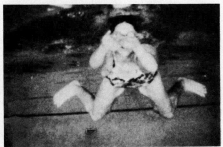
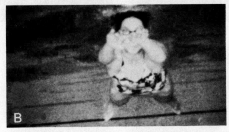

FIGURE 33–3. *Continued.*

tion in technique would be to shorten the pull-through phase—that is, to begin the recovery phase earlier. This would lead to more strokes per distance but relatively fewer periods of supraspinatus hypovascularity. Good technique would allow the elbow to clear the water and the trunk to roll away in recovery (approximately 90-degree body roll). In freestyle swimming the swimmer tries to remain flat for streamlining. If the head and shoulder are carried too high, the hips and legs drop lower in the water and cause greater drag effect. Sprinters tend to hydroplane more than other swimmers. Some of this effect is improved by trunk rotation with each stroke.

Butterfly swimmers with painful shoulders can modify their technique by breathing on every stroke instead of on every other stroke in order to keep the head up. Shortening follow-through is also useful. It is important to not let the arms enter the water too far outside the shoulder width.

In the breast stroke arm pull with no bend in the elbows is a common error to be corrected. Dropping the elbows and putting them into the ribs frequently causes a disruption of the continuous arm motion, and the swimmer sinks lower into the water while trying to breathe too long.[1]

The most common error in backstroke is pull-through with a straight elbow. This frequently creates a straight-line pull rather than an S-shaped pattern.[1]

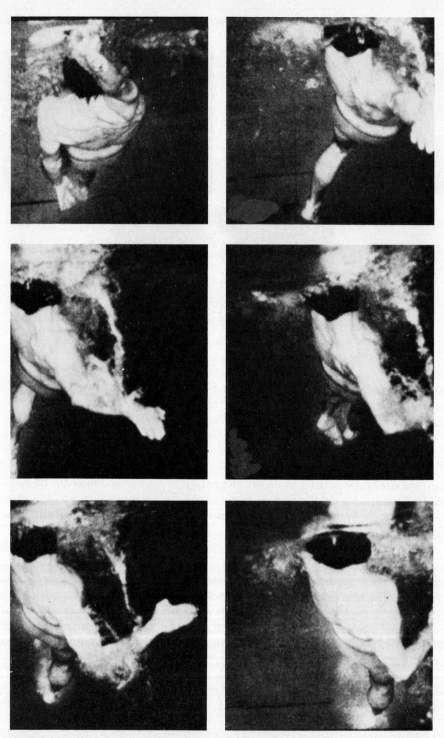

FIGURE 33–4. Backstroke. (Reprinted, with permission, from Councilman, J., *The Science of Swimming*, New Jersey, Prentice Hall, 1968.)

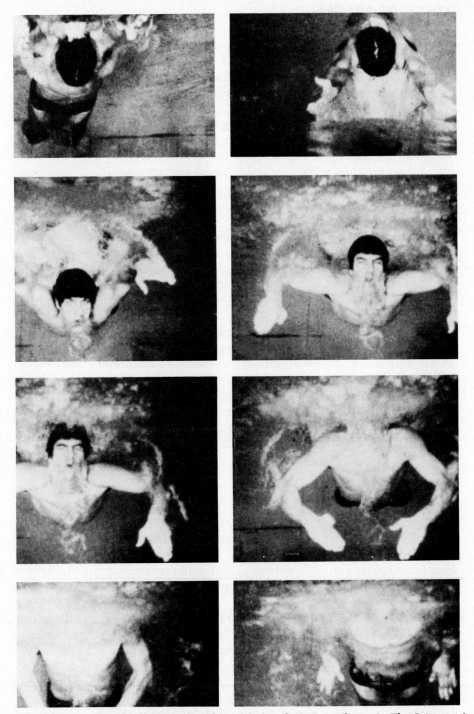

FIGURE 33–5. Butterfly. (Reprinted, with permission, from Councilman, J., *The Science of Swimming*, New Jersey, Prentice Hall, 1968.)

OTHER PROBLEMS

In the backstroke stretch and subluxation of the shoulder are observed. These are more of a problem at the flip turn and again at the pull-through phase under water. This pattern is termed "hesitation shoulder," with shoulder subluxation occurring at the flip turn. Medial epicondylitis is also associated with the backstroke, with an increased medial elbow tensile force occurring at the pull-through phase.

In the breast stroke, knee injuries such as bursitis, sprain, and meniscal pathology are also seen.

EXAMINATION

A dull aching pain in the subacromial or subdeltoid area is characteristically described by the patient. Pain is not located above the clavicle or below the elbow. If it is, other causes should be considered. The phases of impingement syndrome are (1) dull ache noted after workout, (2) pain that occurs during and after workout and leads to decreased distance, and (3) inability to participate.

On examination there may be palpable tenderness at the anterolateral edge of the acromion or over the biceps groove. Typically pain is reproduced on forceful abduction overhead, across-the-chest adduction, and resisted forward flexion. Examination of the patient in a supine position with abduction and external rotation is necessary to evaluate anterior instability. Either apprehension or frank instability is seen. Glenoid labrum tears may be suspected if on passive forward and backward motion of the humeral head a clicking or pop is noted that reproduces the patient's pain.

TREATMENT

Early treatment of the swimmer's shoulder includes (1) warm-up consisting of running in place (to raise body temperature) followed by flexibility exercises, (2) "warm-down" stretch exercises, (3) "icing down" after practice, (4) anti-inflammatory medication (preferably aspirin or non-steroidal anti-inflammatories), and (5) possibly stroke alteration and weight training.

Steroid injections should be resorted to infrequently. The consequence of collagen breakdown after injection in a training athlete is worrisome. If an injection is deemed necessary, strict rest for ten days subsequently is suggested.

Rest and exercise out of water may become necessary with injuries that are unresponsive to more conservative treatment. When the swimmer experiences night pain, alterations in the sleeping position are useful. These include (1) sleeping supine with the affected arm up on a pillow, (2) sleeping in a side-lying position propped up on pillows, or (3) if sleeping on the opposite nonaffected shoulder, cradling of a pillow under the affected arm.

Roentgenographic evaluation is necessary beginning with anteroposterior and axillary lateral views. A West Point view is useful in the subluxating shoulder. Also useful in the evaluation of lesions of the labrum is arthrotomography. For the older athlete with rotator cuff pathology, arthrography is useful.

Surgery to relieve impingement in swimmers produces only marginal or disappointing results. Postoperative return to past high levels of athletic performance is rare. The primary procedure is resection of the coracoacromial ligament (the arch).[4] Surgery for subluxation of the shoulder, however, is useful in the backstroke. The Putti-Platt procedure is recommended.[3] Arthroscopy also has a role in chronic shoulder pain. Labral tears can be resected arthroscopically. Rotator cuff pathology can also be visualized from within the joint as well as from the subacromial bursa using the arthroscope.

CONDITIONING

Only recently have the training techniques used in the United States emphasized out-of-water strengthening programs similar to those utilized by the East Germans. Unfortunately, some strengthening programs stress only specific "prime movers" for each stroke. Weight training, stretching, and swimming drills must include not only anterior muscles but also rotator cuff, trapezius, and rhomboid muscles. The goal of a strengthening program must be to mimic the swimmer's shoulder stroke performance as closely as possible. Therefore, high-speed, high-resistance exercises are important. Slow-speed high-resistance exercises build both muscle and strength but not speed.[5] Ideal exercises have the muscle working at maximal resistance through its full range of isokinetic movement. Simple free weights or Nautilus-type machines alone may be inadequate. Indian clubs, pushups (prone and sitting), wheelbarrow drills, and ergometrics are also useful. Flexibility exercises should be included because shoulder extension enhances arm recovery in freestyle swimming. Passive stretch and isometrics can also be used. Stretching should be performed not just as a warm-up exercise but as part of a regular out-of-water workout.

SUMMARY

Shoulder pain is the most frequent complaint of competitive swimmers. The violent force of the pull-through with adduction and internal rotation leads to impingement syndromes. The mechanism of stroke production causing pathology is similar in freestyle swimming, the backstroke, the butterfly, and the breast stroke. Awareness of proper stroke production and corrections that can be made to minimize impingement syndromes are essential. Conservative treatment can produce good results. Stroke modification also may be necessary. Surgery should be used as a last resort, since the results do not consistently allow return to high-level swimming.

REFERENCES

1. Councilman, J.: The Science of Swimming. Englewood Cliffs, Prentice Hall, 1968.
2. Rathbun, J. B., and MacNab, I.: The microvascular pattern of the rotator cuff. J Bone Joint Surg 52B:540, 1970.
3. Kennedy, J., Hawkins, R., and Krissoff, W. B.: Orthopedic manifestations of swimming. Am J Sports Med 6:309, 1978.
4. Richardson, A., Jobe, F. W., and Collins, H. P.: The shoulder in competitive swimming. Am J Sports Med 8:159, 1980.
5. Penny, J., and Smith, C.: The prevention and treatment of swimmer's shoulder. Can J Appl Sport Sci 5, 1980.

SUGGESTED READINGS

1. Fowler, P.: Swimming problems. Am J Sports Med, 7:141, 1979.
2. Hunter, I., Clancy, W., and Andrews, J.: Common Orthopedic Problems of Female Athletes. AAOS Instructional Course Lectures. St. Louis, C V Mosby Company, 1982, pp. 126–151.
3. Pettrone, F.: Swimmer's shoulder. Athletes in Action 2:2, 3, 1983.

INDEX

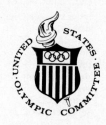

Note: Italics indicate illustrations and t indicates tables.

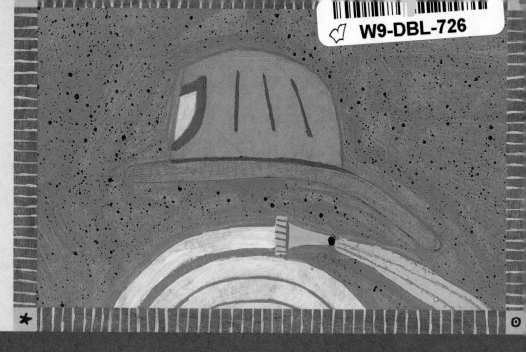

HISTORIA-CIENCIAS SOCIALES PARA CALIFORNIA
NUESTRAS COMUNIDADES

WILLIAM E. WHITE, PH.D.
AUTOR DEL PROGRAMA

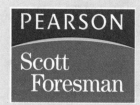

PEARSON

Scott
Foresman

OFICINAS EDITORIALES
Glenview, Illinois
Parsippany, Nueva Jersey
Nueva York, Nueva York

OFICINAS DE VENTA
Boston, Massachusetts
Duluth, Georgia
Glenview, Illinois
Coppell, Texas
Sacramento, California
Mesa, Arizona

ISBN: 0-328-17409-2

Contenido

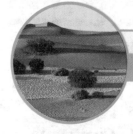

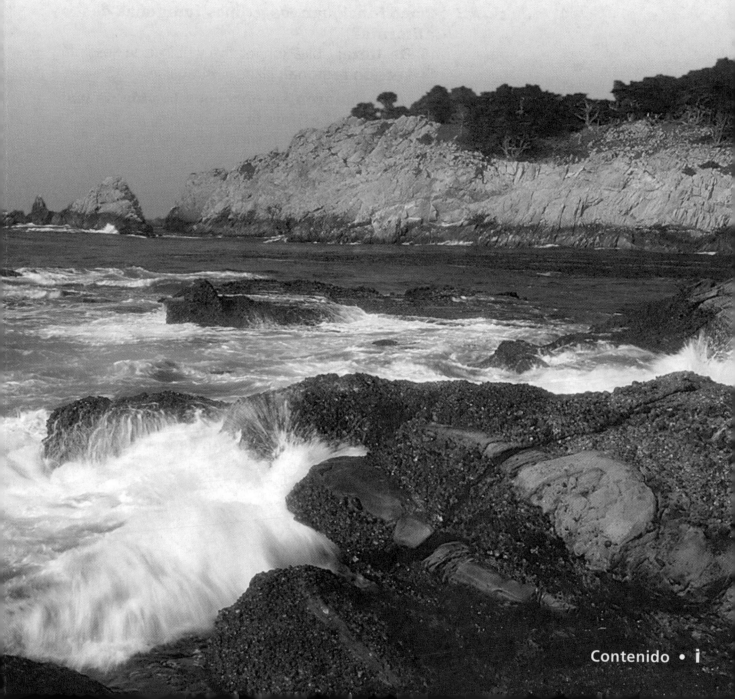

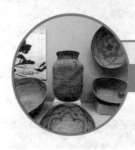
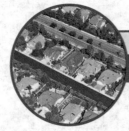

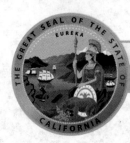

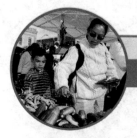

Un libro sobre nuestras comunidades

¿Nunca te has preguntado cómo era hace muchos años el área donde vives? ¿Crees que era diferente de como es hoy? ¿Han cambiado la gente y los edificios?

Este libro es *tu* libro. Trata de las muchas áreas que nuestro estado tiene, incluida en la que vives tú. Trata también de cómo algunas cosas de esos lugares han cambiado con el tiempo, mientras que otras han permanecido igual. Al igual que el área donde vives, tu libro es especial en muchos aspectos.

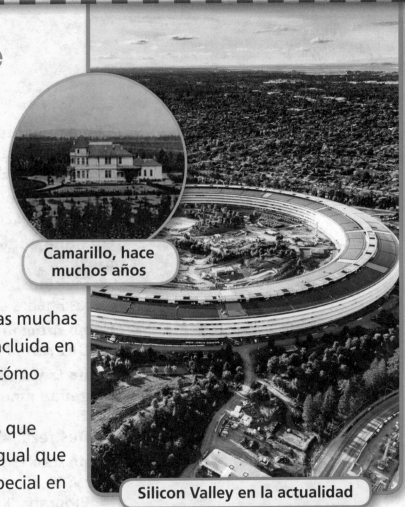

Camarillo, hace muchos años

Silicon Valley en la actualidad

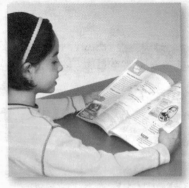

En primer lugar, escribirás, encerrarás en círculos y subrayarás palabras de tu libro. También completarás líneas cronológicas y harás marcas en los mapas.

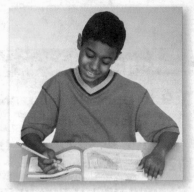

En segundo lugar, cada unidad de tu libro empieza con un Diario de estudio. En él escribirás lo que ya sabes acerca de tu comunidad, así como lo que vas aprendiendo sobre ella.

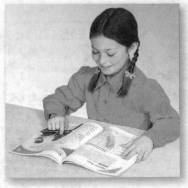

Por último, tu libro tiene muchas fotografías y dibujos de personas y lugares de nuestras comunidades. En algunas ilustraciones verás cosas del pasado. En otras verás cómo son las cosas hoy en día.

Lo que aprenderás

Tu libro empieza con la descripción del terreno y el agua en diferentes áreas de California. Por ejemplo, algunas áreas tienen montañas, mientras que otras tienen desiertos. En cada lugar crecen y vive distintas plantas y animales. La gente ha aprendido a utilizar las cosas que hay en el área donde vive para fabricar lo que necesita para vivir.

Aprenderás que los indígenas de California fueron los primeros habitantes de California. Los distintos grupos tenían su propio modo de vida, que variaba de acuerdo con las características propias del área donde vivían. Los indígenas de California usaban lo que encontraban para preparar comida, construir viviendas y fabricar ropa y herramientas. Hoy en día, algunos indígenas de California conservan el modo de vida que tenían hace muchos años, aunque su vida también ha cambiado de otras maneras.

Muchas otras personas se han mudado a California a lo largo de su historia. Incluso hoy en día siguen viniendo. Esas personas se mudaron de otros estados o de otros países. Vinieron por diferentes razones. Unos vinieron a explorar. Otros, a trabajar en la construcción de las líneas de ferrocarril. Otros más vinieron buscando oro. Una vez aquí, hicieron nuevas vidas y abrieron negocios en diferentes partes de California. Algunos de esos negocios existen en la actualidad.

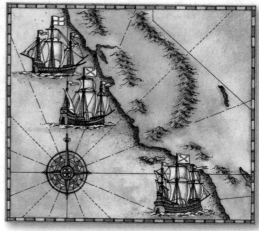

Algunos europeos inicialmente navegaron a lo largo de la costa de lo que hoy es California durante el siglo XVI.

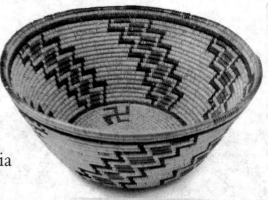

Los indígenas de California han usado los materiales que hay en las áreas donde viven para hacer las cosas que necesitan, como esta canasta.

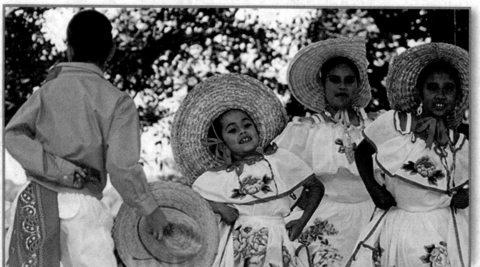

Habitantes de Los Ángeles bailan en celebración del Cinco de Mayo, un día festivo mexicano.

¿Cómo logra llevarse bien toda la gente que ha venido a California? Porque han acordado seguir ciertas reglas que les ayudan a vivir y trabajar juntos. Las reglas pueden estar relacionadas con la seguridad, la justicia o con el cuidado de la tierra y el agua de California. Leerás acerca de la gente que ayuda a manejar nuestros vecindarios, nuestro estado y nuestro país.

A pesar de que el área en que vivimos tiene muchos productos y servicios que mejoran nuestras vidas, aun así necesitamos cosas de otros lugares. Aprenderás cómo los habitantes de California trabajan juntos y con personas de otros estados u otros países para conseguir las cosas que necesitamos.

Estos estudiantes escuchan a un narrador de cuentos indígena de California.

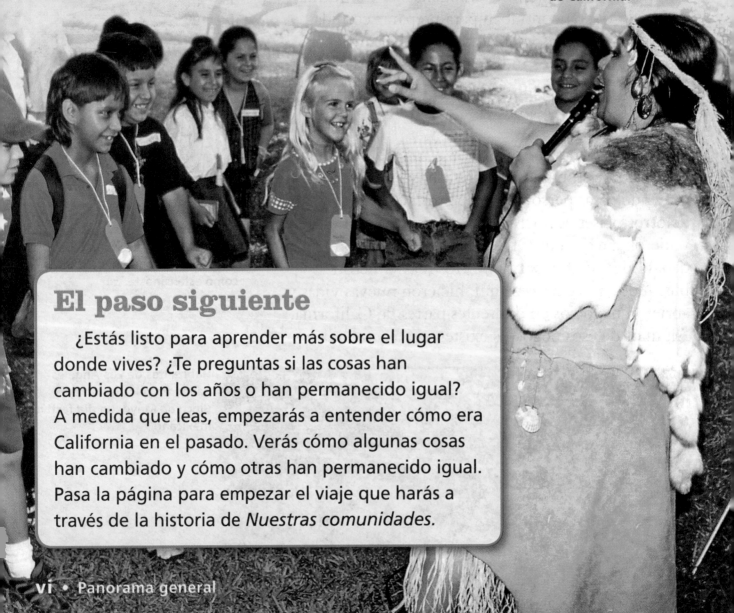

El paso siguiente

¿Estás listo para aprender más sobre el lugar donde vives? ¿Te preguntas si las cosas han cambiado con los años o han permanecido igual? A medida que leas, empezarás a entender cómo era California en el pasado. Verás cómo algunas cosas han cambiado y cómo otras han permanecido igual. Pasa la página para empezar el viaje que harás a través de la historia de *Nuestras comunidades.*

Diario de estudio

En esta unidad aprenderás las características de la tierra de tu área y de otras áreas de California. Aprenderás cómo la gente ha usado la tierra para satisfacer sus necesidades. Completa las actividades que aparecen en estas páginas a medida que leas la unidad.

Lo que sé sobre...

la tierra de California:

_____

El ambiente de California

Sombrea cada región del mapa usando un color distinto. Cuando termines, sombrea la leyenda. Luego escribe un recurso de cada región.

Recurso de la costa:

_____

Recurso de la montaña:

_____

Recurso del valle:

_____

Recurso del desierto:

_____

Leyenda del mapa

Costa   Montaña

Valle   Desierto

Encierra en un círculo la región de California en la que vives. Escribe tres detalles de su geografía.

- Desierto
- Costa
- Montaña
- Valle

1. _____

_____

2. _____

_____

3. _____

_____

Dibuja un recurso de California que deba ser protegido. Escribe una oración que explique por qué la gente debería ayudar a proteger ese recurso.

_____

_____

_____

_____

Escribe un detalle que explique por qué son importantes la represa y el canal.

Represa Shasta

_____

_____

Canal de Panamá

_____

_____

He aprendido...

_____

_____

🐻 **H-SS 3.1.1** Identifican las características geográficas de sus regiones locales (por ejemplo, desiertos, montañas, valles, colinas, áreas costeras, océanos, lagos).

¿Cómo son la tierra y el agua de tu área?

CONÉCTATE ¿Qué apariencia tienen la tierra y el agua donde tú vives? ¿Ves montañas, el océano, un desierto o algo más? Hagamos un recorrido por nuestro estado para aprender más acerca de él.

Vistazo previo
Vocabulario

región *(s.)* área grande de tierra que tiene características parecidas

geografía *(s.)* características de la superficie de un lugar

Actividad de vocabulario Fíjate en la lista de palabras que está abajo. Encierra en un círculo las palabras que creas que son ejemplos de geografía.

casa	desierto	montaña
valle	colina	invierno
playa	verduras	lago

🔊 Lectura: Idea principal y detalles

La *idea principal* es la idea más importante de un párrafo. Los *detalles* dicen más cosas acerca de la idea principal. Subraya la oración que dice la idea principal del párrafo de la página 4.

▷

¿Dónde vives?

    ¿Sabías que California tiene cuatro regiones principales de tierra? Una **región** es un área grande de tierra que tiene características parecidas. Las regiones a menudo se nombran por sus accidentes geográficos más comunes, tales como una montaña o un desierto. Las regiones de nuestro estado son las del desierto, del valle, de la costa y de la montaña. Cuando estudiamos la geografía de California, aprendemos más acerca de sus regiones. La **geografía** se refiere a las características de la superficie de un lugar.

1. Idea principal y detalles **Escribe tres detalles que digan algo más acerca de la idea principal.**

Idea principal

California tiene cuatro regiones principales de tierra.

valle

Detalle

Detalle

Detalle

Detalle

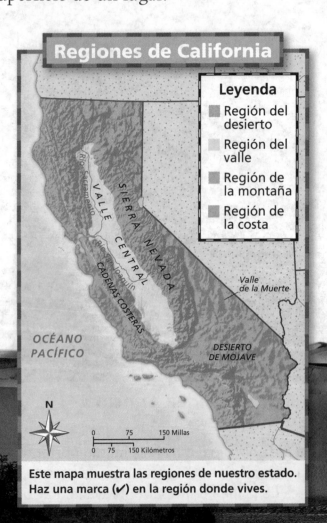

Regiones de California

Leyenda
- Región del desierto
- Región del valle
- Región de la montaña
- Región de la costa

Río Sacramento

VALLE CENTRAL

SIERRA NEVADA

Río San Joaquín

CADENAS COSTERAS

Valle de la Muerte

OCÉANO PACÍFICO

DESIERTO DE MOJAVE

N

0   75   150 Millas
0   75   150 Kilómetros

Este mapa muestra las regiones de nuestro estado. Haz una marca (✔) en la región donde vives.

El Valle de la Muerte se encuentra en la región del desierto de California.

Región del desierto

La región del desierto cubre la mayor parte del sureste de California. En esta región encontrarás el gran desierto de Mojave. Allí los veranos son calientes y secos. Los inviernos pueden ser fríos. Hay áreas planas y bajas. El Valle de la Muerte es el punto más bajo en América del Norte. A pesar de que hay muy poca agua, en esta región pueden crecer árboles, arbustos y cactus.

2. Idea principal y detalles
¿Cómo describirías la región del desierto?

_____

_____

_____

_____

En los desiertos de nuestro estado crecen plantas poco comunes. La planta alta que aparece aquí es un árbol de Josué.

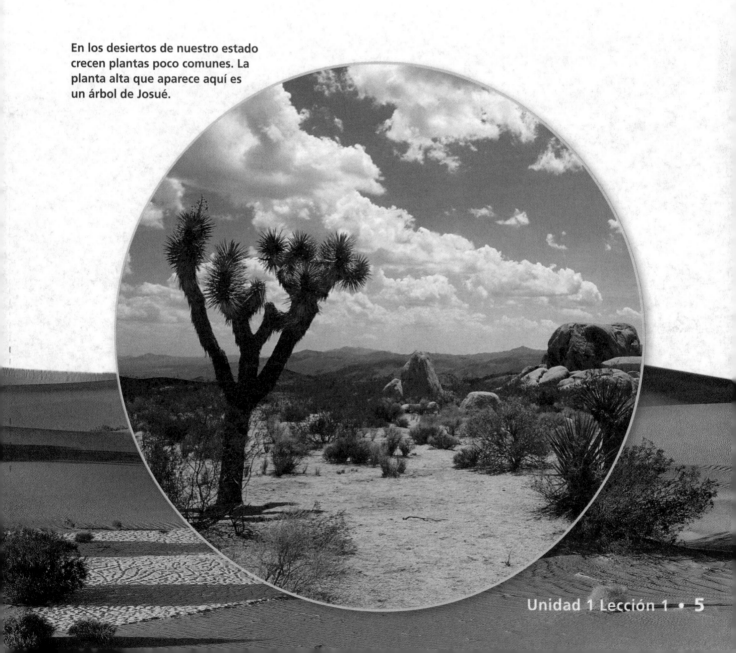

Región del valle

Los valles de San Joaquín y de Sacramento forman la región del valle de California. Un valle es un área larga de tierra baja que se encuentra entre colinas o montañas. La región del valle es plana. Las montañas se elevan en los lados del este y del oeste. En esta región se cultivan muchos tipos de frutas y verduras. Los ríos San Joaquín y Sacramento atraviesan la región del valle.

3. ¿En qué se parecen las regiones del valle y del desierto? *Comparar y contrastar*

El río Sacramento atraviesa la región del valle de California. ¿Puedes ver la ciudad de Sacramento en la parte superior izquierda?

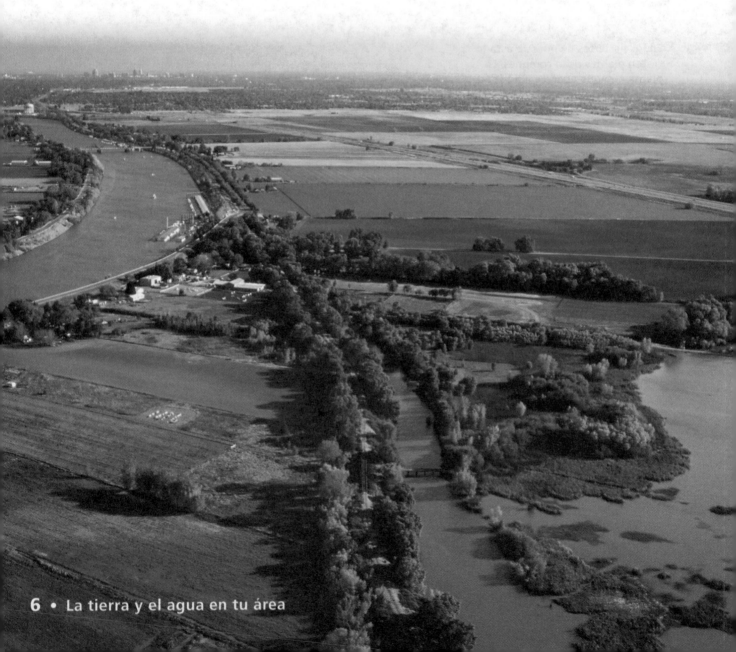

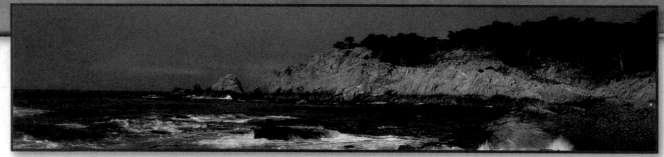

La Reserva Estatal Point Lobos se encuentra en la región de la costa de California.

Región de la costa

La región de la costa de California se encuentra a lo largo del océano Pacífico. La costa tiene más de 800 millas de largo. A lo largo de la costa norte se pueden ver montañas y acantilados. Las famosas secoyas gigantes de nuestro estado crecen allí. La tierra de la región de la costa central es buena para la agricultura. A lo largo de la costa central también se pueden encontrar montañas y dunas, o grandes colinas de arena. Los humedales, o áreas cenagosas, se encuentran en los alrededores de la bahía de San Francisco. En estos humedales viven algunas plantas y animales poco comunes. En algunas partes de la costa sur hay colinas, playas y montañas.

Región de la montaña

La mayoría de las montañas de California están en las partes norte y este del estado. La región de la montaña también tiene muchos lagos. La mayor parte del agua de California que se usa para beber y para irrigar cultivos proviene de esta región. La región de la montaña tiene grandes bosques, así como muchos parques estatales y nacionales, entre ellos el Parque Nacional Yosemite. Las cataratas Yosemite y Ribbon, que se encuentran en ese parque, son de las más altas del mundo.

4. Idea principal y detalles
Escribe tres accidentes geográficos que podrías ver en la región de la costa.

_____

_____

5. Idea principal y detalles
Encierra en un círculo una razón por la que la región de la montaña es importante para los habitantes de California.

Resumen

California tiene cuatro regiones principales: desierto, valle, costa y montaña. Describe algunos accidentes geográficos que tiene tu región. ¿En qué se diferencian de los accidentes geográficos de otras regiones de nuestro estado?

Mapas físicos

Aprende más Un mapa físico es una herramienta útil para aprender geografía. Muestra los accidentes geográficos o las características físicas de una región. Estos accidentes geográficos pueden incluir desiertos, valles o montañas. Un mapa físico también puede mostrar la vegetación que crece en una región. La leyenda del mapa indica los colores que se usan para mostrar los distintos tipos de vegetación. Por ejemplo, el café claro representa la vegetación que crece en la región del desierto.

Usa el siguiente mapa para responder las preguntas.

Inténtalo

1. Traza una línea a lo largo del río San Joaquín. *Identificar*

2. En el mapa, encierra en un círculo el Valle de la Muerte. *Localizar*

3. ¿Qué tipo de vegetación hay en la Sierra Nevada? *Interpretar*

_____

_____

4. Al mirar el mapa, ¿qué crees que es una bahía? *Analizar*

_____

_____

_____

Vegetación de California

OREGÓN

Leyenda
- Arbustos, cactus y árboles pequeños
- Bosque de árboles de hoja perenne
- Pradera
- Bosque mixto
- Frontera internacional
- Límite estatal

CADENAS COSTERAS

Río Sacramento

VALLE CENTRAL

SIERRA NEVADA

Río San Joaquín

Lago Tahoe

NEVADA

Bahía de San Francisco

Valle de la Muerte

ARIZONA

DESIERTO DE MOJAVE

Río Colorado

OCÉANO PACÍFICO

Lago Salton

DESIERTO DE SONORA

0   75   150 Millas
0   75   150 Kilómetros

N

MÉXICO

H-SS 3.1.2 Investigan la manera en que la gente ha utilizado los recursos de la región y ha modificado el ambiente físico (por ejemplo, una represa construida río arriba modificó el cauce del río o la línea costera).

¿Cómo ha usado la gente la tierra en tu región?

CONÉCTATE La gente usa las cosas que están a su alrededor para trabajar y fabricar cosas útiles. ¿Qué usarías tú si quisieras construir una casa en un árbol o sembrar una planta?

Vistazo previo
Vocabulario

recurso *(s.)* cualquier cosa que satisface las necesidades de la gente

ambiente *(s.)* la tierra, el agua y el aire en que viven las personas, los animales y las plantas

represa *(s.)* pared construida para contener el agua

inundación *(s.)* corriente súbita de agua que cubre lo que normalmente es tierra seca

canal *(s.)* vía de navegación estrecha que ha sido cavada a lo largo de una porción de tierra

proteger *(v.)* defender a alguien o algo de algún peligro o amenaza

Actividad de vocabulario Encierra en un círculo la palabra de arriba que sea un sinónimo de *vigilar* o *cuidar*.

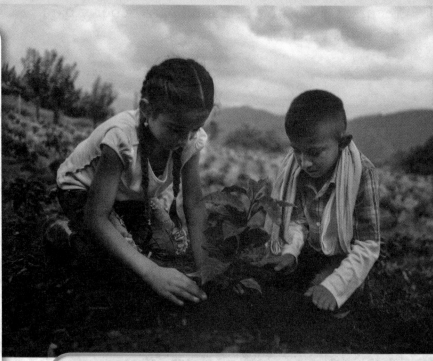

Lectura: Idea principal y detalles

Destreza de lectura

La *idea principal* dice de qué se trata un párrafo. Los *detalles* dicen más cosas acerca de la idea principal. Subraya los detalles del párrafo de la página 10.

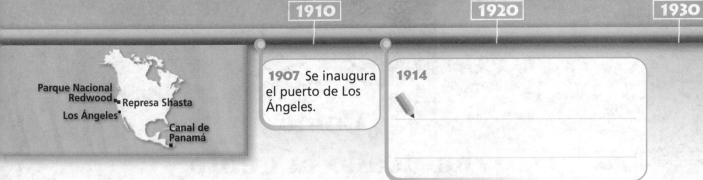

Parque Nacional
Redwood — Represa Shasta
Los Ángeles
Canal de
Panamá

1907 Se inaugura el puerto de Los Ángeles.

1914

Tierra, agua y bosques

California tiene muchos tipos de recursos. Un **recurso** es cualquier cosa útil que satisface las necesidades de la gente. La tierra de la región del valle es fértil, lo que hace que el área sea buena para el cultivo. La tierra es un recurso importante, como también lo son los bosques. Casi la mitad de nuestro estado está cubierto de bosques. Productos como el papel y la madera para casas y muebles se sacan de los bosques y sus árboles. Los ríos y lagos también son recursos. Nos proveen agua para beber y para regar los cultivos.

1. Idea principal y detalles

Nombra un recurso de California. Luego explica su uso.

Los bosques de California, como el Parque Nacional Klamath, mostrado aquí, son uno de los muchos recursos de nuestro estado.

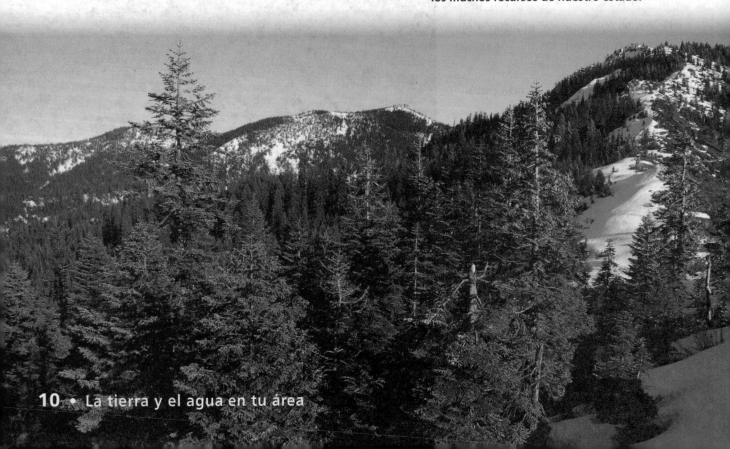

1945 Termina la construcción de la represa Shasta.

1968 Se inaugura el Parque Nacional Secoya.

Modificar la tierra

La gente puede modificar su ambiente. El **ambiente** lo constituyen la tierra, el agua y el aire en que viven la gente, los animales y las plantas. La construcción de la represa Shasta, en el río Sacramento, terminó en 1945. Una **represa** es una pared que se construye para contener el agua. La represa Shasta es una de las más grandes de los Estados Unidos.

Las represas, como la represa Shasta, generan energía eléctrica y proveen agua para los cultivos. Al contener el agua de río tras una pared, las represas también pueden prevenir las inundaciones. Una **inundación** ocurre cuando una corriente súbita de agua cubre lo que normalmente es tierra seca.

2. ¿Qué pasaría si no se construyeran represas?

Predecir

La construcción de la represa Shasta empezó en 1938 y terminó en 1945. La represa está hecha de concreto.

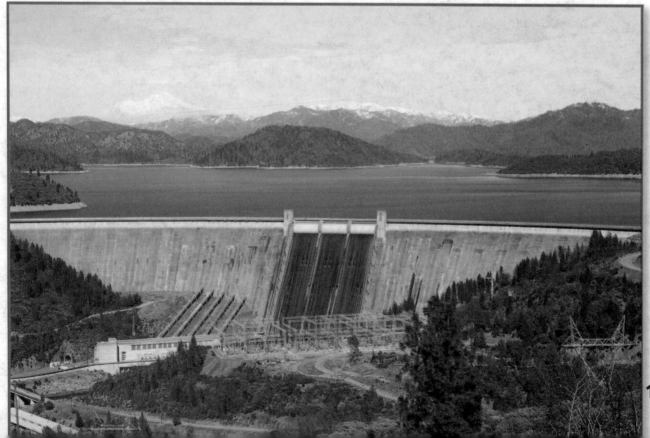

11

Mejores viajes

Los puertos y los canales se construyen para que a la gente le resulte más fácil enviar productos por barco. El puerto de Los Ángeles fue inaugurado en 1907 para poder recibir barcos grandes. Los canales pueden hacer más rápido el viaje por agua. Un **canal** es una vía de navegación estrecha que ha sido cavada a lo largo de una porción de tierra.

El canal de Panamá se terminó de construir en 1914. El canal de Panamá atraviesa una parte del territorio del país llamado Panamá. Esta porción de tierra separa el océano Atlántico del océano Pacífico. La construcción del canal de Panamá hizo más rápida la navegación entre la costa este y la costa oeste de los Estados Unidos. Como resultado, el puerto de Los Ángeles creció en tamaño.

Así es el puerto de Los Ángeles hoy en día.

3. **¿Cómo ayudó el canal de Panamá a que el puerto de Los Ángeles creciera en tamaño?**

Causa y efecto

_____

_____

_____

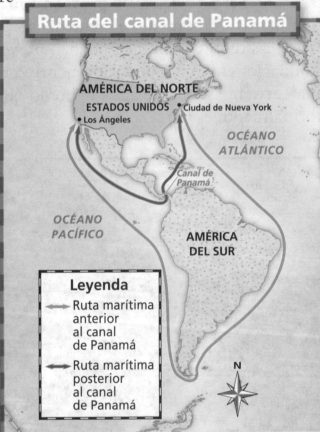

Ruta del canal de Panamá

AMÉRICA DEL NORTE

ESTADOS UNIDOS • Ciudad de Nueva York
• Los Ángeles

OCÉANO ATLÁNTICO

Canal de Panamá

OCÉANO PACÍFICO

AMÉRICA DEL SUR

Leyenda

→ Ruta marítima anterior al canal de Panamá

→ Ruta marítima posterior al canal de Panamá

N

Este mapa muestra las rutas marítimas antes y después de la contrucción del canal de Panamá. En la leyenda del mapa, encierra en un círculo el símbolo que representa la ruta más corta.

Un ambiente saludable

A veces la gente modifica el ambiente y eso crea problemas. La gente, por ejemplo, puede enfermarse debido a la contaminación. La contaminación ensucia el ambiente. Hace que el aire que respiramos o el agua que bebemos no estén limpios. Muchos piensan que es importante que protejamos nuestro ambiente. **Proteger** significa defender a alguien o algo de algún peligro o amenaza. La gente puede ayudar obedeciendo las reglas que protegen el ambiente.

Mucha gente ha trabajado para proteger el ambiente. Hace más de 100 años, un hombre llamado John Muir quiso proteger los recursos de California. Se aseguró de que todo el mundo se enterara de la belleza de nuestro estado. Aunque murió en 1914, su esfuerzo contribuyó a crear parques como el Parque Nacional Secoya, establecido en 1968.

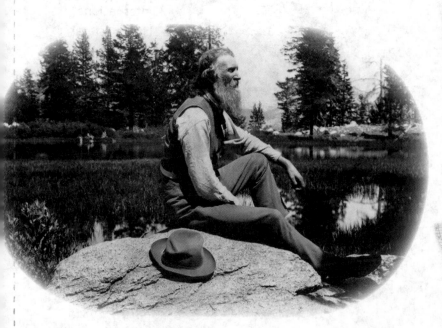

John Muir ayudó a proteger la belleza natural de nuestro estado.

4. Idea principal y detalles

Encierra en un círculo una manera en que la gente puede proteger el ambiente.

Las secoyas de California crecen en Muir Woods. Al bosque se le dio el nombre de Muir Woods en honor a John Muir.

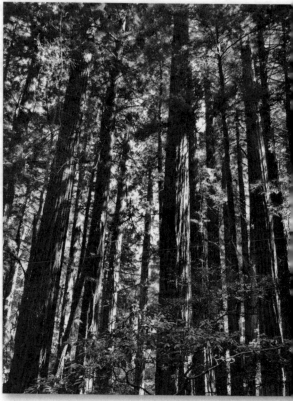

Resumen

California tiene muchos recursos. ¿Cómo ha modificado la gente el ambiente para usar sus recursos?

Mapas de recursos

Aprende más Un mapa de recursos muestra los recursos de un área. California es un estado rico en recursos naturales. Los símbolos del mapa que aparece abajo representan los múltiples recursos que se encuentran en nuestro estado. La leyenda del mapa te dice qué representan los símbolos. Busca el símbolo de naranjas en la leyenda. Representa naranjales, o granjas de árboles de naranja. El mapa te muestra dónde se pueden encontrar los numerosos naranjales de California.

Usa el mapa para responder las siguientes preguntas.

Inténtalo

1. ¿Qué dos recursos se encuentran a lo largo de la costa? *Identificar*

_____

_____

2. Dibuja un cuadro alrededor de la región en que se cultivan almendras.
   Identificar

3. ¿En qué mitad del estado se cultivan naranjas? *Identificar*

_____

4. Encierra en un círculo un recurso de tu región. *Aplicar*

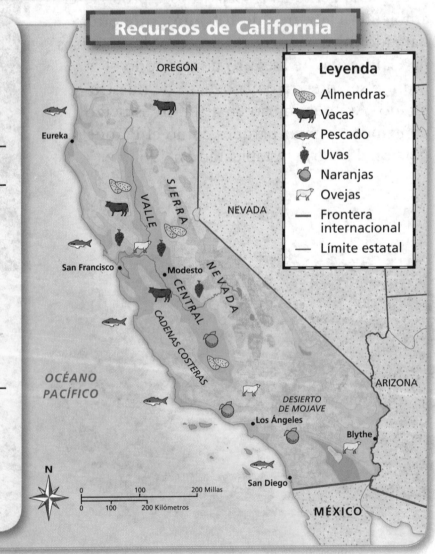

Recursos de California

OREGÓN

Eureka

SIERRA

VALLE

NEVADA

San Francisco

Modesto

CENTRAL

NEVADA

CADENAS COSTERAS

OCÉANO PACÍFICO

ARIZONA

DESIERTO DE MOJAVE

Los Ángeles

Blythe

San Diego

MÉXICO

Leyenda

- Almendras
- Vacas
- Pescado
- Uvas
- Naranjas
- Ovejas
- — Frontera internacional
- — Límite estatal

N

0   100   200 Millas
0   100   200 Kilómetros

Diario de estudio

En esta unidad aprenderás sobre los grupos indígenas de California que viven en tu región y en otras regiones. Te enterarás de las tierras que habitaron, de sus creencias y sistemas de orden social, y de lo que sucedió cuando se encontraron con otras personas que habían llegado a California. Completa las actividades que aparecen en estas páginas a medida que leas la unidad.

Lo que sé sobre...

los grupos indígenas de California:

Costumbres de los indígenas de California

En cada uno de los círculos escribe una costumbre de los indígenas de California.

Costumbres de los indígenas de California

Completa estas secciones a medida que leas la unidad.

Escribe un dato acerca de cada grupo indígena de California.

Montaña

Valle

Costa

Desierto

Escoge dos palabras de la siguiente lista y escribe una oración usando ambas palabras.

- **leyes**
- **gobierno tribal**
- **constitución**
- **economía**
- **reservación**

Escribe la información que falta en esta línea cronológica.

SIGLO XVIII

1767

1775

He aprendido...

H-SS 3.2.1 Describen identidades nacionales, creencias religiosas, costumbres y varias tradiciones folclóricas.

¿En qué se parecen y en qué se diferencian los indígenas de California de tu región?

CONÉCTATE ¿De dónde vino tu familia? Pudo haber venido de Asia, Europa, América del Sur o África. Los indígenas americanos vivían aquí mucho antes de que llegaran personas de otras tierras.

Vistazo previo
Vocabulario

costumbre *(s.)* modo en que se hacen las cosas

folclor *(s.)* relatos y costumbres de un grupo de personas

tradición *(s.)* modo especial en que un grupo de personas hace algo y que ha sido transmitido a otros

ceremonia *(s.)* actividad importante que se hace por una razón especial

Actividad de vocabulario Encierra en un círculo la palabra de arriba que pueda ser un sinónimo de *tradición*.

Lectura: Comparar y contrastar

Comparar es señalar en qué se parecen dos o más cosas. *Contrastar* es señalar en qué se diferencian dos o más cosas. La palabra clave *como* nos da una pista que indica el parecido entre dos o más cosas. Palabras o frases clave que se usan con frecuencia, como *diferente*, *pero* y *sin embargo*, indican diferencias. Subraya esas palabras clave a medida que leas la lección.

Indígenas de América del Norte

América del Norte era el hogar de diferentes grupos indígenas americanos antes de que los europeos llegaran. Cada grupo tenía sus propias **costumbres,** es decir, modos en que hacían las cosas. Los grupos indígenas de América del Norte hoy en día todavía tienen sus propias costumbres.

Estos distintos grupos indígenas americanos hablaban diferentes idiomas, comían diferentes alimentos y construían diferentes tipos de viviendas. Los indígenas americanos de la Zona Boscosa del Este sembraban maíz y frijoles, y cazaban venados. Algunos construían *wigwams*, o casas hechas de madera y corteza. Los indígenas americanos de las Grandes Llanuras vivían la mayor parte del tiempo en chozas hechas de tierra. Cazaban búfalos y usaban la piel para hacer ropa y viviendas. Durante las expediciones de cacería usaban tipis hechos de piel de búfalo.

Algunos indígenas americanos del Desierto del Suroeste vivían en casas de piedra o de barro. Sembraban maíz, a pesar de que en el desierto no había mucha agua. Para los grupos que habitaban el Noroeste del Pacífico la búsqueda de alimentos no era un problema. Comían mucho pescado y mariscos porque vivían cerca del océano Pacífico. También cazaban ballenas y focas en el océano.

1. Comparar y contrastar

Escribe dos diferencias importantes que había entre los indígenas americanos de la Zona Boscosa del Este y los de las Grandes Llanuras.

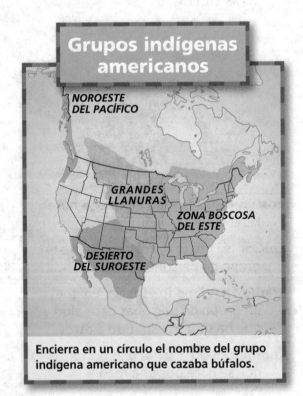

Grupos indígenas americanos

NOROESTE DEL PACÍFICO

GRANDES LLANURAS

ZONA BOSCOSA DEL ESTE

DESIERTO DEL SUROESTE

Encierra en un círculo el nombre del grupo indígena americano que cazaba búfalos.

Grupos indígenas de California

Los numerosos grupos indígenas de California tenían diferentes modos de vida. Unos, como los modocs, los pomos y los yukis, vivían en el norte de California. Cazaban venados y alces, y pescaban. Sin embargo, los chumash vivían en el sur de la costa central de California y la mayoría comía pescado, mariscos, otros animales marinos y aves. Los washos vivían cerca del lago Tahoe, en la Sierra Nevada. Se alimentaban de venados y antílopes, y los usaban para hacer ropa y para construir sus viviendas. Los mojaves y los yumas vivían en el Desierto del Suroeste. Cultivaban y cazaban en la tierra seca.

2. **Completa la siguiente tabla.**

Idea principal y detalles

Grupo	Dónde vivían
Modoc	
	Lago Tahoe
Chumash	

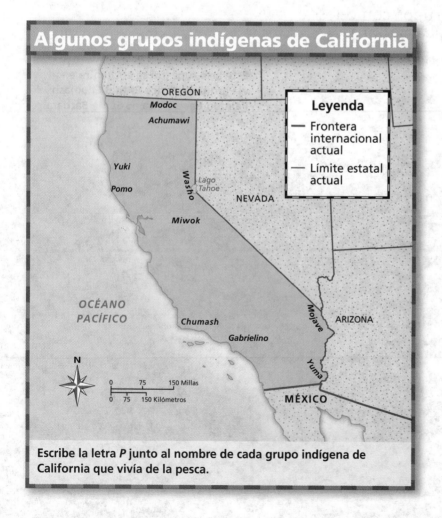

Algunos grupos indígenas de California

OREGÓN
Modoc
Achumawi

Leyenda
— Frontera internacional actual
— Límite estatal actual

Yuki
Pomo
Washo
Lago Tahoe
NEVADA
Miwok

OCÉANO PACÍFICO
Chumash
Gabrielino
Mojave
ARIZONA
Yuma

N

0   75   150 Millas
0   75   150 Kilómetros

MÉXICO

Escribe la letra *P* junto al nombre de cada grupo indígena de California que vivía de la pesca.

Transmitir su historia

En el pasado, la mayoría de los indígenas de California no tenía un lenguaje escrito. En su lugar, transmitían su historia a través del **folclor.** El folclor son los relatos y las costumbres de un grupo de personas. Compartían su pasado a través de mitos y leyendas. Los mitos son relatos que explican los fenómenos de la naturaleza, y las leyendas son relatos acerca de personas del pasado. Hoy en día los indígenas de California continúan transmitiendo el folclor, los mitos y las leyendas.

Los indígenas de California tienen tradiciones para celebrar su historia. Una **tradición** es un modo especial en que un grupo de personas hace algo y que ha sido transmitido a otros. Por ejemplo, algunos grupos como los chumash y los gabrielinos pintaban o tallaban dibujos en las piedras. Los dibujos a menudo muestran sucesos importantes.

3. Comparar y contrastar

Escribe dos cosas que tenían en común la mayoría de los grupos indígenas de California del pasado.

_____

_____

_____

_____

Este arte rupestre se encuentra en el Parque Histórico Estatal Chumash Painted Cave, cerca de Santa Bárbara.

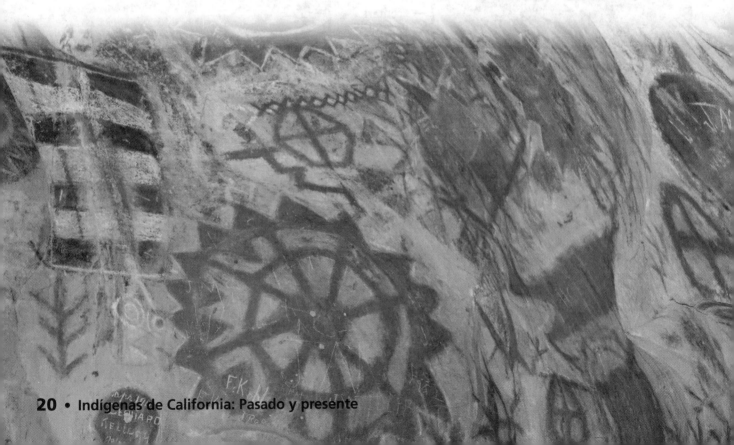

Creencias

Muchos grupos indígenas de California creían en espíritus, y muchos todavía siguen creyendo en ellos. Creían que los espíritus los ayudaban, pero también podían ocasionarles problemas. Ciertos líderes especiales guiaban al grupo durante las ceremonias. Una **ceremonia** es una actividad importante que se hace por una razón especial. Por ejemplo, algunos líderes de los indígenas de California pueden realizar una ceremonia en preparación de una buena caza.

Los indígenas de California hoy en día

Nuestro estado actualmente es el hogar de muchos indígenas de California. Algunos viven en extensiones de tierra que son propiedad del grupo al que pertenecen. Otros se han mudado a las ciudades en busca de trabajo. Hoy en día la mayoría viste y vive de la misma manera que el resto de los estadounidenses. Pero algunos todavía realizan ceremonias tradicionales. Mantienen vivas sus costumbres para las generaciones futuras.

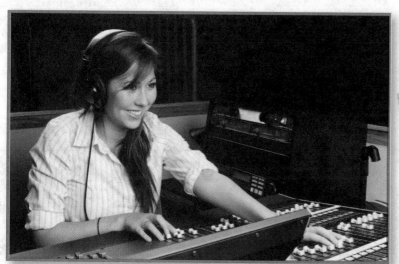

Hoy en día, aproximadamente 242,000 indígenas americanos viven en California.

4. ¿Para qué realizaría un líder una ceremonia? *Causa y efecto*

_____

_____

_____

5. Comparar y contrastar
En el texto, encierra en un círculo los modos en que los indígenas de California del presente se parecen a los indígenas de California del pasado.

Resumen

Los indígenas americanos tenían sus propias costumbres y tradiciones antes de que los europeos llegaran. Algunas de ellas continúan practicándose hoy en día. ¿Cuáles son algunas de las costumbres y tradiciones que tienen los indígenas de California?

Tablas

Aprende más Una tabla facilita comparar y contrastar información. La tabla que está abajo te da información acerca de cuatro diferentes grupos indígenas de California. El encabezado de cada columna indica qué información hay en esa columna. El encabezado de la primera columna es *Grupo*, y muestra el nombre de los distintos grupos. La información acerca de cada grupo está en las otras columnas. Para encontrar información sobre un grupo, ubica ese grupo en la primera columna; mueve el dedo hacia las columnas de la derecha y encontrarás la información acerca de ese grupo. Usa la tabla y contesta las preguntas que están abajo.

Inténtalo

1. Subraya la región donde vivían los chumash.

   Identificar

2. Si quisieras saber si algún grupo construía viviendas subterráneas, ¿bajo qué encabezado buscarías? Encierra en un círculo el encabezado. *Identificar*

3. ¿En qué se diferenciaban los alimentos de los washos y los de los miwoks?

   Interpretar

   _____

   _____

   _____

La vida de los indígenas de California

Grupo	Región	Alimentos	Viviendas
Chumash	Costa	Pescado, aves, animales marinos	Grandes, en forma de cúpula
Miwok	Valle	Bellotas, venado	En forma de cono, parcialmente subterráneas
Washo	Montaña	Venado, antílope	Hechas con piel de venado y antílope
Yuma	Desierto	Semillas, frutas, pescado, maíz, frijoles	Cuadradas, cubiertas de arena

Tradiciones vivas

Muchos y distintos grupos indígenas de California viven en nuestro estado. La música, el arte y la narración de cuentos han sido parte de sus creencias, costumbres y tradiciones.

Grupos

Este mapa muestra las distintas regiones donde vivían muchos grupos indígenas de California.

Fíjate en las grandes letras rojas del mapa. Luego fíjate en las letras de la siguiente lista para ver qué grupo vivía en cuál de las regiones. Muchos de estos grupos todavía viven allí.

A. Achumawi
B. Cahuilla
C. Chumash
D. Costanoan
E. Hupa
F. Luiseño
G. Maidu

H. Miwok
I. Mojave
J. Pomo
K. Shasta
L. Yokuts
M. Yuma
N. Yurok

Leyenda del mapa

= Costa
= Desierto
= Montaña
= Valle

Encierra en un círculo el nombre de un grupo indígena de California que viva en tu región o cerca de ella.

Arte y música

Costa

Obras de arte

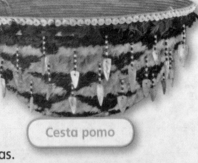
Cesta pomo

Las cestas son importantes para la cultura pomo. Los pomos todavía enseñan el arte de hacer cestas. Hacer una sola cesta puede tomar varios meses. Algunos cesteros usan plumas de aves como pájaros carpinteros, azulejos o patos. También añaden cuentas hechas de conchas de almeja. Algunas cestas pomos son tan pequeñas como la yema de un dedo.

Valle

Música en el valle

La música era importante para muchos indígenas del valle. Los miwoks hacían flautas y silbatos de huesos de ave. También hacían palos musicales partiendo a lo largo por la mitad un trozo de madera. Los palos musicales suenan al agitarlos.

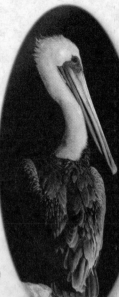
Instrumentos hechos de huesos de ave

Montaña

Madera y huesos

Los indígenas de la montaña usaban muchos recursos para hacer sus instrumentos musicales y sus joyas. Los hupas tallaban silbatos de madera o de huesos de animales. Hacían sonajas uniendo pezuñas de venado a mangos de madera. Los maidus usaban huesos de animales para hacer joyas. A veces les ponían conchas de mar y plumas a sus collares y aretes.

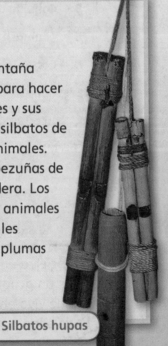
Silbatos hupas

Desierto

Muñecos de arcilla

Muchos indígenas del desierto hacían cerámica. La cerámica incluye ollas y platos hechos de arcilla. Los indígenas del desierto primero moldeaban la arcilla húmeda para darle forma de ollas, platos o recipientes. Después secaban la arcilla con fuego. Los mojaves también usaban arcilla para hacerles muñecos a sus hijos. Decoraban los muñecos para que parecieran personas de verdad. Hasta les ponían pelo humano.

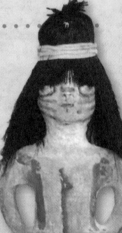
Muñeco mojave de arcilla

Vuelve al texto y encierra en un círculo dos recursos que los indígenas de California usaban para hacer silbatos.

Creencias y costumbres

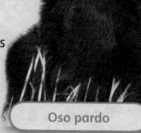

Sonaja pomo

Costa

Sonajas hechas de capullos

Los líderes especiales de los pomos, también llamados chamanes, usaban sonajas de curación. Las sonajas se hacían con capullos. Un capullo es la especie de funda que la oruga hace para cubrir su cuerpo. Los capullos se unían a un mango de madera. Los líderes especiales agitaban la sonaja sobre la persona enferma.

Valle

El poder del oso

Los animales y sus espíritus eran importantes para algunos indígenas del valle. Muchos yokuts veneraban a los animales que estaban conectados con su grupo familiar.

Oso pardo

Algunos yokuts tenían líderes especiales llamados médicos osos. Creían que esos líderes recibían sus poderes de los osos y que incluso podían convertirse en osos.

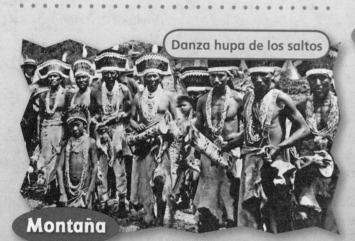

Danza hupa de los saltos

Montaña

Curanderos y bailarines

Los líderes especiales de los hupas realizaban dos danzas importantes. Una era la Danza de la piel de venado blanco. La otra era la Danza de los saltos. Los hupas creían que esas danzas mantenían saludable a su pueblo. También creían que las danzas los ayudarían a tener éxito en la caza y en la pesca.

Desierto

Canciones de las aves

Las canciones de las aves son una tradición importante para los cahuillas. Estas canciones relatan su historia. Las canciones eran parte de muchas ceremonias. A menudo esta canciones tomaban varios días en ser interpretadas. Las canciones de las aves siguen siendo parte de las ceremonias hoy en día. Las canciones conectan a los cahuillas con su pasado.

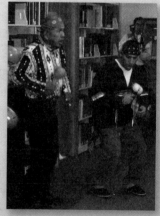

Alvino Silva *(izquierda)* interpreta una canción de las aves.

> Subraya en el texto dos cosas que un líder especial hacía.

Folclor

La narración de cuentos sigue formando parte de la vida de muchos indígenas de California. Los ancianos de cada grupo transmiten sus tradiciones y su historia a los jóvenes narrando cuentos.

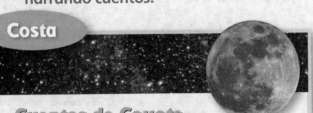

Narrador de cuentos indígena americano

Costa

Cuentos de Coyote

Muchos indígenas de California narran cuentos de Coyote. Éste es un cuento de los pomos.

Hace mucho tiempo, el mundo estaba oscuro. Así que Coyote juntó un poco de pasto e hizo una pelota muy compacta. Luego le pidió a Halcón que llevara la pelota hasta el cielo y le prendiera fuego. Esta pelota se convirtió en el Sol. Pero a ratos se apagaba, ya que el Viento del Norte soplaba al Sol, haciéndolo cruzar el cielo. Así que Coyote envió a Halcón al cielo con otra pelota de pasto. Pero esta pelota estaba húmeda, y no prendió fuego con el mismo brillo que la primera pelota. La segunda pelota se convirtió en la Luna. Por eso es que cuando hay Luna llena, los nietos de Coyote recuerdan la pelota húmeda y aúllan: "La luz de la luna es muy débil".

Montaña

Cómo nació el monte Shasta

Algunos indígenas de la montaña narran un cuento que explica cómo nació el monte Shasta. Se dice que hace muchos años la cima del monte lanzaba cenizas y vapor de vez en cuando.

El Viejo de las Alturas vivía al otro lado del cielo. Un día decidió visitar la Tierra. Para ello dejó caer hielo y nieve hasta que formó un montón tan alto que casi tocaba el cielo. Entonces el Viejo de las Alturas hizo su viaje a la Tierra saltando de nube en nube. Pronto llegó al montón, y en la punta hizo un gran hoyo. El Viejo se mudó al hoyo y ahí construyó su casa. Por eso es que cuando los shastas veían que la punta del montón de nieve lanzaba cenizas y vapor, decían: "El Viejo de las Alturas está en casa".

Monte Shasta

Encierra en un círculo las dos cosas que según el cuento estaban hechas con pelotas de pasto.

Valle

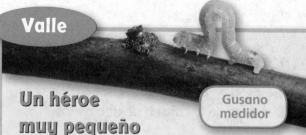

Gusano medidor

Un héroe muy pequeño

Los miwoks narran un cuento de una montaña en el valle Yosemite. Esa montaña hoy se conoce con el nombre de El Capitán.

· · · · · · · · · · · · · · · · · · ·

Dos ositos hermanos se quedaron dormidos sobre una roca. Mientras dormían, la roca creció hasta convertirse en una montaña. La mamá osa estaba preocupada porque no encontraba a sus cachorros. Por fin los otros animales se dieron cuenta de que los hermanos estaban en la cima de la montaña. Muchos animales grandes y fuertes trataron de saltar o trepar hasta la cima de la montaña, pero ninguno logró ayudar. Hasta que, finalmente, un pequeño gusano medidor trepó lentamente hasta la cima. Le llevó mucho tiempo. Pero el gusanito les mostró a los osos hermanos cómo bajar la montaña sin que se hicieran daño.

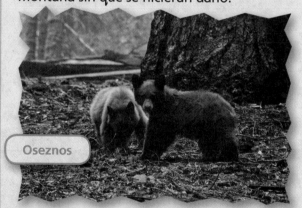

Oseznos

Desierto

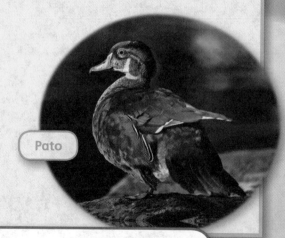

El río Colorado

Grandes relatos

Los mojaves cuentan cosas de los Primeros Tiempos, que ocurrieron hace mucho tiempo. Narran estos cuentos a su grupo y los llaman los Grandes Relatos.

· · · · · · · · · · · · · · · · · · ·

En los Primeros Tiempos sólo había personas. No había animales ni cultivos para comer. Así que el espíritu Mastamho enterró en la tierra una ramita de sauce. Cuando sacó la ramita, el agua brotó sobre la tierra. Esa agua se convirtió en el río Colorado. Estaba repleto de patos y peces. Entonces Mastamho les enseñó a los mojaves a cultivar sembrando semillas. También les enseñó a hacer fuego. Después les enseñó a hacer ollas para cocinar.

Pato

Subraya en el cuento dos cosas que Mastamho les enseñó a los mojaves.

¿Cuál es la cultura de los indígenas de California?

En el círculo del centro escribe el nombre de la región donde vives. En cada uno de los otros círculos escribe un detalle acerca de la cultura de uno de los grupos de la región donde vives.

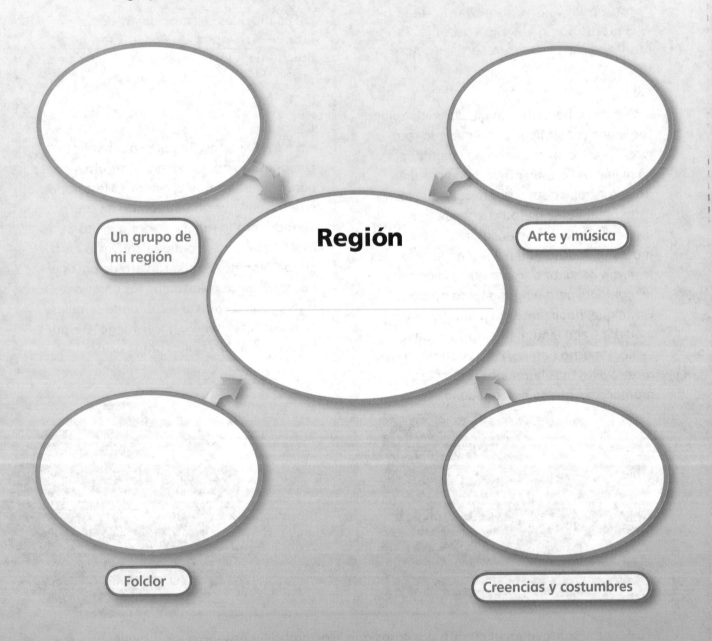

Un grupo de mi región

Arte y música

Región

Folclor

Creencias y costumbres

H-SS 3.2.2 Discuten cómo la geografía física, incluido el clima, influyó en la manera en que las naciones de indígenas locales se adaptaron a su ambiente natural (por ejemplo, cómo obtenían alimentos, vestimenta y herramientas).

Lección 2

¿Cómo han vivido los indígenas de California en su ambiente?

CONÉCTATE ¿Cómo afecta el lugar donde vives el modo en que vives? Los indígenas de California comían los alimentos que hallaban en las áreas donde vivían. Construían viviendas con madera, pasto y otras plantas que crecían a su alrededor.

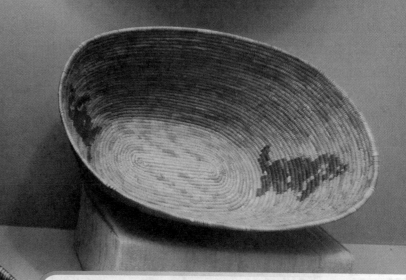

Vistazo previo

Vocabulario

tiempo *(s.)* temperatura y condiciones del aire en un lugar y en un momento dados

adaptarse *(v.)* cambiar para acomodarse a condiciones nuevas

clima *(s.)* tiempo que un área suele tener cada año

Actividad de vocabulario Escribe una oración con una de las palabras del vocabulario que describa el clima de tu región.

_____

_____

Lectura: Causa y efecto

Una *causa* es la razón por la que algo sucede. Un *efecto* es lo que sucede como resultado de la causa. A medida que leas la lección, subraya las partes del texto que digan por qué a los achumawis se les llamaba "indígenas del río Pit".

29

Ambientes diferentes

California tiene montañas, valles, desiertos y costas. Normalmente, cada una de esas áreas tiene un ambiente diferente. Esto significa que las plantas, los animales, los accidentes geográficos y el tiempo de un área son diferentes que los de las otras áreas. El **tiempo** consiste en la temperatura y las condiciones del aire en un lugar y en un momento dados. Los indígenas de California tuvieron que adaptarse a su medio ambiente. **Adaptarse** implica cambiar para acomodarse a las condiciones nuevas.

Alimentos

Los indígenas de California comían los alimentos que encontraban a su alrededor. Los achumawis vivían en la región de la montaña. Comían bellotas y venados. Se les llamaba "indígenas del río Pit" porque cavaban hoyos (*pits*) para atrapar a los venados que cazaban. Los pomos vivían en la región de la costa. Recolectaban alimentos como semillas, bellotas y bayas.

1. Llena el cuadro del efecto que está abajo. *Causa y efecto*

Causa:

> Las regiones de California tienen distintos ambientes.

Efecto:

2. ¿Qué tipos de alimentos comían los pomos? Explica por qué. *Idea principal y detalles*

_____

_____

_____

_____

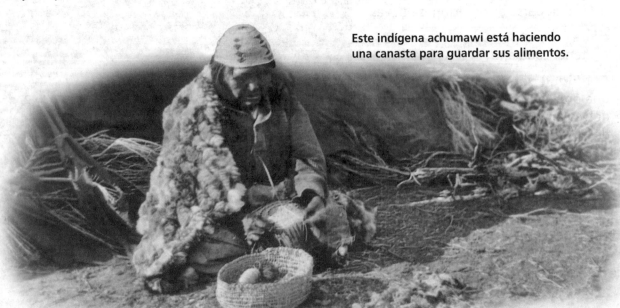

Este indígena achumawi está haciendo una canasta para guardar sus alimentos.

Viviendas

Los indígenas de California también adaptaron su forma de vivir según el clima del área, o área climatológica, donde vivían. El **clima** es el tiempo que un área suele tener cada año. Los modocs habitaban la región de la montaña. Vivían en casas que brindaban calor porque los inviernos son fríos y nevados. Los miwoks, de la región del valle, vivían en casas hechas con ramas, arbustos pequeños o pasto. Los yumas, de la región del desierto, hacían casas con ramas y arbustos pequeños; las cubrían con tierra o arena para mantenerlas frescas bajo el sol ardiente.

Los hupas, que vivían en la región de la montaña, construían casas con madera de cedro.

Vestimenta y herramientas

Los indígenas de California usaban plantas y piel de animales para hacer sus ropas. Algunos grupos comerciaban con otros grupos para obtener aquellos artículos que querían o necesitaban. Los washos, que vivían en la región de la montaña, cazaban venados. Usaban la piel de venado para hacer camisas y pantalones. Usaban los cuernos de venado como herramientas para cavar y cortar. Los chumash vivían en la región de la costa. Las mujeres chumash llevaban faldas hechas con algas marinas que encontraban en la costa. Los indígenas de California que vivían en el desierto, como los mojaves y los yumas, vestían ropa ligera para mantenerse frescos.

3. ¿Cómo afectó el clima las viviendas que los yumas construían? *Causa y efecto*

_____

_____

4. Encierra en un círculo las oraciones que describan la ropa que los indígenas de California hacían con materiales de su región.

Idea principal y detalles

Resumen

Los indígenas de California lograron vivir en muchos tipos de ambientes. ¿Cómo afectó el clima el modo en que vivían?

Mapas de climas

Aprende más En un mapa de climas se usan distintos colores para mostrar las áreas climatológicas de distintas regiones. El mapa de climas que aparece abajo muestra las diferentes áreas climatológicas de California. La leyenda del mapa explica qué color corresponde a cada área climatológica. Por ejemplo, el color verde corresponde a un clima de inviernos templados y lluviosos con veranos calientes y secos. Usa el mapa para contestar las siguientes preguntas.

Inténtalo

1. ¿Cuántas áreas climatológicas se muestran en el mapa?

Identificar

2. ¿Cómo es el área climatológica de Sacramento?

Interpretar

3. Encierra en un círculo las palabras de la leyenda del mapa que describan el área climatológica de Eureka.

Identificar

4. ¿Qué color corresponde al área climatológica del lugar donde vives? *Aplicar*

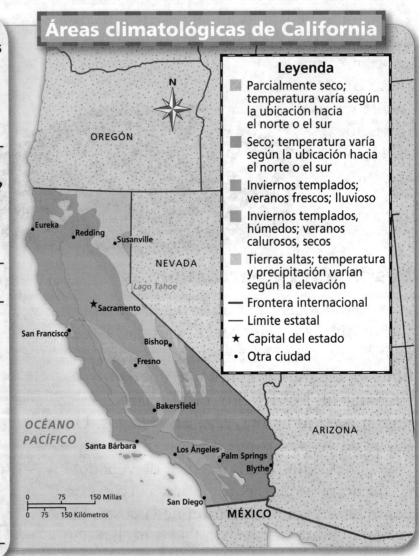

Áreas climatológicas de California

Leyenda

- Parcialmente seco; temperatura varía según la ubicación hacia el norte o el sur
- Seco; temperatura varía según la ubicación hacia el norte o el sur
- Inviernos templados; veranos frescos; lluvioso
- Inviernos templados, húmedos; veranos calurosos, secos
- Tierras altas; temperatura y precipitación varían según la elevación
- — Frontera internacional
- — Límite estatal
- ★ Capital del estado
- • Otra ciudad

Vivir en la tierra

Los indígenas de California usaban plantas, animales y otros recursos naturales de su región para hacer lo que necesitaban para vivir.

Ambientes

Cada región de California tiene un ambiente y un clima diferentes.

Encierra en un círculo el nombre de la región en que vives.

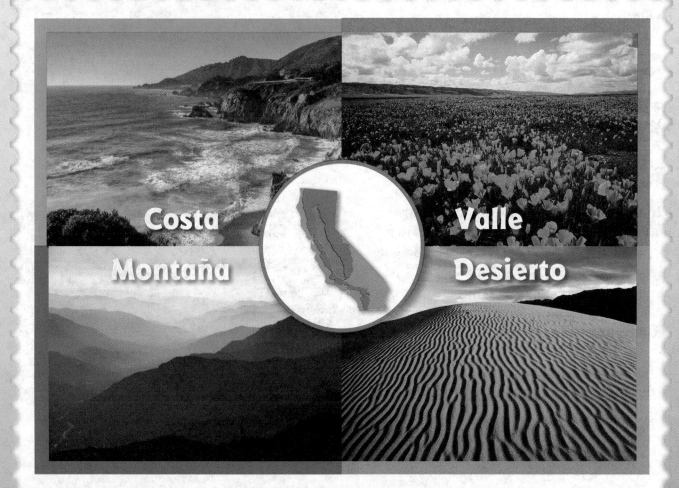

Costa

Valle

Montaña

Desierto

Viviendas

Costa

Casas hechas de plantas y madera

Los indígenas de la costa construían sus casas con plantas y árboles de su región. Los yuroks hacían sus casas con madera de secoya. Los pomos primero armaban una estructura con postes de madera y luego la cubrían con ramas de roble o de sauce. Por último, cubrían sus casas con hierba de junco.

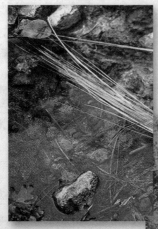

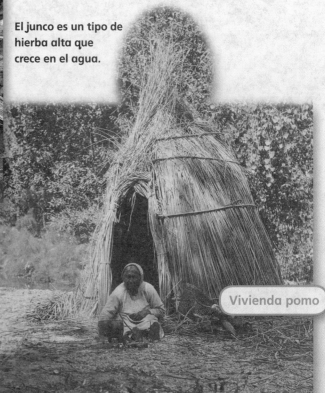

El junco es un tipo de hierba alta que crece en el agua.

Vivienda pomo

Montaña

Casas construidas bajo tierra

Los hupas cavaban agujeros profundos en la tierra para construir sus viviendas. Después hacían estantes de tierra comprimida junto a las paredes subterráneas. El techo y las paredes superiores estaban hechas de tablones de madera de cedro de la región. En el centro de cada casa había un hoyo para el fogón, que se usaba para cocinar y calentar la casa.

¿Qué usaban los indígenas de la costa y los de la montaña para construir sus viviendas?

_____

_____

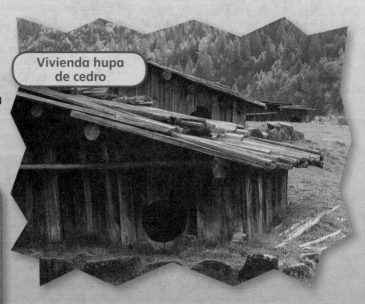

Vivienda hupa de cedro

Viviendas

Valle

Casas hechas de hierba

Los yokuts y los miwoks construían casas en forma de cono. Primero cavaban una zanja no muy profunda y hacían una estructura de postes. Luego entretejían ramas de árbol en los postes. Después ataban manojos de hierba seca a las ramas. Por último, hacían el techo con corteza de árboles de cedro o de pino.

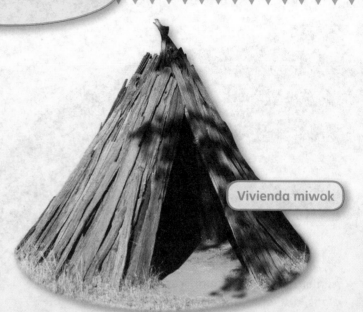

Vivienda miwok

Desierto

Vivienda de verano, vivienda de invierno

¿Qué tipo de vivienda construirías si vivieras en un lugar caluroso y seco? Los indígenas del desierto hacían sus casas con arbustos y madera. Construían parte de sus viviendas bajo tierra para protegerse del caliente sol. Para mantenerse abrigados durante el invierno, los mojaves amontonaban lodo sobre sus casas.

Desierto de Mojave

En el texto, encierra en un círculo un recurso usado en el valle y otro recurso usado en el desierto para la construcción de viviendas.

Alimentos

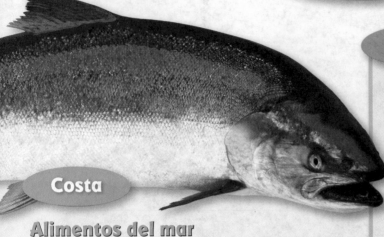

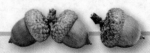

Valle

Comer bellotas

Alimentos: Bellotas, mariscos, plantas, raíces, saltamontes, alces, aves, antílopes

Muchos indígenas del valle comían bellotas. ¿Cómo las comían? Primero ponían las bellotas en un hueco que se hacía en una piedra y las molían. Después remojaban las bellotas molidas para que supieran mejor. Por último, las cocinaban y obtenían una sopa espesa.

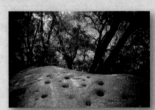

Huecos para moler bellotas

Costa

Alimentos del mar

Alimentos: Pescado, mariscos, aves marinas, algas, antílopes, focas, ballenas, uvas, miel

Los indígenas de la costa obtenían la mayor parte de sus alimentos del mar. Se metían al agua y usaban una red grande para atrapar peces. Recolectaban almejas, mejillones, cangrejos y langostas, y atrapaban aves marinas en redes grandes.

Muchos indígenas de California comían bellotas, semillas, venados, pescado, nueces, bayas, osos y liebres. ¿Qué otros alimentos comían en cada región?

Bellotas molidas

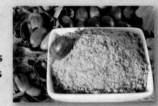

Montaña

Saltamontes asados

Alimentos: Uvas, alces, mapaches, ardillas, codornices, patos, saltamontes, semillas

¿Has atrapado alguna vez un saltamontes? Los maidus atrapaban saltamontes y se los comían. Primero, usaban ramas de árbol para hacer que los saltamontes cayeran en hoyos llenos de agua. Después los sacaban de los hoyos con cestas. Por último, los asaban antes de comérselos.

Desierto

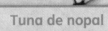

Tuna de nopal

Bocadillos de cactus

Alimentos: Maíz, calabacines, frijoles, calabazas, nopal, carnero cimarrón, insectos

El nopal era un alimento importante para los indígenas del desierto. Comían la tuna, que es la fruta del nopal. Algunas veces la secaban al sol para que se mantuviera fresca por más tiempo.

Encierra en un círculo los nombres de dos regiones donde los indígenas de California comían saltamontes.

Vestimenta

Costa

Plumas y pieles

En invierno, los indígenas de la costa usaban ropa hecha con plumas y con piel de animales. Primero, secaban las pieles de venado, conejo o nutria marina. Luego le daban forma de bata o de cobija. Los luiseños también hacían zapatos con pieles de animales.

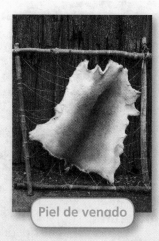
Piel de venado

Valle

Ropa de hierba y pieles

La mayoría de los indígenas del valle hacían su ropa con plantas y piel de animales. Las mujeres yokuts hacían ropa con juncos y corteza de sauce. Durante el invierno, los hombres y las mujeres usaban batas y vestidos hechos con pieles de animales.

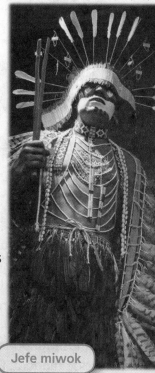
Jefe miwok

Montaña

Ropa de conchas marinas

Los indígenas de la montaña a menudo usaban conchas marinas para hacer ropa. Muchas mujeres hupas usaban faldas tejidas con yuca y conchas. También hilaban cáscaras de piñón con yuca para hacer delantales. Para las ceremonias especiales decoraban los delantales y las faldas con pedazos de concha de almeja y de otros moluscos. Los hupas decoraban sus tocados para la cabeza con plumas de aves como búhos y pájaros carpinteros.

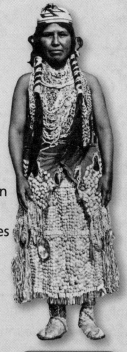
Mujer hupa

En el texto, encierra en un círculo los tipos de recursos que los indígenas de California utilizaban para hacer ropa.

Desierto

Batas en el desierto

Muchas mujeres indígenas del desierto usaban delantales hechos con corteza de árbol. Los indígenas del desierto a menudo usaban sandalias hechas con fibras tejidas de la planta de yuca. Las sandalias les protegían los pies cuando caminaban sobre la áspera tierra. Los inviernos son fríos incluso en el caluroso desierto. Muchos indígenas del desierto usaban batas hechas con piel de liebre para mantenerse calientes.

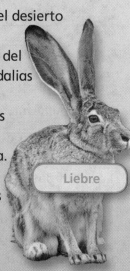
Liebre

Herramientas

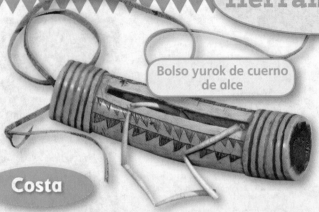

Bolso yurok de cuerno de alce

Valle

Herramientas de pesca y caza

Punta de arpón de obsidiana

Costa

Muchos tipos de herramientas

Los indígenas de la costa usaban muchos recursos de su región para hacer herramientas. Utilizaban fibras de plantas como el algodoncillo para hacer cuerda. Los chumash tallaban platos y cuencos de madera. Los yuroks hacían bolsos de cuerno de alce y conchas marinas.

Muchos indígenas de California eran cesteros hábiles. Hacían las cestas con distintas partes de plantas. Tenían muchos usos.

Los indígenas del valle usaban madera, piedras y plantas para hacer herramientas de pesca y caza. Los miwoks hacían arpones de pesca tallados en madera. Las puntas de arpón eran de una piedra dura y vidriosa llamada obsidiana. Los indígenas del valle hacían redes de pesca con fibras de plantas.

Cesta timbisha

Montaña

Pescar en el río

Hombre mojave con arco y flechas

Desierto

Herramientas hechas con plantas y arcilla

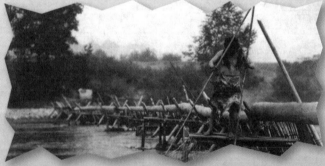

Represa hupa en el río Trinity

Los indígenas de la montaña usaban diferentes herramientas de pesca. Los hupas pescaban con redes. Durante el verano, cuando el nivel del agua del río estaba bajo, construían una enorme represa de madera que cruzaba el río. Luego se sentaban en la represa y tiraban grandes redes al agua para atrapar peces.

Los indígenas del desierto utilizaban diversos recursos para hacer herramientas. Algunos hacían cestas con juncos y hierba. Los mojaves hacían ollas de arcilla. También hacían arcos y flechas de madera.

Subraya en el texto seis herramientas u otras cosas útiles que los indígenas de California hacían con madera.

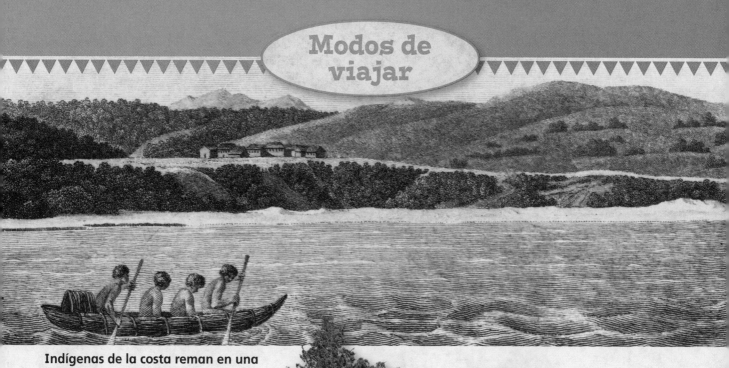

Modos de viajar

Indígenas de la costa reman en una balsa en la bahía de San Francisco.

Costa

Viajar en canoa

Los indígenas de California usaban balsas y canoas para viajar por agua. Las balsas eran manojos de juncos atados. Los chumash construían botes de cedro. Los yuroks hacían canoas escarbando el interior de troncos de árboles.

Montaña

Canoas de secoya

Las canoas eran un importante medio de transporte para los indígenas de la montaña. Los hupas hacían canoas con troncos de secoya. Usaban las canoas en el río Trinity.

Secoyas

Valle

Otros modos de viajar

Los indígenas del valle no usaban canoas. Muchos de ellos nadaban. Los que no sabían nadar viajaban en troncos empujados por los que nadaban. Algunos indígenas del valle también usaban balsas para transportar personas y provisiones por río.

Desierto

Ir con la corriente y flotar

Los yumas y los mojaves vivían cerca de ríos pero no hacían canoas. A menudo usaban balsas para dejarse llevar por la corriente río abajo. Algunas veces dejaban que las provisiones flotaran en troncos huecos. Muchos indígenas del desierto nadaban junto a grandes palanganas llenas de ropa y sábanas que echaban a flotar en los ríos.

En el texto, encierra en un círculo los diferentes modos que los indígenas de California tenían de viajar por agua.

¿Cómo vivían los indígenas de California?

Completa la oración de la caja que está abajo en el centro escribiendo el nombre de la región en que vives. Luego escribe en las otras cajas una lista de datos sobre los indígenas de California de tu región.

Alimentos

Vestimenta

Idea central

Los indígenas de California de la región del (de la) _____ usaban los recursos para hacer las cosas que necesitaban.

Viviendas

Herramientas

Modos de viajar

H-SS 3.2.3 Describen la economía y los sistemas de gobierno, especialmente aquellos que tienen constituciones tribales, y su relación con los gobiernos federal y estatal.

¿Cómo funcionan los grupos indígenas de California?

CONÉCTATE ¿Hay reglas en tu casa? Muchos grupos indígenas americanos tienen un plan escrito que explica las reglas a sus miembros.

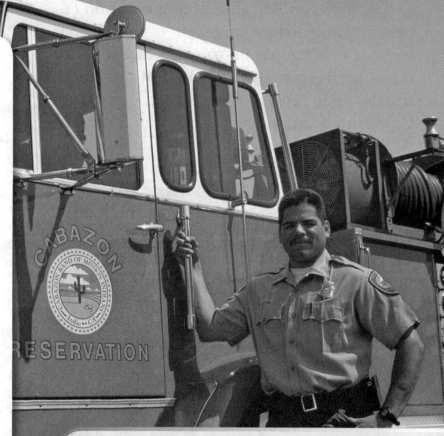

Vistazo previo
Vocabulario

reservación *(s.)* extensión de tierra que pertenece a un grupo indígena americano

gobierno *(s.)* personas que dirigen un estado o un país, o las leyes de un estado o un país

leyes *(s.)* reglas hechas por un gobierno

constitución *(s.)* plan escrito para gobernar

economía *(s.)* manera en que las cosas se fabrican y se compran y venden en un país, una región, un estado o un área local

Actividad de vocabulario Escoge las palabras del vocabulario que mejor completan esta oración:

Las _____ de un país están hechas por las personas que dirigen el _____ .

🔊 Lectura: Comparar y contrastar

Recuerda que *comparar* significa describir en lo que se parecen dos o más cosas. *Contrastar* significa describir en lo que se diferencian. Subraya la oración de la página 42 que compare o que contraste dos cosas.

Tierras de los indígenas americanos

Hoy en día algunos indígenas americanos viven en reservaciones o en rancherías, que son reservaciones más pequeñas. Una **reservación** es una extensión de tierra que pertenece a un grupo indígena americano.

Cómo funcionan los gobiernos tribales

Las reservaciones de indígenas americanos tienen gobiernos tribales. El **gobierno** son las personas que dirigen un estado o un país, o las leyes de un estado o un país. Las **leyes** son las reglas hechas por un gobierno. Los gobiernos tribales están separados del gobierno estatal de California y están supervisados por el gobierno de los Estados Unidos. Dos tipos de gobierno indígena americano son el consejo tribal y el consejo general. Su función es hacer las leyes de una reservación. Al igual que nuestras ciudades y nuestros estados, algunas reservaciones tienen sus propias fuerzas policiales, que se aseguran de que se obedezcan las leyes, así como servicios de bomberos. Algunas también tienen sus propios tribunales y jueces.

Este policía indígena de California trabaja en una reservación cerca de Indio.

1. 🎯 Comparar y contrastar

¿En qué se diferencian las reservaciones a las rancherías?

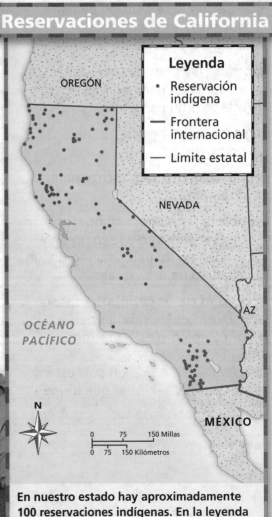

Reservaciones de California

Leyenda
- • Reservación indígena
- — Frontera internacional
- — Límite estatal

OREGÓN

NEVADA

AZ

OCÉANO PACÍFICO

N

MÉXICO

| 0 | 75 | 150 Millas |
| 0 | 75 | 150 Kilómetros |

En nuestro estado hay aproximadamente 100 reservaciones indígenas. En la leyenda del mapa, encierra en un círculo el símbolo que representa una reservación.

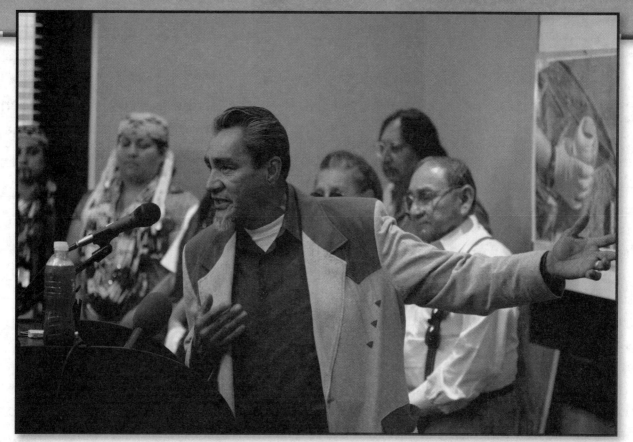

Un miembro del consejo tribal indígena de California habla sobre la condición del río Klamath en el norte de California.

Algunos gobiernos tribales de indígenas americanos hacen leyes de la misma manera que nuestro gobierno estatal. Esas leyes garantizan la seguridad de las personas. También aseguran que las personas tengan derecho al voto y a tener tierras.

Planes escritos de gobierno

Muchos gobiernos tribales, tal como el cahuilla, tienen su propia constitución. Una **constitución** es un plan escrito para gobernar. Esas constituciones tienen un preámbulo, al igual que las constituciones de los Estados Unidos y de California. Un preámbulo es una introducción. Esas constituciones también tienen partes llamadas artículos, que dan más detalles acerca de las leyes.

2. ¿Qué función tienen los consejos tribales y generales?

Idea principal y detalles

3. Comparar y contrastar
¿En qué se parecen la constitución cahuilla y la Constitución de los Estados Unidos?

Las reservaciones ganan dinero

Los indígenas de California ayudan a la economía de nuestro estado de muchas maneras. Una **economía** es la manera en que las cosas se fabrican y se compran y venden en un país, una región, un estado o un área local. Algunos grupos administran granjas o tiendas. Muchos grupos reciben visitantes en sus reservaciones y rancherías. Los visitantes gastan dinero para poder acampar en el área o para comprar objetos de arte o artesanías, como canastas y joyas. También llegan para entretenerse con las danzas, los cantos o las narraciones de historias. Cuando pescan, grupos como los yuroks guardan una parte de la pesca y venden el resto a personas que no viven en la reservación.

4. Escribe tres cosas que pueden comprar los visitantes de una reservación o una ranchería.

Idea principal y detalles

_____

_____

_____

Este hombre hupa cuida árboles jóvenes en un invernadero.

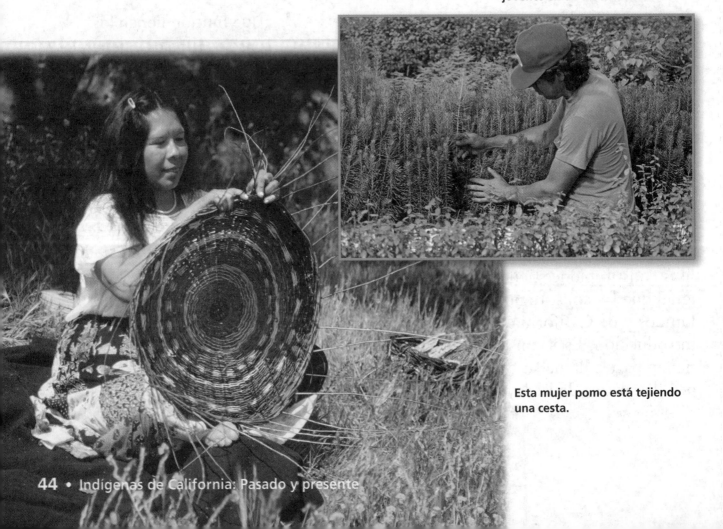

Esta mujer pomo está tejiendo una cesta.

Ayudar a la economía

El dinero que las personas gastan en las reservaciones y rancherías ayuda a nuestra economía. Esto les permite a los indígenas de California gastar ese dinero fuera de la reservación o la ranchería. En los pueblos cercanos compran la cosas que necesitan y quieren, o pagan ciertas actividades, como el servicio de un banco. A su vez, los negocios de los pueblos pagan dinero a nuestro gobierno estatal y al gobierno de los Estados Unidos. Entre otras cosas, el gobierno utiliza el dinero para construir o mejorar escuelas, carreteras y parques.

5. Describe el flujo de dinero que sale de una reservación o ranchería. *Secuencia*

_____

_____

_____

_____

_____

Flujo del dinero entre los grupos indígenas de California y las ciudades de California

entretenimiento

frutas y verduras

objetos de arte y artesanías

Los visitantes en la reservación o ranchería gastan dinero en . . .

actividades que la gente no puede hacer en la reservación, como el servicio de un banco

Los indígenas de California visitan los pueblos locales y gastan dinero en . . .

HOSPITAL

TIENDA

cosas que la gente no puede comprar en la reservación

En el diagrama, encierra en un círculo los lugares donde los habitantes de una reservación gastan dinero.

Resumen

Los gobiernos tribales usan constituciones para establecer las reglas de las reservaciones. ¿En qué se parecen los gobiernos tribales a los gobiernos estatal y nacional?

Ubicación relativa y ubicación absoluta

Aprende más Puedes describir dónde la mayoría de los lugares se encuentran usando ubicación relativa o ubicación absoluta. La ubicación relativa te indica dónde está un lugar comparado con la ubicación de otro lugar. Se quisieras describir la ubicación relativa del edificio del consejo tribal, dirías que está cerca del lote de estacionamiento.

La ubicación absoluta te indica con mayor exactitud la ubicación de un lugar. Puedes usar un mapa con cuadrícula para buscar la ubicación relativa o la absoluta. Cada cuadrado tiene una letra y un número basados en el lugar donde la columna de letras se encuentra con la columna de números. La ubicación absoluta del edificio del consejo tribal es C1. Usa el siguiente mapa con cuadrícula para contestar las preguntas.

Inténtalo

1. Encierra en un círculo el lugar cuya ubicación absoluta sea A1. *Identificar*

2. ¿Cuál es la ubicación relativa del lote de estacionamiento en relación al edificio del consejo tribal y al museo tribal? *Interpretar*

_____

_____

_____

3. ¿Cuál es la ubicación absoluta de los árboles? *Identificar*

_____

4. Dibuja una casa en el lugar cuya ubicación relativa está entre el estanque y la granja. *Aplicar*

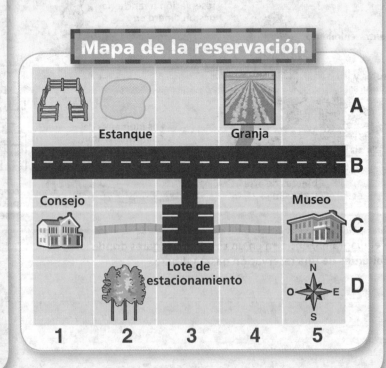

Mapa de la reservación

Estanque   Granja   A

B

Consejo   Museo   C

Lote de estacionamiento   D

1   2   3   4   5

Planear y trabajar

Los indígenas de California han combinado su modo de vida con maneras nuevas de gobernarse y de llevar a cabo sus negocios.

Naciones indígenas de California

¿Sabías que muchos indígenas de California pertenecen a un grupo indígena de California, a nuestro estado y a nuestro país?

Algunos indígenas de California pertenecen a una nación indígena de California. El gobierno de los Estados Unidos llegó a acuerdos con grupos indígenas americanos de la misma manera que lo hizo con otras naciones. Más de 100 de estas naciones se encuentran en California.

Los Estados Unidos

Montaña
Tribu del valle Hoopa (Hupa)

Valle
Grupo Tuolumne de indígenas miwoks

Costa
Grupo Santa Ynez de indígenas chumash

Desierto
Grupo Agua Caliente de indígenas cahuillas

California

Subraya la nación indígena de California que se encuentra en tu región.

Costa

De líder a comité administrativo

Hace muchos años, cada poblado chumash tenía un líder llamado *wot*. El *wot* podía ser hombre o mujer, y era quien tomaba las decisiones importantes para el grupo.

Hoy en día muchos chumash viven en la reservación Santa Ynez. Tienen su propia constitución. Estos chumash eligen, o escogen, a cinco personas, que formarán parte de un comité administrativo. El comité toma decisiones sobre asuntos de importancia para los chumash. Todo adulto chumash tiene voz en las decisiones que el comité toma.

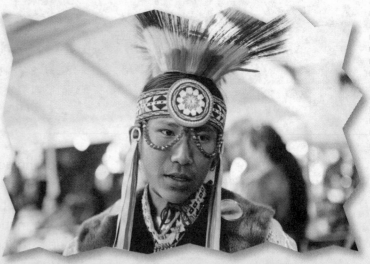

Hombre chumash de hoy en la ropa tradicional

Valle

Reuniones en la Casa Redonda

En el pasado, casi todos los grupos miwoks tenían un líder. El líder asignaba labores durante la cosecha de bellotas, resolvía problemas, recibía a invitados y se encargaba de las ceremonias. A veces el líder se reunía con la gente en la Casa Redonda.

Hoy en día muchos miwoks viven en rancherías. Cada grupo tiene una constitución. La mayoría de las rancherías eligen un consejo tribal. El consejo trabaja para mejorar cosas como escuelas y servicios de salud. El consejo de la ranchería Tuolumne a veces se reúne en la Casa Redonda.

> Encierra en un círculo los nombres de los grupos pequeños que son elegidos por algunos chumash y miwoks.

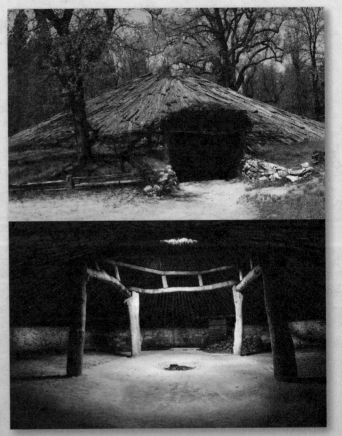

Exterior e interior de la Casa Redonda de un consejo miwok

Montaña

Trabajar juntos

Hace mucho tiempo, los hupas vivían en siete poblados en el valle Hoopa. Cada poblado tenía su propio líder. Los habitantes de los poblados trabajaban como grupo. Se reunían para celebrar ceremonias especiales. También se unían cuando tenían que defenderse.

Hoy en día los hupas manejan las distintas partes de su gobierno. Han tenido una constitución por más de cincuenta años. Los hupas eligen un consejo tribal. Operan sus propios hospitales, cuerpos de policía y de bomberos, y escuelas.

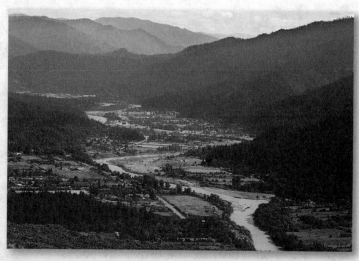

Vista de la reservación indígena del valle Hoopa

Escribe una marca junto a las regiones donde viven grupos que tienen una constitución.

Desierto

Líderes cahuillas

En cada grupo cahuilla había una persona llamada *nét*, que se aseguraba de que las canciones y las ceremonias fueran llevadas a cabo correctamente. También era quien tomaba decisiones importantes para el grupo.

Actualmente hay nueve grupos, o bandas, cahuillas. Cada banda elige su propio consejo tribal. El consejo tribal hace las reglas de la banda. La constitución del grupo de Agua Caliente establece las funciones de su consejo tribal. Una de esas funciones es proteger los recursos naturales de las tierras del grupo.

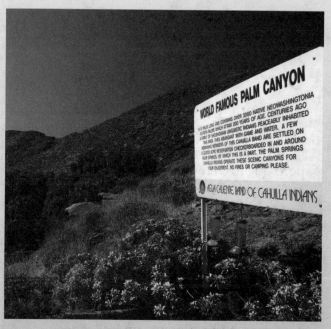

Una de las funciones de los consejos tribales cahuillas es proteger los recursos naturales, como Palm Canyon.

Economía

Costa

Nuevos usos de la tierra

Los luiseños han encontrado nuevas maneras de usar la tierra donde, hace mucho tiempo, pescaban, cazaban y recolectaban alimentos. Un grupo luiseño dirige un área para acampar en su reservación, cerca de San Diego. El río San Luis Rey, que atraviesa la reservación, se usa para actividades como flotación en tubo, natación y pesca. Los visitantes van a la reservación para disfrutar de esas actividades.

Otro grupo luiseño se ha dedicado a cultivar huertos en su reservación. El grupo cultiva y vende naranjas, limones amarillos y aguacates. Estas actividades ayudan a la economía.

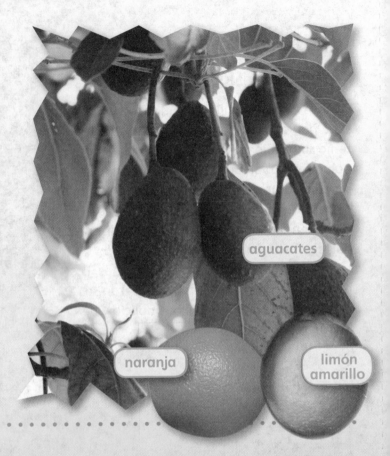

aguacates

naranja

limón amarillo

Valle

Big Time

Cada otoño los miwoks celebran *Big Time* (el Gran Momento), o Festival de la Bellota. El *Big Time* es una oportunidad para que los miwoks les enseñen sus tradiciones a otras personas. También los ayuda a ganar dinero con los visitantes que llegan a ver el festival. Muchas personas visitan la ranchería Tuolumne para presenciar el Festival de la Bellota. Se divierten viendo a los bailarines, comprando objetos de arte y artesanías, comiendo o participando en los juegos.

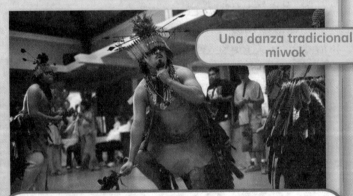

Una danza tradicional miwok

Escribe de qué dos maneras los visitantes ayudan a las economías de los luiseños o los miwoks.

_____

_____

Montaña

Peces etiquetados

La pesca siempre ha sido parte del modo de vida de los hupas. Actualmente los hupas, junto con el gobierno de California, dirigen un criadero de peces. Un criadero es el lugar donde se protege a los peces jóvenes que han salido del huevo. Después los peces son liberados en arroyos y ríos. Los hupas les ponen unas pequeñas etiquetas para poder seguirles el rastro. Una vez que crecen, los peces son capturados y vendidos. Esta actividad ayuda a la economía de la región.

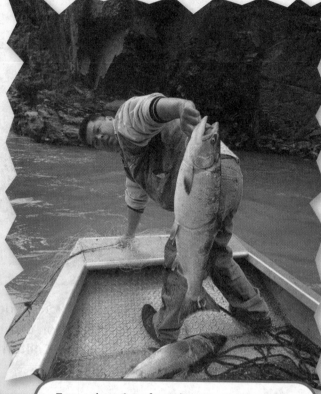

Un empleado de un criadero de peces hupa muestra los salmones que ha pescado en el río Trinity.

En cada párrafo subraya una oración que explique cómo los hupas y los cahuilla de Agua Caliente ayudan a la economía de su región.

Desierto

Vistas del cañón

Los baños termales de Palm Springs han sido una parte importante de la historia de los Agua Caliente, un grupo cahuilla. Los baños suministraban agua al grupo. Después se convirtieron en una forma de ganar dinero. Hoy en día los cahuillas dirigen un centro de recreación cercano a los baños termales. Los visitantes se hospedan en el centro, o simplemente recorren los cañones cercanos. Los cahuillas siguen protegiendo los cañones donde, hace mucho tiempo, se dedicaban a la caza y a la recolección de alimentos.

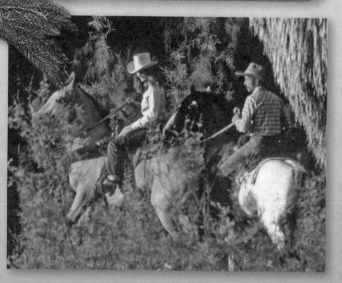

Visitantes recorren a caballo los cañones en las tierras de los Agua Caliente.

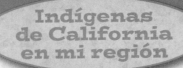

¿Qué es importante sobre la economía y el gobierno de los indígenas de California en mi región?

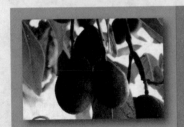 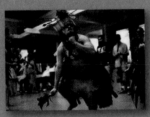 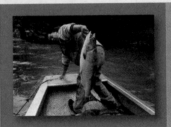 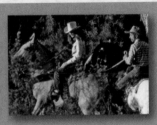

Costa   **Valle**   **Montaña**   **Desierto**

Encierra en un círculo la fotografía de arriba que muestre tu región. Basándote en la fotografía, a continuación escribe una oración que diga algo acerca de la economía de los indígenas de California en tu región.

_____

_____

Escribe dos datos sobre el actual gobierno de los indígenas de California en tu región.

1. _____

_____

2. _____

_____

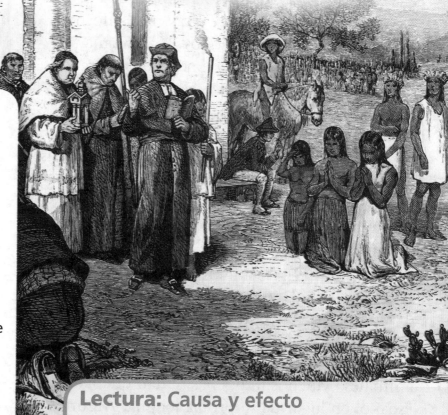

H-SS 3.2.4 Discuten la interacción entre los nuevos colonos y los indígenas que ya estaban establecidos en la región.

¿Cómo cambiaron los europeos la vida de los indígenas de California?

IMAGINA LA ESCENA ¿Qué harías si te estuvieras mudando a una nueva casa y encontraras que ya hay alguien viviendo en ella? Eso fue lo que ocurrió cuando los europeos llegaron a vivir a América del Norte. La tierra donde querían vivir ya era el hogar de muchos grupos indígenas americanos.

Vistazo previo
Vocabulario

interactuar *(v.)* hablar con otras personas y trabajar con ellas

colono *(s.)* alguien que llega a un nuevo lugar para vivir allí

cooperar *(v.)* trabajar juntos

conflicto *(s.)* lucha o desacuerdo

misión *(s.)* asentamiento establecido por un grupo religioso donde se le enseña religión y otros modos de vida a la población indígena

religión *(s.)* sistema de fe y de culto

Actividad de vocabulario Dibuja una línea que una las dos palabras del vocabulario que tienen casi el mismo significado.

Lectura: Causa y efecto

Recuerda que una *causa* es la razón por la que algo sucede. Un *efecto* es lo que sucede como resultado de la causa. Subraya la oración de la página 54 que explique el efecto que tuvieron en los indígenas de California las enfermedades que los colonos españoles trajeron.

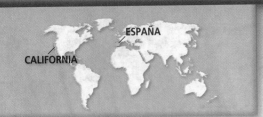
1767 España envía a Gaspar de Portolá para que administre sus tierras en California.

1775 Un grupo de indígenas de California destruye una misión.

Llegan los españoles

Los españoles llegaron en el siglo XVIII a lo que hoy es California. Muchos buscaban tierras y riquezas. En esa época, aproximadamente 300,000 indígenas de California vivían en la región. Los españoles empezaron a interactuar con los indígenas de California. **Interactuar** significa hablar con otras personas y trabajar con ellas. En 1767 España envió a Gaspar de Portolá para que administrara sus tierras en California.

La llegada de más colonos a California cambió el modo de vida de muchos indígenas de California. Un **colono** es alguien que llega a un nuevo lugar para vivir allí. Algunos colonos españoles querían que los indígenas construyeran **misiones** y trabajaran en ellas. Las misiones son asentamientos establecidos por grupos religiosos donde se enseñaba religión y otro modo de vida a la población indígena. **Religión** es un sistema de fe y de culto.

Muchos indígenas de California habían vivido de la caza y la recolección de alimentos desde mucho antes de que los españoles llegaran. Pero algunos colonos españoles los obligaron a trabajar en sus granjas y a cuidar sus animales. Muchos indígenas tenían que hablar español en lugar de su propia lengua. Algunos se enfermaron con enfermedades que los colonos habían traído consigo de España. Esto causó que la población de indígenas de California disminuyera.

1. Escribe un efecto para la causa que está abajo. *Causa y efecto*

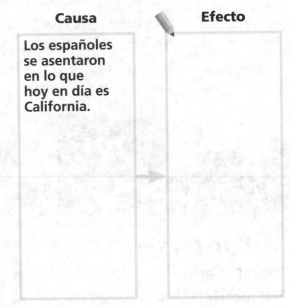

Causa	Efecto
Los españoles se asentaron en lo que hoy en día es California.	

SIGLO XIX

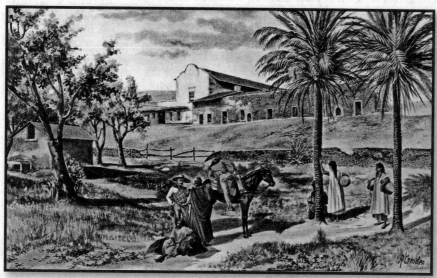

Algunos colonos españoles obligaron a muchos indígenas de California a trabajar en las granjas de las misiones.

Tratar de llevarse bien

Los colonos españoles a veces se llevaban bien con los indígenas de California. Otras veces, no. El comercio era un aspecto en el que se llevaban bien. Cuando comerciaban, **cooperaban** entre sí, es decir, trabajaban juntos.

Durante el siglo XIX, los colonos españoles querían tener más tierras. Una de las razones por las que los colonos querían más tierras era para sus animales. Ésas eran las tierras donde los indígenas de California habían vivido durante mucho tiempo. La necesidad de tierras pronto desembocó en un conflicto entre los colonos y los indígenas de California. Un **conflicto** es una lucha o un desacuerdo. En 1775 un grupo de indígenas se defendío y destruyó una misión en San Diego.

2. Comparar y contrastar

Subraya una situación en la que los indígenas de California y los colonos españoles se llevaban bien y otra en la que no.

Resumen

La vida de muchos indígenas de California cambió con la llegada de los europeos. ¿Cómo interactuaron estos dos grupos?

Diarios: Padre Pedro Font

Aprende más Una fuente primaria es la descripción de un suceso por alguien que estuvo presente cuando el suceso ocurrió. Las fuentes primarias pueden ser diarios, cartas, documentos, entrevistas e incluso pinturas o fotografías. La fuente primaria que se muestra abajo es del diario del padre Pedro Font. Los diarios nos cuentan los pensamientos y los sentimientos de personas que vivieron hace mucho tiempo.

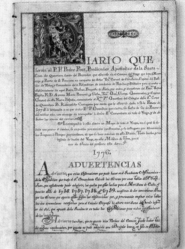

El padre Pedro Font viajó a California con otros colonos españoles a finales del siglo XVIII. En su diario escribió acerca de los encuentros que tuvo con diferentes grupos de indígenas americanos. Lee la anotación de diario del padre Font. Luego contesta las preguntas.

1. Subraya las cosas que los indígenas cajuenches llevaron para intercambiarlas con los españoles.

Identificar

2. ¿Por qué decidieron quedarse en el lago el padre Font y los otros colonos?

Analizar

_____

_____

_____

Para que los caballos y las mulas, que estaban en malas condiciones, pudieran refrescarse con el buen pasto que hay alrededor de este estanque, decidimos quedarnos aquí. Muchos indígenas de la nación cajuenche, que viven desde aquí y río abajo, se acercaron gozosos al campamento trayendo consigo muchas sandías, calabazas y otras provisiones [suministros de comida], que intercambiaron por cuentas.

—7 de diciembre de 1775

Interactuar con otros

Los indígenas de California interactuaron con los colonos y con otros que llegaron a su área. Algunos de sus encuentros fueron amistosos. Otros, no.

Intercambio de regalos y comercio

Los indígenas de California y los colonos cooperaban intercambiando regalos o comerciando entre sí.

A veces los indígenas de California recibían a los colonos tras sus largos viajes y les ofrecían alimentos como nueces, frutas, verduras o pescado. A cambio, ellos recibían herramientas de metal de los colonos. Los indígenas de California también estaban interesados en las telas y la ropa europea. Algunos indígenas de California comerciaban con piel de castor con los colonos.

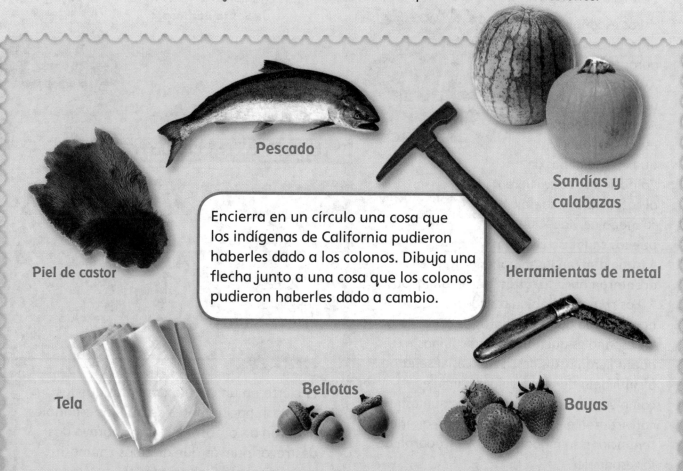

Pescado

Sandías y calabazas

Piel de castor

Encierra en un círculo una cosa que los indígenas de California pudieron haberles dado a los colonos. Dibuja una flecha junto a una cosa que los colonos pudieron haberles dado a cambio.

Herramientas de metal

Tela

Bellotas

Bayas

57

Algo huele a pescado

¿Sabías que probablemente uno de los primeros regalos que los indígenas de California les hicieron a los europeos fue pescado? Ocurrió en 1542, cuando las embarcaciones de Juan Rodríguez Cabrillo navegaban cerca de la costa. Unos chumash salieron en canoas para recibirlos a él y a su tripulación, que venían de España, y les llevaron pescado como alimento.

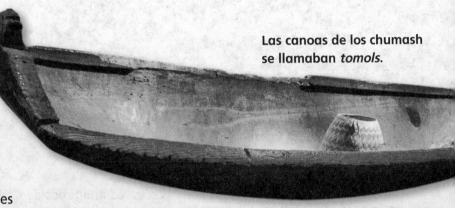

Las canoas de los chumash se llamaban *tomols*.

Los chumash en las misiones

Los españoles regresaron a California durante el siglo XVIII para construir asentamientos. Algunos colonos españoles querían que los indígenas de California se convirtieran al catolicismo y cambiaran su modo de vida. Querían que los chumash vivieran y trabajaran en las misiones. Algunos aceptaron hacerlo, otros fueron obligados.

Los chumash habían cazado y pescado en esta área durante cientos de años. Pero los españoles querían que los chumash aprendieran otras destrezas. Les enseñaron a cultivar la tierra y a cuidar animales como vacas y caballos. Algunos chumash se convirtieron en vaqueros. Otros no querían renunciar a su modo de vida y escaparon de los españoles.

Los indígenas de California lavaban su ropa en estos lavaderos de la misión de Santa Bárbara.

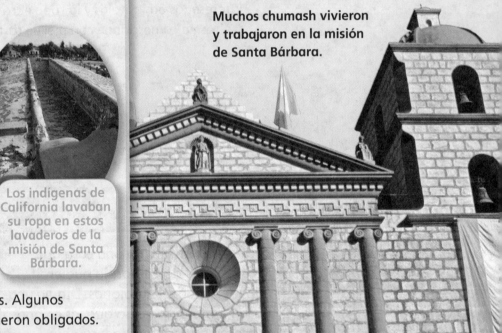

Muchos chumash vivieron y trabajaron en la misión de Santa Bárbara.

Encierra en un círculo dos cosas que los chumash hacían antes de que los españoles llegaran a California. Luego subraya dos destrezas nuevas que algunos chumash aprendieron de los españoles.

Desierto

Ellos fueron los guías

¿A quién le pedirías que te guiara por el desierto? Los mojaves conocían la manera de cruzar el desierto de Mojave. Seguían caminos que habían usado por muchos años. En 1776 algunos mojaves guiaron al padre Francisco Garcés, un sacerdote español, y a su grupo a través del desierto. Esto ayudó a que los españoles aprendieran a viajar por tierra desde México hasta sus misiones en California. En 1826 los mojaves ayudaron a guiar a Jedediah Smith, un comerciante de pieles estadounidense, por los caminos del desierto de Mojave.

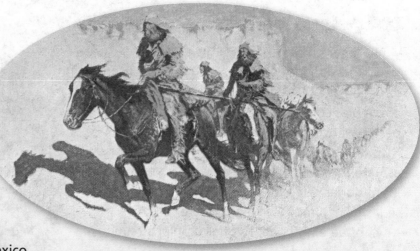

Con la ayuda de los mojaves, Jedediah Smith y su grupo fueron los primeros estadounidenses en llegar a California por tierra desde el este.

Una disputa por pieles

Jedediah Smith escribió en su diario que los mojaves lo trataron con mucha amabilidad. También describió los melones y las calabazas asadas que le dieron. Pero los problemas surgieron cuando llegaron los tramperos de pieles. Un trampero es alguien que caza animales para obtener su piel. Los mojaves pensaban que los tramperos no mostraban respeto por los animales que atrapaban. Sólo usaban la piel del animal y desperdiciaban el resto.

Los tramperos y los mojaves

En 1827 los mojaves y algunos tramperos comenzaron a pelear. Los mojaves les pidieron a los tramperos un caballo a cambio de ayudarlos a atrapar castores. Los tramperos no estaban de acuerdo con ese intercambio y comenzaron a pelear. Las peleas entre los tramperos y los mojaves duraron cerca de veinte años.

Los castores viven a lo largo del río Colorado, en la región del desierto. Estuvieron a punto de desaparecer porque los tramperos atraparon demasiados castores durante el siglo XIX.

Encierra en un círculo el nombre de las personas a quienes los mojaves ayudaron a cruzar el desierto.

Obligados a mudarse

El primer encuentro de los yokuts con los españoles se dio en 1772. Fueron amigables con los españoles, pero a principios del siglo XIX, algunos colonos regresaron con soldados españoles. Necesitaban más trabajadores para las misiones que tenían en la costa. Los españoles se llevaron a muchos yokuts a esas misiones. Muchos de ellos tuvieron que cambiar su modo de vida.

Los yokuts vivían en el valle de San Joaquín. Ahí se dedicaban a la caza y la recolección de alimentos.

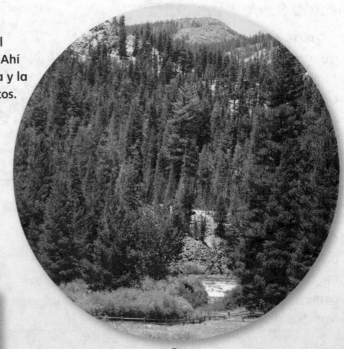

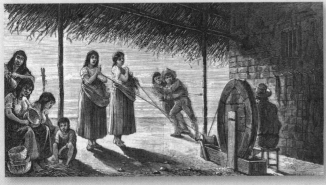

Los indígenas de California hacían soga en las misiones.

Un modo de vida distinto

Muchos yokuts eran infelices en las misiones. Fueron forzados a aprender una nueva religión. Ya no podían cazar, pescar o recolectar alimentos. En su lugar, los sacerdotes españoles los obligaron a trabajar en las granjas. Muchos yokuts se volvieron hábiles entrenadores de caballos y manejadores de ganado. Vivían amontonados en pequeñas cabañas. Cientos de yokuts se enfermaron y murieron. Sin embargo, algunos lograron escapar de las misiones y vivieron en libertad lejos de la costa.

> Subraya dos cosas en el texto que cambiaron el modo de vida de los yokuts.

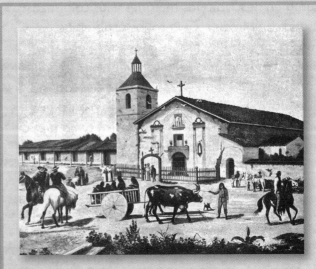

La misión de Santa Clara de Asís fue una de las misiones donde los yokuts fueron llevados a trabajar y a vivir.

Montaña

Escondidos

Las montañas alrededor del valle Hoopa aislaban a los hupas que vivían allí de cualquier visitante. Durante muchos años ni los colonos europeos, ni los estadounidenses pudieron llegar tan al norte, donde se encuentra este valle. Los hupas pescaban en el río Trinity y cazaban en los bosques del valle. Finalmente, en 1828, los hupas conocieron a un grupo de estadounidenses encabezado por Jedediah Smith. Después también conocieron a tramperos de pieles que pasaban por las montañas.

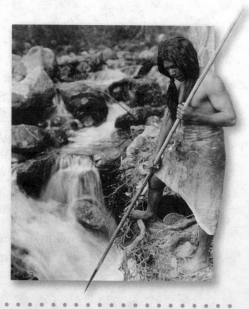

A veces los hombres hupas pescaban con arpón.

El oro lo cambia todo

En 1848 se descubrió oro en California. Muy pronto llegaron cientos de mineros a la zona. Gran parte del territorio en que se establecieron era donde vivían los hupas. Los mineros buscaban oro, por lo que cortaron muchos árboles y echaron desperdicios al río. Sus acciones hicieron que a los hupas se les hiciera difícil la caza de ciervo y la pesca.

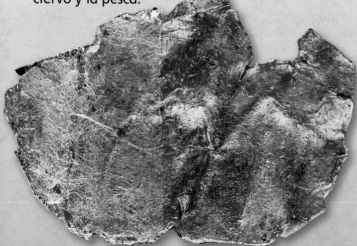

Éste es uno de los primeros pedazos de oro que fue hallado en California.

¡Hay oro en las colinas!

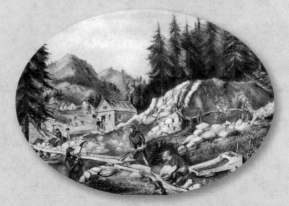

El descubrimiento de oro atrajo a miles de colonos a las tierras de los indígenas de California.

Encierra en un círculo dos de las cosas de abajo que a los hupas se les hizo difícil hacer después de la llegada de los mineros.

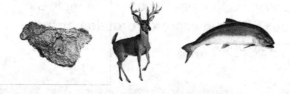

La pérdida de sus tierras

Más colonos llegaron después de que California se convirtiera en estado en 1850. Querían tierras para sus propias granjas, haciendas, pueblos y negocios. Algunos colonos atacaron a grupos indígenas de California. Querían sacarlos de las tierras donde habían vivido por cientos de años. Algunos grupos se defendieron. Hacia finales del siglo XIX, algunos indígenas de California vivían en reservaciones. Muchos otros se quedaron sin tierras.

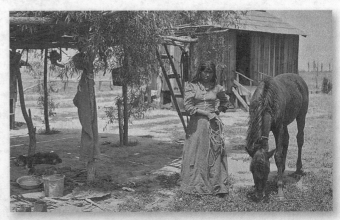

Algunos yokuts vivían cerca del lago Tulare, en el valle de San Joaquín, hasta principios de la década de 1930.

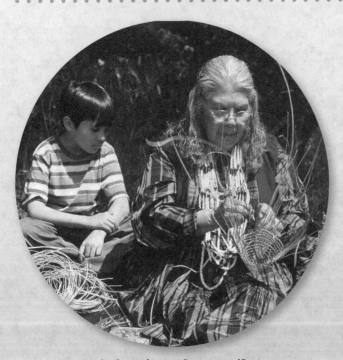

Una mujer hupa le enseña a uno niño a tejer una cesta.

Los indígenas de California en el presente

Actualmente los indígenas de California viven en reservaciones, en ciudades y en pueblos de nuestro estado. Están orgullosos de sus tradiciones y las comparten con los demás. Interpretan canciones y danzas. Hablan en la lengua de su grupo y se la enseñan a sus hijos. Las artesanías que hacen son tradicionales y también nuevas. Los indígenas de California en todo nuestro estado continúan celebrando su pasado al mismo tiempo que miran hacia el futuro.

> Escribe una manera en que los indígenas de California expresan orgullo por sus tradiciones.

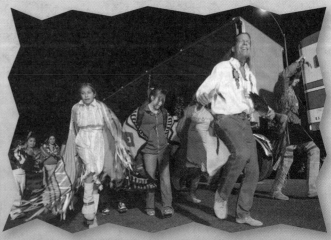

Danza tradicional indígena americana en un festival en California.

Para aprender más, puedes visitar un museo de tu pueblo o ciudad.

Costa

Si quieres aprender a excavar y extraer con cuidado objetos del pasado, apúntate al programa *"Dig It"* del **Museo del Suroeste del Indígena Americano (Southwest Museum of the American Indian)** en Los Ángeles. Aprenderás que los objetos enterrados nos pueden decir muchas cosas acerca de los indígenas y los colonos que llegaron.

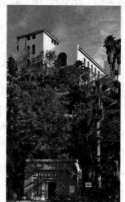

Desierto

¿Te has preguntado cómo los indígenas hacían fuego sin fósforos? ¿Qué comían? ¿Cómo cocinaban sus alimentos? En el **Museo Indígena de Antelope Valley (Antelope Valley Indian Museum)** en el desierto de Mojave, cerca de Lancaster, encontrarás las respuestas, e incluso podrás moler maíz.

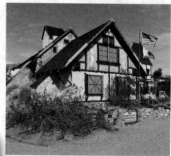

> Encierra en un círculo una cosa que te gustaría ver o hacer en uno de los museos. Subraya el nombre del museo.

Valle

En el área de taller del **Museo Indígena del Estado de California (California State Indian Museum)** en Sacramento, puedes probar a usar herramientas de los indígenas. También puedes ver sus casas, instrumentos de caza, instrumentos musicales y una canoa.

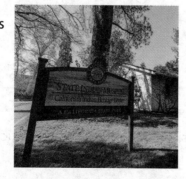

Montaña

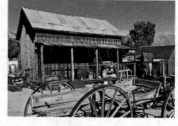

¿Sabías que algunas de las cestas más hermosas del mundo han sido hechas por los indígenas de California? Si visitas el **Museo de California del Este (Eastern California Museum)** en Independence, podrás ver una colección de cestas hechas por los paiutes y los shoshones.

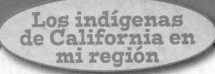

¿Qué sucedió en mi región?

Encierra en un círculo el grupo indígena de California más cercano a la región donde tú vives. Luego, escoge tres sucesos importantes que ocurrieron entre los colonos y el grupo indígena de California que encerraste en el círculo. Por último, en las cajas que están abajo escribe los sucesos en el orden en que ocurrieron.

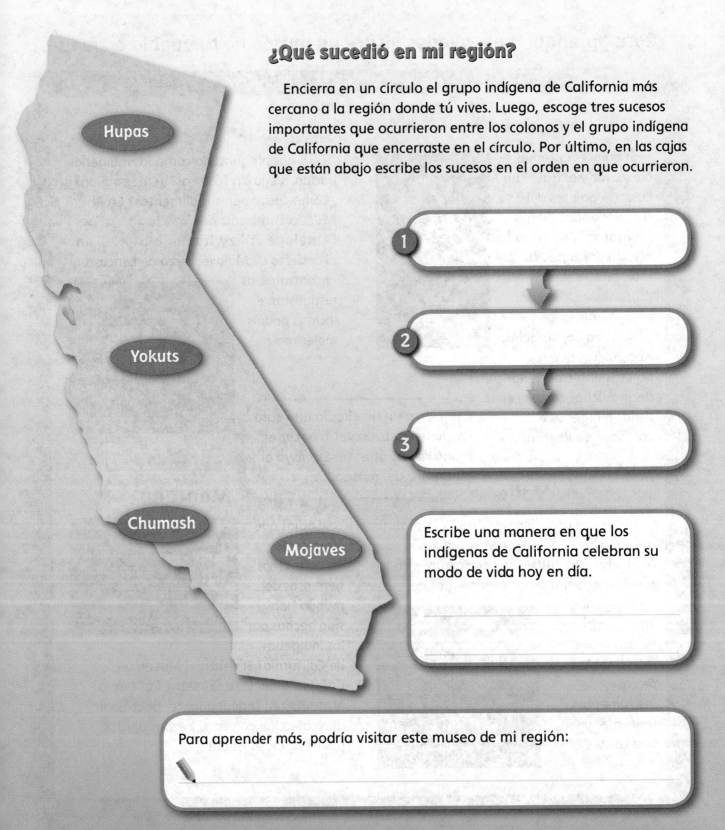

1

2

3

Escribe una manera en que los indígenas de California celebran su modo de vida hoy en día.

Para aprender más, podría visitar este museo de mi región:

Diario de estudio

En esta unidad aprenderás a ordenar correctamente la secuencia de algunos sucesos históricos de California. Verás cómo los lugares cambiaron conforme distintos grupos de gente se mudaban a las diferentes áreas. Completa las actividades que aparecen en estas páginas a medida que leas la unidad.

Lo que sé sobre...

los asentamientos en California:

_____

La gente que exploró o se asentó en California

Escribe la información que falta a continuación.

Tres personas que exploraron California fueron	Muchos trabajadores vinieron a California porque	Muchos pobladores vinieron a California porque

Escoge uno de los siguientes productos. Di por qué es importante para California.

- oro
- computadoras
- ferrocarril transcontinental
- naranjas
- películas

_____

_____

_____

_____

_____

Haz un dibujo de la persona más interesante de la unidad y escribe algo sobre ella.

Escribe la información que falta en esta línea cronológica.

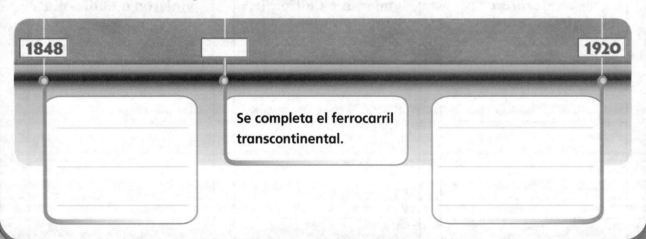

1848		1920

Se completa el ferrocarril transcontinental.

He aprendido...

H-SS 3.3.1 Investigan acerca de los exploradores que llegaron aquí, de los nuevos pobladores y de la gente que sigue llegando a la región, incluidas las contribuciones y tradiciones culturales y religiosas.

¿Quiénes han llegado a tu región?

IMAGINA LA ESCENA ¿Por qué ha llegado mucha gente a vivir a tu región? Los europeos llegaron por primera vez a lo que hoy es California en el siglo XVI. Les siguieron personas de muchos lugares. Todos llegaron por distintas razones. ¿Cómo colaboraron a que tu región sea lo que es actualmente?

Vistazo previo

Vocabulario

explorador *(s.)* alguien que viaja a nuevos lugares para saber más acerca de ellos

cultura *(s.)* artes, creencias, conductas e ideas de un grupo de gente

Actividad de vocabulario *Explorar* significa viajar a nuevos lugares para saber más acerca de ellos. Subraya la palabra de arriba que signifique "alguien que explora".

Personajes

Juan Rodríguez Cabrillo
Sebastián Vizcaíno
Francis Drake
John Sutter

Lectura: Secuencia

A menudo los escritores incluyen fechas para mostrar una *secuencia*, u orden, de los sucesos. En el primer párrafo de la página 69 encierra en un círculo las fechas relacionadas con los exploradores que llegaron a California. Usa la línea cronológica en la parte superior de cada página para seguir los sucesos.

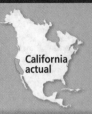

California actual

1542 Juan Rodríguez Cabrillo explora lo que hoy es la bahía de San Diego.

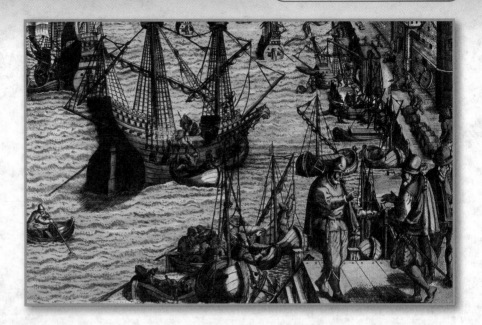

Un barco europeo de finales del siglo XVI inicia un viaje.

En busca de nuevas tierras

Los exploradores europeos navegaron los mares en busca de nuevas tierras en los siglos XVI y XVII. Un **explorador** es alguien que viaja a nuevos lugares para saber más acerca de ellos. A veces los gobernantes accedían a pagar esos viajes. Los exploradores a menudo tenían que darles una parte de lo que encontraran. A veces los exploradores mismos pagaban sus viajes. Esperaban hacerse ricos con el comercio y con las tierras que exploraban, y así pagar los gastos de sus viajes.

Muchos exploradores europeos viajaron a las Américas. Buscaban tierras o riquezas como oro y plata. También andaban en busca de una nueva ruta comercial entre Europa y Asia. Una razón por la que los exploradores de España llegaron a las Américas fue para difundir la religión católica romana.

1. Escribe un aspecto importante en que los exploradores de España se diferenciaban de otros exploradores europeos.

Comparar y contrastar

_____

_____

_____

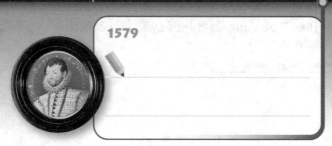

1579

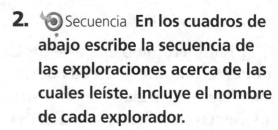

1602 Sebastián Vizcaíno explora y da nombre a la bahía de Monterey.

Los exploradores llegan a California

Los exploradores europeos llegaron a California durante los siglos XVI y XVII. Tres de ellos fueron Juan Rodríguez Cabrillo y Sebastián Vizcaíno, de España, y Francis Drake, de Inglaterra. En 1542 Cabrillo navegó desde México hasta la actual bahía de San Diego. Fue uno de los primeros europeos que divisó California. Drake desembarcó en una bahía situada al norte de lo que hoy es la bahía de San Francisco en 1579. Más tarde esa bahía fue bautizada como bahía Drake. Vizcaíno exploró y dio nombre a la bahía de Monterey en 1602.

2. Secuencia **En los cuadros de abajo escribe la secuencia de las exploraciones acerca de las cuales leíste. Incluye el nombre de cada explorador.**

Primero

Después

Por último

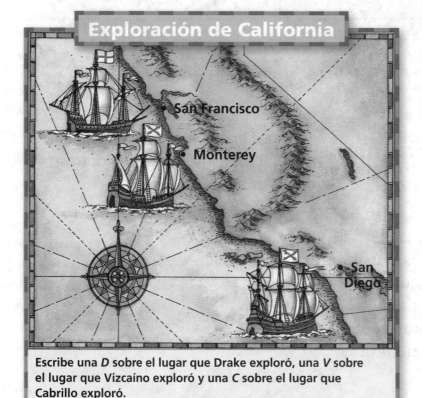

Exploración de California

San Francisco

Monterey

San Diego

Escribe una *D* sobre el lugar que Drake exploró, una *V* sobre el lugar que Vizcaíno exploró y una *C* sobre el lugar que Cabrillo exploró.

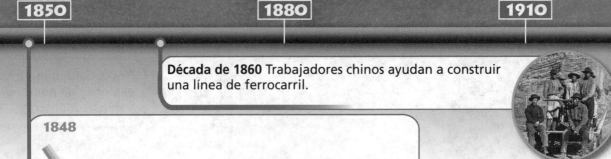

Década de 1860 Trabajadores chinos ayudan a construir una línea de ferrocarril.

1848

El oro trae crecimiento

El número de habitantes de California aumentó durante la década de 1840. En 1839 John Sutter se mudó a California, donde fundó un asentamiento agrícola. En 1848 su vida cambió para siempre. Alguien que trabajaba para Sutter descubrió oro en una parte de su propiedad que quedaba cerca de lo que hoy es Sacramento. La noticia del descubrimiento se difundió. En poco tiempo miles de personas de todo el mundo llegaron a la zona con la esperanza de hacerse ricas.

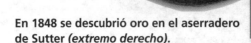

En 1848 se descubrió oro en el aserradero de Sutter *(extremo derecho)*.

3. **¿Qué motivó a mucha gente a ir a California después de 1848?**

Idea principal y detalles

_____

_____

El ferrocarril trae crecimiento

El ferrocarril transcontinental trajo aun más nuevos pobladores a California. El ferrocarril ayudó a conectar la costa este con la costa oeste. Facilitó el viaje de esa distancia tan larga. Durante la década de 1860, muchos trabajadores chinos llegaron para ayudar en la construcción de la línea del ferrocarril transcontinental. Una vez terminada la construcción, algunos de ellos se quedaron para dedicarse a la agricultura o para abrir negocios.

4. **¿De qué modo cambió California con el ferrocarril transcontinental?**

Causa y efecto

_____

_____

2004 California tiene una población aproximada de 35 millones de habitantes.

La diversa población de California

La población de California ha aumentado mucho desde el siglo XIX. En 2004 su población era de aproximadamente 35 millones de habitantes. Tiene más habitantes que cualquier otro estado del país. La gente ha llegado a trabajar en sectores como la agricultura, la electrónica y las fuerzas armadas.

Muchos hispanos, asiáticos, europeos y otros grupos han traído la cultura de su tierra natal a California. **Cultura** son las artes, las creencias, las conductas y las ideas de un grupo de gente. Los californianos han adoptado muchos aspectos de esas culturas. Puedes verlo en los festivales que tienen lugar a lo largo y ancho de nuestro estado.

5. Subraya las oraciones del texto que indiquen por qué en nuestro estado celebramos diferentes festivales.

Causa y efecto

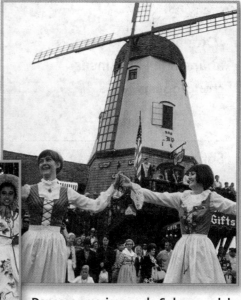

Daneses americanos de Solvang celebran el Festival de los Días Daneses.

Mexicoamericanos de Los Ángeles celebran el 16 de septiembre.

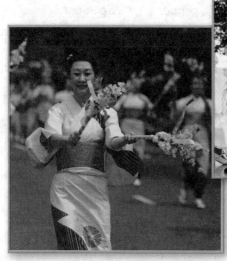

Japoneses americanos de San Francisco celebran el Festival de Cerezos Floridos.

Resumen

Muchos grupos de personas han llegado a California por diferentes razones. Compara y contrasta las razones por las que llegaron los primeros europeos con las de las personas que llegan hoy en día a California.

Líneas cronológicas

Aprende más Una línea cronológica te ayuda a seguir distintos sucesos. Muestra las fechas en que los sucesos ocurrieron. Sigue estos pasos cuando leas una línea cronológica:

1. Estudia el título para saber de qué trata la línea cronológica.
2. Establece qué período de tiempo abarca la línea cronológica.
3. Lee la línea cronológica de izquierda a derecha. El suceso que está en el extremo izquierdo es el más antiguo. El suceso que está en el extremo derecho es el más reciente.

Las líneas cronológicas que están abajo comparan sucesos que ocurrieron en California con sucesos que ocurrieron en los Estados Unidos durante el mismo período de tiempo. Estudia las líneas cronológicas y luego contesta las preguntas.

Inténtalo

1. ¿Qué período de tiempo abarcan las dos líneas cronológicas? *Identificar*

   _____

2. Subraya el suceso más antiguo. *Interpretar*

3. Encierra en un círculo el año en que California se convirtió en el trigésimo primer estado. *Identificar*

4. ¿Qué suceso ocurrió en California dos años después de que los Estados Unidos entraran en guerra con México? *Aplicar*

   _____

   _____

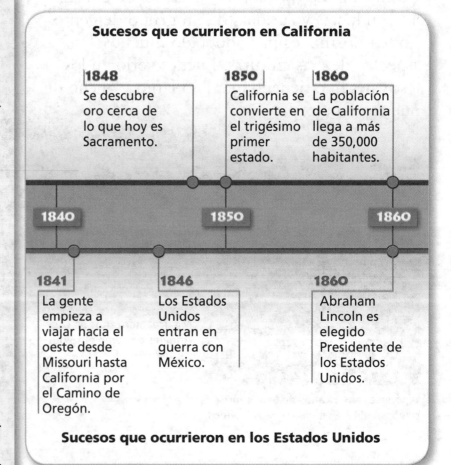

Sucesos que ocurrieron en California

1848 Se descubre oro cerca de lo que hoy es Sacramento.

1850 California se convierte en el trigésimo primer estado.

1860 La población de California llega a más de 350,000 habitantes.

1840   1850   1860

1841 La gente empieza a viajar hacia el oeste desde Missouri hasta California por el Camino de Oregón.

1846 Los Estados Unidos entran en guerra con México.

1860 Abraham Lincoln es elegido Presidente de los Estados Unidos.

Sucesos que ocurrieron en los Estados Unidos

H-SS 3.3.2 Describen las economías que establecieron los colonos y su influencia en la economía de hoy en día, haciendo énfasis en la importancia de la propiedad privada y de la libre empresa.

¿Cómo afectaron los primeros colonos la economía de tu región?

IMAGINA LA ESCENA

¿Piensas en el oro cuando te comes una dulce y jugosa naranja de California? Probablemente no. La fiebre por encontrar oro impulsó la agricultura de California. ¿Cómo ayudaron los buscadores de oro y otros colonos a establecer la economía de California?

Vistazo previo

Vocabulario

posesión *(s.)* tener algo que te pertenece sólo a ti

propiedad *(s.)* algo de lo que alguien es dueño

trabajador *(s.)* alguien que trabaja

bien *(s.)* algo que se produce o se cultiva y luego se vende

servicio *(s.)* trabajo que alguien hace para otros y que normalmente es pagado

Actividad de vocabulario Utiliza una de las palabras del vocabulario para completar esta oración:

Una _____ es algo de lo que alguien es dueño, como una bicicleta.

Personajes

James Marshall
Levi Strauss

Lectura: Causa y efecto

Recuerda que una *causa* es por lo que algo ocurre. Un *efecto* es lo que ocurre como resultado de la causa. Cuando leas la página 74, subraya las palabras *como resultado*, que indican un efecto.

73

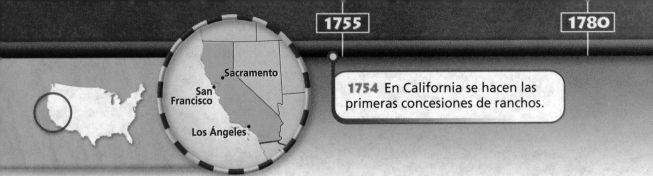

1755   1780

1754 En California se hacen las primeras concesiones de ranchos.

Concesiones de ranchos

A partir de 1754, los funcionarios españoles y mexicanos concedieron, o dieron, a la gente tierras llamadas ranchos para que las ocupara, las cultivara y creara nuevos negocios. A esas personas se les dio completa **posesión** de las tierras, o sea que les pertenecían sólo a ellas. Como resultado, las tierras pasaron a ser su **propiedad** privada, que es algo de lo que alguien es dueño.

Los primeros negocios y el comercio

En el siglo XIX mucha gente llegó a California para empezar negocios. El padre Antonio Cruzado, de España, plantó en 1804 lo que se convirtió en el primer naranjal de California. Hoy en día California es el mayor productor de frutas del país.

En 1848 un **trabajador,** o persona que trabaja, llamado James Marshall descubrió oro mientras trabajaba en un aserradero cerca de lo que hoy es Sacramento, California. Poco después, durante lo que se llamó la Fiebre del Oro, cerca de 100,000 personas llegaron a California en busca de oro. Casi nadie lo encontró, pero muchos se quedaron a vivir como trabajadores o abrieron negocios.

Levi Strauss se mudó a San Francisco en 1853, después de la Fiebre del Oro. Más tarde, él y otra persona se dieron cuenta que los mineros necesitaban pantalones resistentes. Como resultado, en 1873 empezaron a producir y vender *blue jeans*.

1. ¿Cómo crees que se sintieron las personas al poseer ranchos? *Predecir*

2. Escribe el efecto de la causa que aparece abajo.

Causa y efecto

Causa		Efecto
Los mineros necesitaban pantalones resistentes.	→	

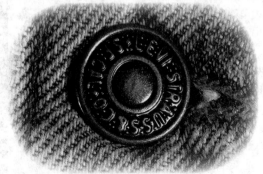

La compañía de Levi Strauss sigue haciendo *blue jeans* hoy en día.

1848 James Marshall descubre oro cerca de lo que hoy es Sacramento, California.

1853 Levi Strauss se muda a California.

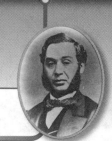

Los negocios siguen creciendo

A través del tiempo, California ha necesitado trabajadores para impulsar el crecimiento de su economía. Esos trabajadores han producido bienes y prestado servicios. Los **bienes** son cosas que se producen o se cultivan y luego se venden. Un **servicio** es un trabajo que alguien hace para otros y que normalmente es pagado. En la década de 1930, mucha gente se mudó aquí en busca de trabajo. Muchos trabajaron en granjas. Hoy en día, nuestro estado es uno de los principales productores de frutas y verduras. Hacia 1920 el área de Los Ángeles se convirtió en el centro de la industria cinematográfica. Lo sigue siendo hoy en día. A partir de la década de 1960, mucha gente se ha mudado al área de la bahía de San Francisco para empezar negocios que producen piezas para computadoras.

3. **¿Cómo ayudaron los trabajadores al crecimiento de California?** *Idea principal y detalles*

En Silicon Valley, en el norte de California, hay muchos negocios de computadoras.

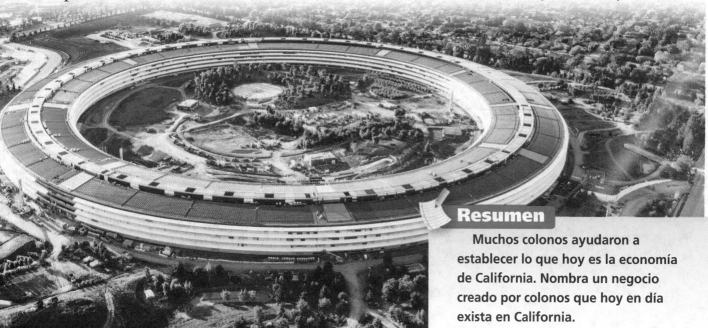

Resumen

Muchos colonos ayudaron a establecer lo que hoy es la economía de California. Nombra un negocio creado por colonos que hoy en día exista en California.

Canciones: "El pésimo minero"

Aprende más Podemos aprender acerca de la vida de los mineros durante la Fiebre del Oro estudiando fuentes primarias. Una de las razones por la que muchos mineros se quedaron en California fue que no pudieron pagarse el viaje de regreso a sus casas. Algunos escribieron canciones acerca de cómo los hacía sentir su situación.

A continuación están los primeros y los últimos versos de la canción "El pésimo minero". *Pésimo* significa "de muy mala calidad". Lee la letra de la canción y luego contesta las preguntas.

1. Subraya la cantidad de tiempo que el pésimo minero ha estado buscando oro. *Identificar*

2. ¿Qué palabras utilizarías para expresar lo que el minero siente al haber dejado su hogar? *Analizar*

_____

_____

_____

_____

El pésimo minero

*Han pasado cuatro largos años desde que llegué a
   esta tierra
a buscar oro entre las piedras y la arena;
y aún sigo siendo pobre, porque a decir verdad,
soy un pésimo minero,
un pésimo minero tras el brillo del oro.*

*O, tierra del oro, cómo me has engañado.
Ahora tendré que dejar mis huesos bajo tu suelo;
adiós pues, dulce hogar, que mis amigos me esperan
   fríos y tiesos,
soy un pésimo minero,
un pésimo minero tras el brillo del oro.*

—de *The Original California Songster*
("El cantor original de California"),
publicado por John A. Stone en 1855

H-SS 3.3.3 Investigan la razón del establecimiento de su comunidad, la manera en que los individuos y las familias contribuyeron a su fundación y desarrollo, y cómo ha cambiado la comunidad con el tiempo; obtienen la información de mapas, fotografías, historias orales, cartas, periódicos y otras fuentes primarias.

¿Cómo ha ayudado la gente a que crecieran los lugares en tu región?

IMAGINA LA ESCENA ¿Qué sabes de los comienzos de los pueblos y las ciudades de California? Por ejemplo, San Diego empezó como una misión. ¿Cómo ayudaron los individuos y las familias que llegaron antes que tú a darle forma al lugar que ahora llamas tu hogar?

Vistazo previo

Vocabulario

comunidad *(s.)* lugar donde un grupo de gente vive, trabaja y se divierte

fundó *(v.)* estableció

Actividad de vocabulario Encierra en un círculo la palabra de arriba que sea un sinónimo de *vecindario*.

Personajes

Junípero Serra

Lectura: Secuencia

Recuerda que una *secuencia* es el orden en que ocurren los sucesos. A veces no tienes fechas que te ayuden a establecer la secuencia de los sucesos. Tendrás entonces que buscar palabras como *primero* y *después* para hallar el orden de los sucesos. Encierra en un círculo esas palabras a medida que leas la página 78.

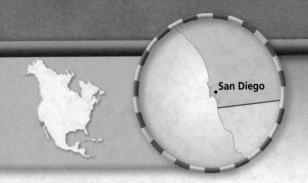

1769 El padre Junípero Serra funda una misión en lo que hoy es San Diego.

Los primeros pueblos

Las comunidades de California fueron establecidas por distintas razones. Una **comunidad** es el lugar donde un grupo de gente vive, trabaja y se divierte. Algunas comunidades empezaron como misiones. En 1769 el padre Junípero Serra **fundó,** o estableció, la primera misión en lo que hoy en día es San Diego, California. Después fundó ocho de las veintiuna misiones que hay en California. Muchas de ellas crecieron hasta convertirse en pueblos o ciudades.

1. Secuencia **Escribe la secuencia de los sucesos de modo que correspondan con el orden en que las misiones crecieron hasta convertirse en pueblos o ciudades.**

1.ᵉʳ suceso

_____

_____

2.º suceso

_____

_____

3.ᵉʳ suceso

_____

_____

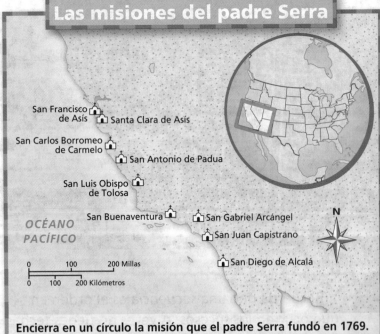

Las misiones del padre Serra

San Francisco de Asís
Santa Clara de Asís
San Carlos Borromeo de Carmelo
San Antonio de Padua
San Luis Obispo de Tolosa
San Buenaventura
San Gabriel Arcángel
San Juan Capistrano
San Diego de Alcalá

OCÉANO PACÍFICO

0   100   200 Millas
0   100   200 Kilómetros

N

Encierra en un círculo la misión que el padre Serra fundó en 1769.

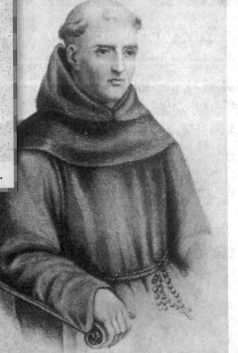

Junípero Serra fundó la misión en lo que hoy es San Diego el 16 de julio de 1769.

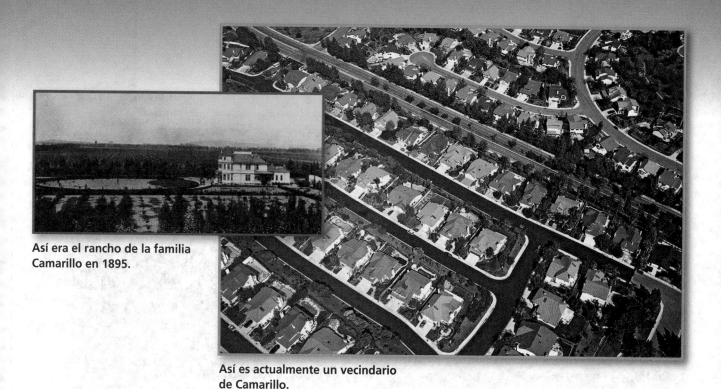

Así era el rancho de la familia Camarillo en 1895.

Así es actualmente un vecindario de Camarillo.

Familias y comunidades

A veces las familias ayudaban a establecer comunidades. Una de ellas fue la familia Camarillo, quien era dueña del Rancho Calleguas. La familia Camarillo cedió tierra para que junto a su rancho se construyeran varias iglesias, una universidad y una escuela secundaria. En 1899 el pueblo recibió el nombre de Camarillo en honor a la familia. Camarillo se encuentra en el sur de California.

Camarillo ha cambiado mucho desde 1899. La población ha aumentado hasta alcanzar más de 60,000 habitantes. Como resultado del aumento de la población, hoy en Camarillo hay muchas casas más. Hoy en día Camarillo tiene también más tiendas y restaurantes que sirven a la comunidad.

2. **¿Cómo ayudó la familia Camarillo a establecer una comunidad?**

Idea principal y detalles

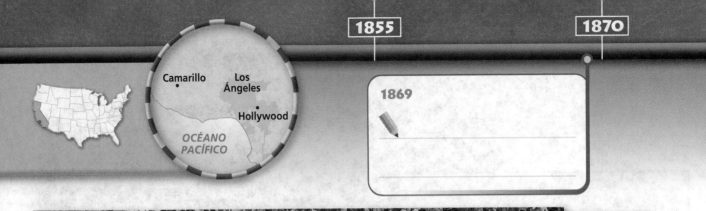

1869

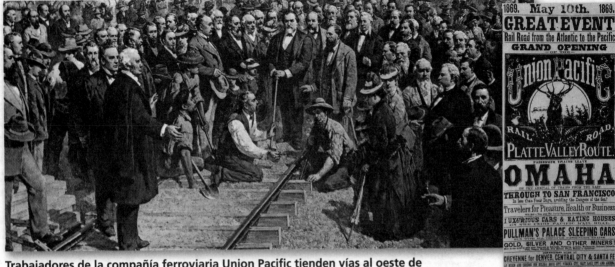

Trabajadores de la compañía ferroviaria Union Pacific tienden vías al oeste de Omaha, Nebraska, que se encontrarán con las vías de la compañía Central Pacific, en Promontory, Utah.

Llega el ferrocarril transcontinental

Mucha gente ayudó a que las comunidades de California crecieran y cambiaran. Miles de trabajadores llegaron a California para ayudar a construir el ferrocarril Central Pacific. Tendieron vías hacia el este, desde Sacramento hasta Promontory, Utah. En 1869 Central Pacific formó parte de la primera línea de ferrocarril que conectó el Este con el Oeste. Este ferrocarril se llamó el ferrocarril transcontinental.

Bienes y gente comenzaron a llegar más rápidamente a California. La gente se establecía en los pueblos cercanos a las vías del ferrocarril para estar cerca de los bienes que llegaban en el tren, y también para enviar los bienes que ellos producían.

3. ¿Cuál fue un efecto que tuvo el ferrocarril Central Pacific en las comunidades de California?

Causa y efecto

1899

1920 Hollywood se convierte en el centro de la industria cinematográfica de nuestro país.

Las comunidades crecen

Hollywood es un área de la ciudad de Los Ángeles. Es otro ejemplo de una comunidad que con el tiempo ha crecido y cambiado. En 1887 un hombre llamado Horace Wilcox fundó allí una comunidad religiosa. Sin embargo, hacia 1920 Hollywood se había convertido en el centro de la producción de películas del país.

La nueva industria cinematográfica ayudó a que el área de Los Ángeles creciera. Actores y directores de cine de todo el mundo llegaron a Los Ángeles a vivir y trabajar. Hoy en día el área de Los Ángeles sigue siendo el centro de la industria cinematográfica.

4. **¿Por qué crees que la industria cinematográfica ayudó a que el área de Los Ángeles creciera?** *Causa y efecto*

_____

_____

_____

_____

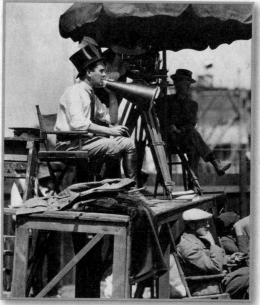

Hacia 1920 Hollywood se había convertido en el centro de la industria cinematográfica de nuestro país.

Resumen

California ha crecido mucho desde los tiempos de los exploradores españoles. ¿De qué modos ayudaron los primeros colonos al desarrollo de las comunidades de California?

Cartas: Andrew Jackson Chase

Aprende más Podemos aprender sobre la historia de los pueblos y ciudades por medio del estudio de las cartas escritas por una persona. Andrew Jackson Chase dejó Stoneham, Massachusetts, y se fue en busca de fortuna a San Francisco, California, durante la Fiebre del Oro. A continuación se muestra una parte de una carta que escribió a su hermano acerca de San Francisco en 1850. Lee el pasaje y luego contesta las preguntas.

29 de marzo de 1850

Tu carta del 8 de diciembre la recibí hace 2 semanas...

Aunque este país tiene tanta riqueza mineral, no aconsejaría a ninguno de mis amigos que deje las comodidades de su hogar para venir aquí. Sin embargo, para los amantes del oro siguen habiendo excelentes perspectivas [posibilidades de hacerse rico] y muchos siguen viniendo a pesar de todos los riesgos [peligros]. Digan lo que digan, el oro que se traerá de las minas esta temporada volverá loco a todo el mundo; y el crecimiento de San Francisco no tiene paralelo [algo similar] en la historia, pero los cambios bruscos de las fortunas son igualmente sorprendentes [impactantes]; aquí no hay estabilidad para nada...

1. Gente de todo el mundo llegaba a California buscando fortuna. Encierra en un círculo las descripciones de cómo fue la vida en California.
   Identificar

2. ¿Crees que era fácil vivir en San Francisco en 1850? ¿Por qué sí o por qué no?
   Analizar

   _____

   _____

   _____

Diario de estudio

En esta unidad aprenderás cómo las reglas y las leyes afectan nuestra vida diaria. También aprenderás cómo funciona el gobierno de los Estados Unidos. Completa las actividades de estas páginas a medida que leas la unidad.

Lo que sé sobre...

el gobierno de los Estados Unidos y las reglas y leyes que obedecemos todos los días:

_____

Defender las creencias

Completa las siguientes oraciones con el nombre correcto en el banco de palabras. Una de las oraciones tiene dos respuestas.

_____ escribió y habló abiertamente en contra de la esclavitud.

_____ ayudaron a redactar la Declaración de Independencia.

_____ habló abiertamente acerca de sus creencias religiosas.

_____ ayudó a liberar a personas esclavizadas.

_____ publicó la Proclamación de Emancipación.

_____ trabajó por los derechos civiles.

Abraham Lincoln

Anne Hutchinson

Benjamin Franklin

Dr. Martin Luther King, Jr.

Frederick Douglass

Harriet Tubman

Thomas Jefferson

Escribe un dato acerca de cada símbolo.

● **Bandera de California**

● **Bandera de los EE.UU.**

● **Estatua de la Libertad**

En la siguiente tabla escribe dos derechos y dos deberes de los ciudadanos.

Derechos	Deberes

Escribe dos detalles acerca del nivel de gobierno que se indica en cada cuadro.

Gobierno municipal

Gobierno del estado de California

Gobierno federal

🐻 **H-CS 3.4.1** Determinan las razones de las reglas, las leyes y la Constitución de los Estados Unidos, el papel del civismo en el fomento de reglas y leyes; y las consecuencias que deben enfrentar las personas que violan las reglas y las leyes.

¿Cómo ayudan las reglas y las leyes a que las personas vivan unidas?

CONÉCTATE Los conductores que se detienen en las señales de tráfico y los ciclistas que llevan casco son ejemplos de cómo la gente cumple las reglas. Las reglas y las leyes ayudan a dar seguridad a las personas. ¿De qué manera hacen posible que las personas vivan y trabajen mejor juntas?

Vistazo previo
Vocabulario

ciudadano *(s.)* miembro de una comunidad

derecho *(s.)* algo que se le garantiza a alguien por ley o por costumbre

deber *(s.)* responsabilidad, o algo que una persona debe hacer

obedecer *(v.)* hacer lo que te dicen que tienes que hacer

Actividad de vocabulario Escribe una oración que describa un deber que tengas en la escuela.

_____

_____

📖 **Lectura:** Causa y efecto

Una *causa* es la razón por la que algo sucede. Un *efecto* dice lo que sucede. A medida que leas acerca de reglas y leyes, hazte preguntas para buscar relaciones de causa y efecto. Escribe una pregunta en estas líneas.

_____

_____

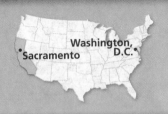

Washington, D.C.
Sacramento

Las leyes y la Constitución

La Constitución de los Estados Unidos explica los poderes que tiene el gobierno nacional. El gobierno nacional es el único que puede hacer leyes para el país. Las leyes protegen a los **ciudadanos,** o miembros de una comunidad. La Constitución también explica a los ciudadanos cuáles son sus **derechos,** o las cosas que por ley o costumbre se le garantiza a alguien. Por ejemplo, los ciudadanos tienen derecho a practicar la religión que escojan.

Los ciudadanos y las leyes

Los ciudadanos ayudan a hacer leyes. ¿Cómo? Eligen a los líderes que hacen las leyes. También pueden decirles a sus líderes cuáles son las leyes que quieren que se establezcan. Algunos líderes hacen leyes para todo el país. Trabajan en el Capitolio Nacional, que queda en Washington, D.C. Los líderes estatales en Sacramento hacen leyes para California.

1. 🎯 Causa y efecto **Usa detalles del texto para completar el siguiente diagrama.**

Causa

| El gobierno nacional hace leyes. |

Efecto

| |

2. **Subraya en el texto cómo los ciudadanos ayudan a hacer leyes.** *Idea principal y detalles*

El Preámbulo establece los objetivos de la Constitución.

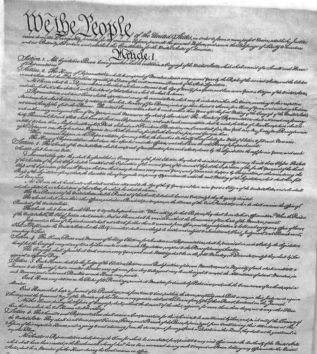

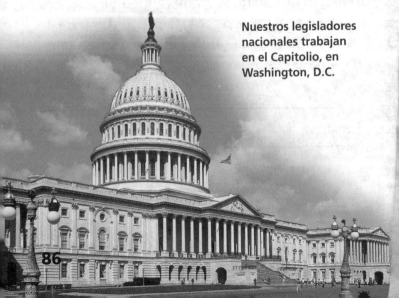

Nuestros legisladores nacionales trabajan en el Capitolio, en Washington, D.C.

Ayudar a la comunidad

Muchos buenos ciudadanos sienten que tienen el deber de hacer lo que es bueno para su comunidad. Un **deber** es una responsabilidad, o algo que una persona debe hacer. Bridget Biddy Mason es un ejemplo de alguien que cumplió con su deber cuando ayudó a los demás. Durante la década de 1800, Mason se hizo rica comprando tierras en Los Ángeles. Luego usó su dinero para dar albergue y comida a los pobres.

Leyes y castigos

La población debe obedecer las leyes y cumplir las reglas. **Obedecer** es hacer lo que te dicen que tienes que hacer. Unas leyes dicen que no se debe robar. Otras dicen que los pasajeros de un carro deberán llevar puesto el cinturón de seguridad. Los que no obedecen las leyes tienen que enfrentar las consecuencias, que son los resultados de ciertas acciones. Una consecuencia son las multas, que es dinero que debe pagarse al gobierno. Las personas que no lleven puesto el cinturón de seguridad pueden terminar pagando una multa.

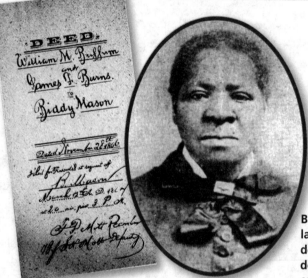

Biddy Mason y la escritura, o el documento oficial, de las tierras que compró.

3. ⊙ Causa y efecto ¿Qué efecto tuvo la riqueza de Biddy Mason en los pobres de California?

4. ⊙ Causa y efecto
Subraya las palabras del texto que indiquen lo que podría ocurrirles a las personas que no obedezcan las leyes.

Resumen

La gente debe cumplir las reglas y obedecer las leyes que el gobierno hace. ¿Por qué se deben cumplir las reglas y obedecer las leyes?

Elizabeth Wanamaker Peratrovich (1911–1958)

Aprende más Elizabeth Wanamaker Peratrovich pertenecía al grupo indígena tlingit. Vivía en la zona sureste de lo que hoy es el estado de Alaska.

Los padres de Elizabeth murieron cuando ella era todavía una niña, y Andrew y Mary Wanamaker la adoptaron. Creció, se casó y tuvo tres hijos.

En 1941 Elizabeth y su familia se mudaron a Juneau, Alaska, donde no trataban bien a los indígenas de Alaska. A ellos no se les permitía entrar a muchos restaurantes y tiendas. Los niños indígenas de Alaska no podían asistir a las escuelas públicas. Peratrovich y su esposo trabajaron para que los indígenas de Alaska obtuvieran derechos.

En 1945 Peratrovich habló ante los líderes del gobierno territorial de Alaska. Los convenció de que aprobaran una ley que diera igualdad de derechos a los indígenas de Alaska. En Alaska se celebra el Día de Elizabeth Peratrovich cada 16 de febrero, fecha en que se aprobó la ley.

Contesta las siguientes preguntas.

1. Encierra en un círculo tres lugares a los que los indígenas de Alaska no podían ir en 1941. *Identificar*

2. ¿Qué efecto tuvieron los esfuerzos de Peratrovich para los indígenas de Alaska? *Interpretar*

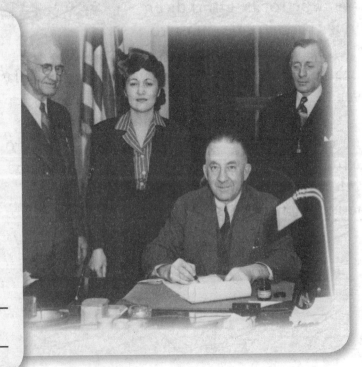

_____

_____

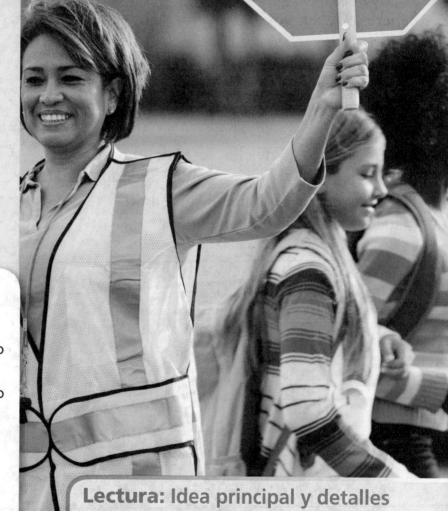

H-CS 3.4.2 Discuten la importancia de la virtud pública y el papel de los ciudadanos, incluida la manera de participar en el salón de clase, en la comunidad y en la vida cívica.

¿Por qué es importante ser un buen ciudadano?

CONÉCTATE Un adulto que ayuda a los estudiantes a cruzar la calle es un buen ciudadano. Un estudiante que ayuda a limpiar un parque también es un buen ciudadano. Los buenos ciudadanos hacen que tu comunidad sea un mejor lugar para vivir. ¿Eres tú un buen ciudadano?

Vistazo previo
Vocabulario

votar *(v.)* expresar tu elección de algo o alguien

voluntario *(s.)* persona que hace algo sin que se le pague o recompense

impuesto *(s.)* dinero que el gobierno recauda para pagar por los servicios que presta

Actividad de vocabulario
Encierra en un círculo la palabra del vocabulario que describa a una persona que podría ayudar en tu escuela.

Lectura: Idea principal y detalles

La *idea principal* dice de qué trata un párrafo. Los *detalles* dicen algo más acerca de la idea principal. Subraya la oración que diga la idea principal del primer párrafo de la página 90.

Derechos de los ciudadanos

Los ciudadanos de los Estados Unidos tienen derechos básicos. Esos derechos están descritos en la Constitución de los Estados Unidos. La libertad de expresión es uno de ellos. Los ciudadanos de los Estados Unidos son libres de expresar cualquier cosa en la que crean. También tienen el derecho a elegir a sus líderes.

Los ciudadanos de los Estados Unidos tienen deberes. Deben **votar,** o expresar su elección de algo o alguien. Los ciudadanos muchas veces votan haciendo una marca en un papel o alzando la mano. Antes de votar, los buenos ciudadanos se informan acerca de las personas que quieren servir en el gobierno. Pueden informarse acerca de ellas leyendo el periódico o escuchando las noticias. Votar cuidadosamente contribuye al mejoramiento de nuestras ciudades, nuestros estados y nuestro país.

1. Completa la siguiente tabla escribiendo la idea principal y otro detalle.

Idea principal y detalles

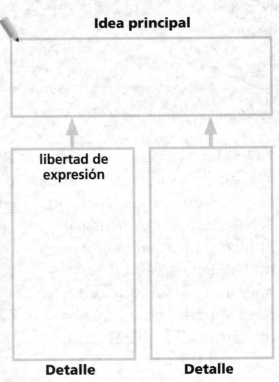

Idea principal

libertad de expresión

Detalle

Detalle

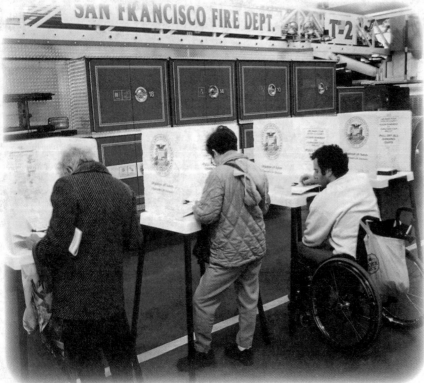

Los ciudadanos votan para elegir a las personas que servirán en el gobierno.

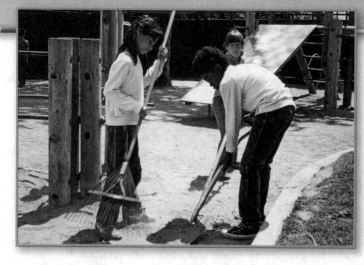

Los buenos ciudadanos
construyen comunidades sólidas.

Ser un buen ciudadano

Los habitantes de una comunidad demuestran de muchas maneras que son buenos ciudadanos. Cumplen las reglas y obedecen las leyes. Respetan los derechos y las propiedades de los demás. Algunos ciudadanos trabajan de voluntarios. Un **voluntario** es aquella persona que hace algo sin que se le pague. Los voluntarios pueden trabajar colocando libros en los estantes de una biblioteca o ayudando a limpiar un patio de recreo.

Las personas también demuestran que son buenos ciudadanos pagando sus impuestos. **Impuesto** es el dinero que el gobierno recauda para pagar por los servicios que nuestra comunidad necesita, tales como protección policíaca, escuelas, parques y carreteras.

Buenos ciudadanos en el salón de clase

Tú también puedes ser un buen ciudadano en el salón de clase. Como estudiante, debes respetar a tus maestros y a los demás estudiantes. Debes cumplir las reglas del salón y participar en las actividades de la clase. Debes ayudar al maestro en todo lo que puedas, así como también a los demás estudiantes.

2. **Enumera algunas maneras en que los voluntarios se diferencian de otros trabajadores.**

Comparar y contrastar

_____

_____

_____

_____

3. **Subraya los detalles del texto que digan algo más acerca de los buenos ciudadanos en el salón de clase.**

Idea principal y detalles

Resumen

Ser un buen ciudadano es importante. Nombra algunas maneras en que puedes demostrar que eres un buen ciudadano.

Entrevistar

Aprende más Por lo regular, una entrevista es una reunión que dos o más personas llevan a cabo para hablar acerca de algo. Puedes entrevistar a alguien que trabaje de voluntario en tu comunidad. Antes de la entrevista tienes que seguir ciertos pasos. Haz una lista de los temas que te interesan y anota las cosas que quieres saber. Haz una lista de buenas preguntas. Recuerda hacer preguntas que empiecen con *quién, qué, cuándo, dónde, por qué* o *cómo.* Escribe o graba las respuestas de la persona que estás entrevistando. Sé educado durante la entrevista. Siempre da las gracias cuando termines.

Lee las notas que están abajo y úsalas en una posible entrevista con una voluntaria. Luego contesta las preguntas.

Inténtalo

1. Encierra en un círculo dos temas de las notas que podrían ayudarte a escribir las preguntas que le harías a la Srta. Rodríguez durante la entrevista. *Analizar*

2. En las líneas que están a la derecha escribe dos preguntas que le harías a la Srta. Rodríguez durante la entrevista. Empieza cada pregunta con *quién, qué, cuándo, dónde, por qué* o *cómo.*

   Hacer preguntas

3. ¿Qué debes hacer cuando termines de entrevistar a la Srta. Rodríguez? *Identificar*

_____

Notas para la entrevista

La Srta. Rodríguez planeó un proyecto para limpiar el parque Orange. Pidió ayuda a otras personas. Muchos ciudadanos llegaron para recoger basura, sacar malas hierbas y sembrar flores. Por su trabajo, la Srta. Rodríguez recibirá el Premio de Civismo Comunitario de este año.

1. ¿Por qué decidió limpiar el parque Orange?

2.

3.

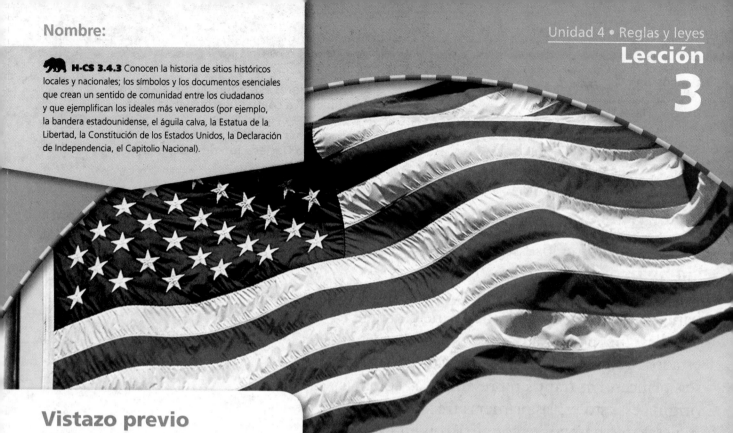

H-CS 3.4.3 Conocen la historia de sitios históricos locales y nacionales; los símbolos y los documentos esenciales que crean un sentido de comunidad entre los ciudadanos y que ejemplifican los ideales más venerados (por ejemplo, la bandera estadounidense, el águila calva, la Estatua de la Libertad, la Constitución de los Estados Unidos, la Declaración de Independencia, el Capitolio Nacional).

Vistazo previo

Vocabulario

símbolo *(s.)* algo que representa otra cosa

libertad *(s.)* poder hacer o decir lo que quieras sin que te limiten

orgullo *(s.)* sentimiento de gran placer y satisfacción que se tiene por algo que tú u otras personas han hecho

sitio histórico *(s.)* edificio, monumento o lugar importante

herencia *(s.)* creencias, valores y costumbres tradicionales de una familia o un grupo

unir *(v.)* juntar para formar una sola cosa

Actividad de vocabulario Encierra en un círculo la palabra de arriba que describe el sentimiento que tendrías si hicieras algo bien.

Personajes

Thomas Jefferson
Benjamin Franklin

¿Qué une a nuestras comunidades y a nuestro país?

CONÉCTATE Piensa en todos los lugares donde ves la bandera de nuestra nación. La ves en las escuelas, en los aeropuertos, en los estadios y en muchos otros lugares. ¿De qué manera nuestra bandera y otras cosas que representan a los Estados Unidos ayudan a que los estadounidenses se sientan unidos?

Lectura: Comparar y contrastar

Comparar y contrastar te ayudará a ver cómo las cosas son similares y cómo son diferentes. Subraya las palabras de la página 94 que digan en qué se parecen la bandera de los Estados Unidos y la bandera de California.

ESTADOS UNIDOS • Ciudad de Nueva York — FRANCIA

1782 Líderes estadounidenses escogen el águila calva como nuestra ave nacional.

1776 Se firma la Declaración de Independencia.

La bandera de los Estados Unidos

La bandera de los Estados Unidos es un **símbolo,** o algo que representa otra cosa. Representa nuestro país, los Estados Unidos. La bandera de los Estados Unidos tiene cincuenta estrellas, una por cada uno de nuestros cincuenta estados. También tiene trece franjas, siete rojas y seis blancas. Las franjas representan las colonias originales, esto es, las primeras trece colonias inglesas que después se convirtieron en estados.

1. **¿Qué representan las cincuenta estrellas y las trece franjas de la bandera de los Estados Unidos?** *Idea principal y detalles*

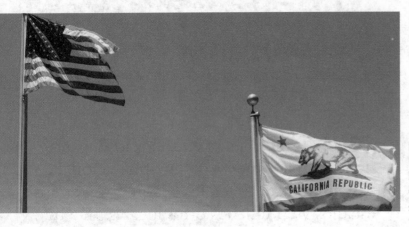

La bandera de los Estados Unidos *(izquierda)* y la bandera del estado de California *(derecha)* son símbolos importantes.

La bandera de California

La Bandera del Oso de California es un símbolo de nuestro estado. California se convirtió en estado en 1850. Los legisladores estatales designaron la Bandera del Oso como bandera de nuestro estado en 1911. La bandera muestra un oso pardo, una estrella roja y las palabras *California Republic*. El oso pardo es un símbolo de fuerza. La estrella fue tomada de la bandera de la Estrella Solitaria de Texas.

2. **¿Por qué crees que el oso pardo es un buen símbolo de fuerza?** *Sacar conclusiones*

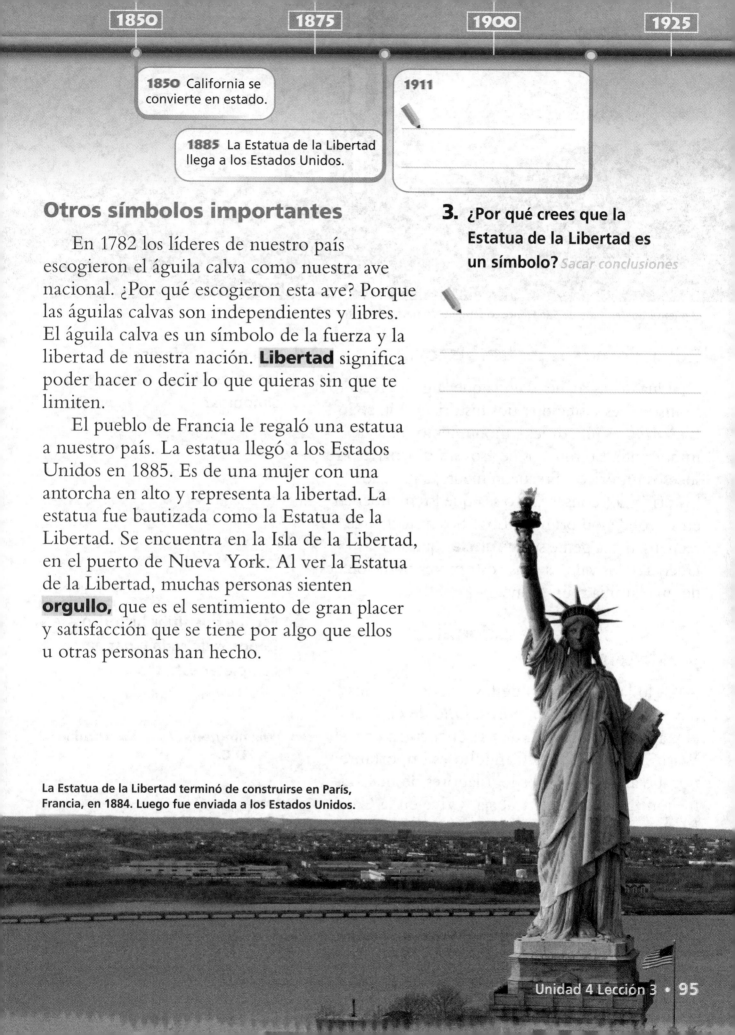

1850 California se convierte en estado.

1885 La Estatua de la Libertad llega a los Estados Unidos.

1911

Otros símbolos importantes

En 1782 los líderes de nuestro país escogieron el águila calva como nuestra ave nacional. ¿Por qué escogieron esta ave? Porque las águilas calvas son independientes y libres. El águila calva es un símbolo de la fuerza y la libertad de nuestra nación. **Libertad** significa poder hacer o decir lo que quieras sin que te limiten.

El pueblo de Francia le regaló una estatua a nuestro país. La estatua llegó a los Estados Unidos en 1885. Es de una mujer con una antorcha en alto y representa la libertad. La estatua fue bautizada como la Estatua de la Libertad. Se encuentra en la Isla de la Libertad, en el puerto de Nueva York. Al ver la Estatua de la Libertad, muchas personas sienten **orgullo,** que es el sentimiento de gran placer y satisfacción que se tiene por algo que ellos u otras personas han hecho.

La Estatua de la Libertad terminó de construirse en París, Francia, en 1884. Luego fue enviada a los Estados Unidos.

3. **¿Por qué crees que la Estatua de la Libertad es un símbolo?** *Sacar conclusiones*

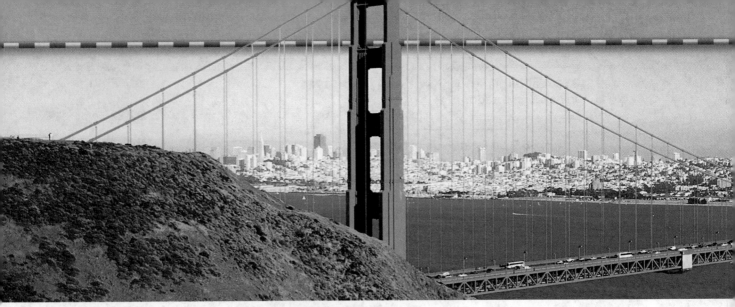

El puente Golden Gate de San Francisco terminó de construirse en 1937.

Recordemos nuestra historia

Una de las maneras en la que la gente recuerda su historia es visitando sitios históricos. Un **sitio histórico** es un edificio, monumento o lugar importante. En muchos de esos sitios ocurrieron sucesos históricos. Frecuentemente, a los sitios históricos los conservan, o sea que los mantienen en su condición original. Los sitios históricos le recuerdan a la gente su **herencia,** que son las creencias, los valores y las costumbres tradicionales de una familia o un grupo.

Sitios históricos nacionales y estatales

A lo largo y ancho de los Estados Unidos hay sitios históricos famosos. Uno de ellos es el Capitolio Nacional, que se encuentra en Washington, D.C. El Capitolio es importante porque allí trabajan los legisladores de nuestra nación. El Presidente trabaja y vive en la Casa Blanca, otro importante sitio histórico de Washington, D.C.

La población de California también valora sus sitios históricos. Las misiones españolas, el Capitolio Estatal, en Sacramento, y el puente Golden Gate son algunos de los muchos sitios históricos que se encuentran en nuestro estado.

4. ¿En qué se diferencian los sitios históricos de los símbolos? *Comparar y contrastar*

_____

_____

_____

_____

5. Escribe dos sitios históricos famosos de cada lugar para completar esta tabla.

Comparar y contrastar

Washington, D.C.	California
1.	1.
2.	2.

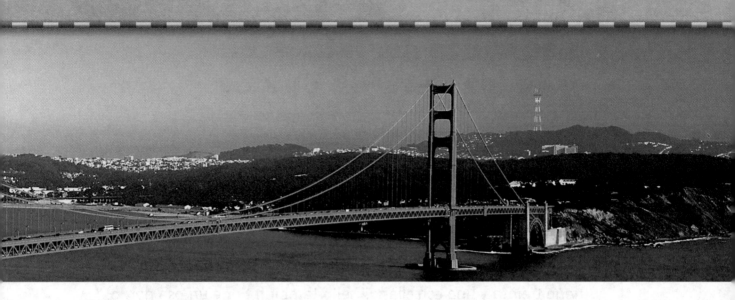

Documentos importantes

Los documentos, o papeles importantes, también pueden ser símbolos. Algunas veces expresan las creencias y los valores para **unir,** o juntar, a la población de un estado o un país. La Declaración de Independencia es un documento nacional importante. Thomas Jefferson escribió casi todo el documento, con la ayuda de Benjamin Franklin y otros. Una creencia, o ideal, que aparece en la Declaración de Independencia es que todas las personas son creadas iguales.

La Constitución de los Estados Unidos y la Constitución de California también expresan creencias importantes. La Constitución de los Estados Unidos incluye la Declaración de Derechos. La Declaración de Derechos establece algunas de nuestras libertades básicas, como la libertad de expresión. La Constitución de California también establece ese derecho.

6. Subraya las palabras en el texto que indican en qué se parecen la Declaración de Independencia y la Constitución de los Estados Unidos. *Comparar y contrastar*

Thomas Jefferson *(izquierda)* escribió la mayor parte de la Declaración de Independencia.

Resumen

Símbolos como banderas, sitios históricos y documentos son importantes para nuestra historia local y para la historia de los Estados Unidos. ¿Qué creencias importantes representan nuestros símbolos nacionales y estatales?

Los sellos de California y de los Estados Unidos

Aprende más Tanto el estado de California como los Estados Unidos tienen sellos. Un sello es una estampa o marca oficial que por lo general tiene un diseño. El Sello del Estado de California se imprime en las leyes que se aprueban en California. El sello fue aprobado en 1849. California fue el estado número treinta y uno en unirse a los Estados Unidos. Por eso es que nuestro sello estatal tiene treinta y una estrellas. El sello también tiene un oso pardo, que representa la fuerza. El agua representa el océano Pacífico.

El Gran Sello de los Estados Unidos se imprime en los documentos que firma el Presidente. También se encuentra en los billetes de un dólar. El sello fue aprobado en 1782. Las 13 franjas rojas y blancas que muestra representan las 13 colonias. El color azul que está encima de las franjas representa tres cosas: ser cuidadoso, siempre terminar la labor iniciada y obedecer las leyes de modo que todos sean tratados justamente.

Un documento tiene estos sellos cuando lo que se expresa en él está de acuerdo o concuerda con las ideas y creencias que el gobierno considera como importantes. Por estas razones, los sellos son importantes símbolos de civismo.

Examina los sellos y luego contesta las siguientes preguntas.

1. Encierra en un círculo un símbolo que se usa tanto en el sello de California como en el de los Estados Unidos. *Identificar*

2. Subraya una oración que explique por qué la impresión de un sello en un documento demuestra civismo. *Interpretar*

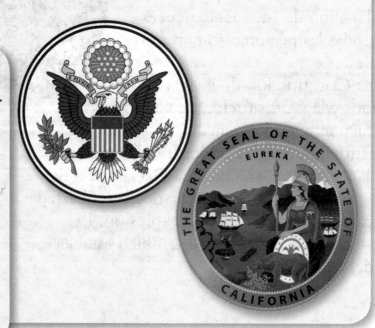

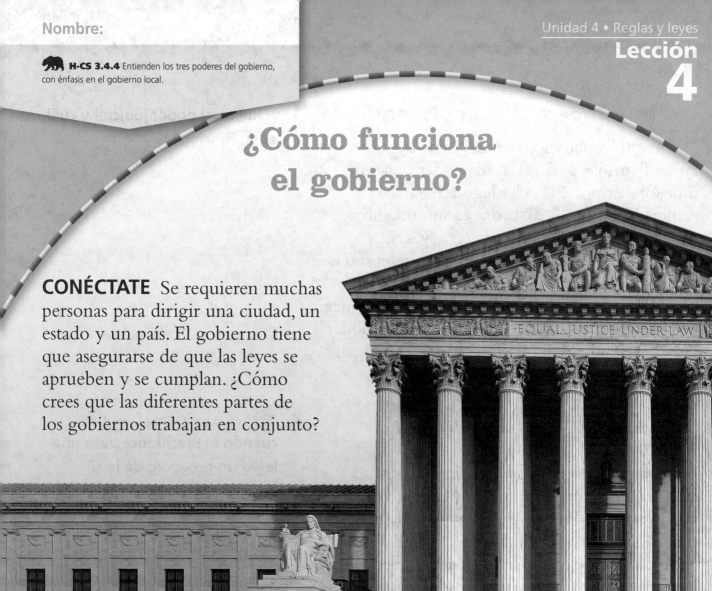

H-CS 3.4.4 Entienden los tres poderes del gobierno, con énfasis en el gobierno local.

¿Cómo funciona el gobierno?

CONÉCTATE Se requieren muchas personas para dirigir una ciudad, un estado y un país. El gobierno tiene que asegurarse de que las leyes se aprueben y se cumplan. ¿Cómo crees que las diferentes partes de los gobiernos trabajan en conjunto?

Vistazo previo
Vocabulario

legislador *(s.)* miembro del gobierno que ayuda a hacer leyes

Congreso *(s.)* grupo legislador, o que hace leyes, del gobierno de los Estados Unidos

vetar *(v.)* rechazar un proyecto de ley que ha sido aprobado por un grupo legislador

alcalde *(s.)* líder de una ciudad o un pueblo

Actividad de vocabulario Encierra en un círculo las palabras de arriba que se podrían aplicar a personas que aparecerían en la categoría *Personajes*.

Lectura: Causa y efecto

Buscar causas y efectos te puede ayudar a entender las conexiones que hay entre distintos sucesos. Una *causa* dice por qué algo sucede. Un *efecto* dice qué ha sucedido. A medida que leas la página 100, subraya los efectos que la gente podría tener en una ley.

▷

99

Los tres poderes del gobierno

Nuestro gobierno nacional tiene tres partes o ramas llamadas poderes. Cada poder tiene una función distinta. El poder legislativo hace y cambia leyes. Los **legisladores** son miembros del gobierno que ayudan a hacer leyes. El **Congreso** es el grupo legislador del gobierno de los Estados Unidos. El poder ejecutivo hace cumplir las leyes. El Presidente dirige este poder. Los jueces de la Corte Suprema dirigen el poder judicial. Ellos se aseguran de que las leyes sigan la Constitución de los Estados Unidos.

El sistema de controles y equilibrios

Cada rama o poder del gobierno controla y equilibra, o limita, lo que los otros poderes pueden hacer. ¿Por qué? Para asegurarse de que ninguno de los otros poderes tenga demasiada autoridad. Por ejemplo, el Presidente puede vetar un proyecto de ley que haya sido aprobado por el Congreso. **Vetar** es rechazar un proyecto de ley que ha sido aprobado por un grupo legislador. Sin embargo, si consigue suficientes votos, el Congreso puede derogar, o anular, un veto. Los jueces de la Corte Suprema pueden derrocar una ley que el Congreso y el Presidente hayan acordado aprobar.

1. ¿Qué es el poder judicial y cuál es su función?

Idea principal y detalles

2. Causa y efecto **¿Qué pasa cuando el Presidente veta una ley o un proyecto de ley?**

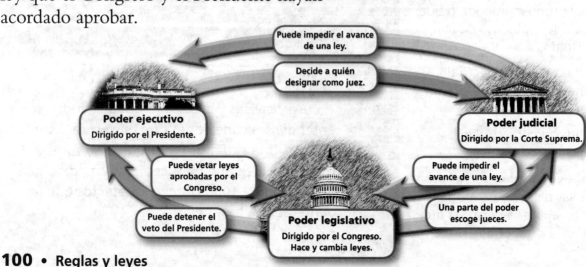

Puede impedir el avance de una ley.

Decide a quién designar como juez.

Poder ejecutivo
Dirigido por el Presidente.

Poder judicial
Dirigido por la Corte Suprema.

Puede vetar leyes aprobadas por el Congreso.

Puede impedir el avance de una ley.

Puede detener el veto del Presidente.

Poder legislativo
Dirigido por el Congreso.
Hace y cambia leyes.

Una parte del poder escoge jueces.

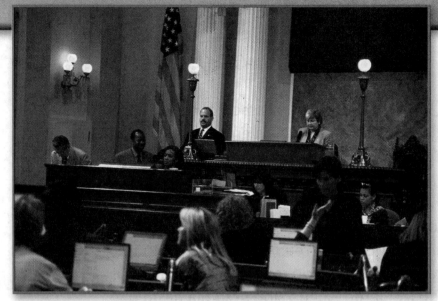

La Asamblea Estatal de California hace leyes para nuestro estado.

Gobiernos locales

Los gobiernos municipales también tienen partes que trabajan en conjunto. Todas las ciudades de California tienen un consejo municipal. Los ciudadanos eligen a los miembros de su consejo municipal. Casi todos los consejos municipales se reúnen en la Alcaldía para hacer leyes locales. También trabajan con el líder de la ciudad. Algunas ciudades tienen un líder comunitario llamado **alcalde.** En las ciudades grandes como Los Ángeles, la población elige a su alcalde. En las ciudades más pequeñas, el consejo municipal elige al alcalde. Otras ciudades de California tienen líderes llamados administradores municipales. El consejo municipal elige a esa persona.

Los consejos municipales y los líderes de la ciudad trabajan en conjunto para tomar buenas decisiones acerca de asuntos locales importantes. Por ejemplo, a menudo deciden dónde construir una escuela o cuándo contratar a más bomberos.

3. Encierra en un círculo los detalles del texto que digan algo más acerca de los gobiernos municipales de California. *Idea principal y detalles*

Resumen

La estructura de nuestro gobierno nacional es distinta a la de nuestro gobierno local. Explica en qué se diferencia la estructura de nuestro gobierno nacional de la de nuestro gobierno local.

Tablas

Aprende más Las tablas facilitan la lectura de la información. En una tabla, la información se organiza en columnas, que se leen de arriba abajo, y en filas, que se leen de izquierda a derecha. El rótulo que va arriba de cada columna agrupa la información de una manera. El rótulo que va a la izquierda de cada fila agrupa la información de otra manera.

La tabla de abajo muestra las reuniones de varios comités municipales. Para averiguar cuándo se reúne un comité, busca su nombre en el lado izquierdo. Luego sigue esa fila hasta que encuentres la columna que indique cuándo y dónde ese comité se reúne. Estudia la tabla y luego contesta las preguntas de abajo.

Inténtalo

1. Encierra en un círculo el día, la hora y el lugar de la reunión del Consejo municipal. *Identificar*

2. Dibuja un cuadro alrededor del nombre del grupo que se reúne el viernes. *Identificar*

3. Escribe en la tabla la hora y el lugar de otra reunión de la Mesa directiva escolar. *Aplicar*

4. A tu familia le gustaría que en el vecindario hubiera un parque para los perros. Subraya el día, la hora y el lugar de la reunión a la que tendría que ir tu familia para presentar esta idea. *Analizar*

Reuniones municipales

Grupo	Lunes	Martes	Miércoles	Jueves	Viernes
Consejo municipal			8–10 P.M. Alcaldía		
Mesa directiva escolar		7–9 P.M. Escuela Secundaria Wagner			
Comité Municipal de Parques				2–3 P.M. Biblioteca principal	
Comisión de Bellas Artes					10–11 A.M. Museo Smith

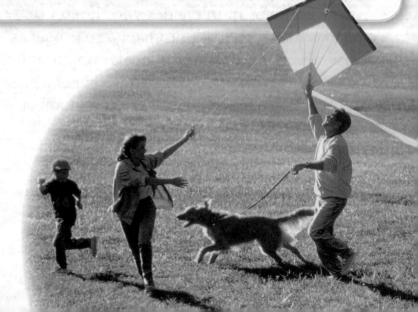

H-CS 3.4.5 Describen la manera en que California, los otros estados y las tribus soberanas de indígenas americanos contribuyen al desarrollo de nuestra nación y participan en el sistema federal del gobierno.

¿Cómo trabajan en conjunto los estados, los indígenas americanos y el gobierno de nuestro país?

CONÉCTATE Nuestro estado tiene mayor población que cualquier otro estado de los Estados Unidos. Como tiene tanta gente, California desempeña un papel importante en el gobierno de nuestro país. ¿Cómo colaboran, o ayudan, los grupos indígenas americanos con nuestro gobierno nacional?

Vistazo previo

Vocabulario

senador *(s.)* miembro del Senado

federal *(adj.)* relacionado con el gobierno de todo el país, es decir, el gobierno nacional

gobernador *(s.)* líder máximo de un estado

cuerpo legislativo *(s.)* grupo de personas que hacen o cambian las leyes

Actividad de vocabulario A veces una palabra contiene otra palabra o parte de ella que significa casi lo mismo. Encierra en un círculo la palabra raíz que veas dentro de *legislativo*. Luego escribe una definición corta.

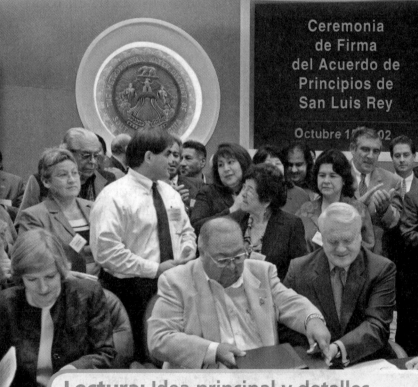

Ceremonia de Firma del Acuerdo de Principios de San Luis Rey

Octubre 1 02

Lectura: Idea principal y detalles

Las *ideas principales* pueden ayudarte a entender de lo que trata un párrafo. Algunos escritores incluyen una oración temática que incluye la idea principal. A medida que leas el primer párrafo de la página 104, subraya la oración que indique la idea principal.

El gobierno de nuestra nación

El Congreso, que es el poder legislativo del gobierno de los Estados Unidos, está compuesto de líderes que provienen de nuestros cincuenta estados. El Congreso tiene dos partes: el Senado y la Cámara de Representantes. El Senado tiene 100 **senadores,** es decir personas que son sus miembros. Cada estado elige a dos senadores. La Cámara de Representantes tiene 435 miembros. El número de representantes de cada estado cambia según la población de su respectivo estado. El Congreso es parte del gobierno **federal,** o nacional. Hace leyes que tienen efecto a nivel nacional, es decir, en todo el país.

Gobierno estatal

El gobierno estatal, o del estado, y el gobierno federal funcionan de manera similar. El **gobernador** es el líder máximo de un estado. El presidente es el líder de nuestro país. El **cuerpo legislativo** es el grupo de personas que hacen y cambian las leyes estatales. El cuerpo legislativo de California tiene dos partes: el Senado Estatal y la Asamblea Estatal.

1. Escribe dos detalles que apoyen la idea principal del primer párrafo. *Idea principal y detalles*

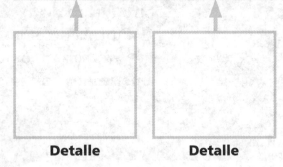

Idea principal

El Congreso está compuesto por líderes de nuestros cincuenta estados.

Detalle   **Detalle**

2. ¿En qué se parecen el gobierno estatal y el gobierno federal?

Comparar y contrastar

_____

_____

_____

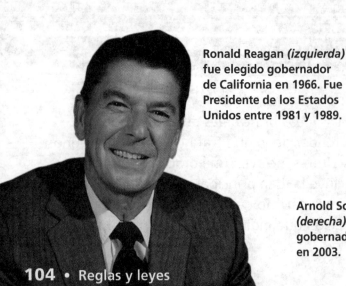

Ronald Reagan *(izquierda)* **fue elegido gobernador de California en 1966. Fue Presidente de los Estados Unidos entre 1981 y 1989.**

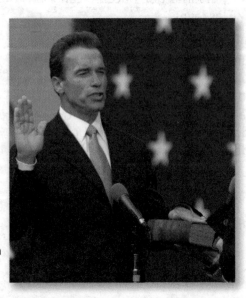

Arnold Schwarzenegger *(derecha)* **fue elegido gobernador de California en 2003.**

Gobiernos indígenas americanos

Por ley federal, el gobierno estatal y el gobierno federal deben satisfacer las necesidades de los indígenas americanos. Sin embargo, muchos grupos indígenas americanos tienen su propio gobierno tribal. Cada gobierno tribal obedece las leyes federales. Los miembros de los gobiernos tribales también eligen a sus líderes.

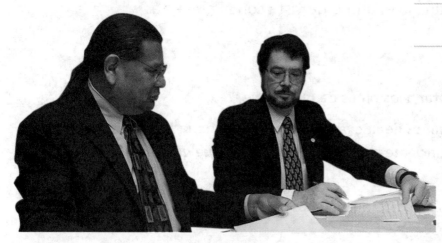

3. Basándote en lo que has leído, ¿qué crees que sucedería si los gobiernos tribales no obedecieran las leyes estatales y federales? *Predecir*

_____

_____

_____

El líder del gobierno tribal de un grupo indígena de California *(a la izquierda)* toma decisiones importantes para el grupo.

Un sistema de gobierno

Los habitantes de nuestro país y los gobiernos tribales de los indígenas americanos contribuyen al funcionamiento de nuestro sistema federal de gobierno. Por ejemplo, los dos senadores de nuestro estado representan a California en el Senado de los Estados Unidos. Trabajan con el Congreso Nacional para hacer leyes sobre impuestos, que es el dinero que se paga al gobierno por los servicios que presta. Los habitantes de California y de otros estados, así como los grupos indígenas americanos, pagan esos impuestos. El gobierno federal usa el dinero de los impuestos para producir papel moneda, así como para prestar servicios, entre ellos el cuidado de parques y monumentos nacionales.

4. Subraya las partes del texto que dicen cómo los grupos indígenas americanos colaboran con el gobierno federal. *Idea principal y detalles*

Resumen

California y otros estados, así como grupos indígenas americanos, colaboran con el gobierno federal. ¿Cómo están conectados el gobierno federal, el gobierno estatal y los gobiernos tribales?

Temas y puntos de vista

Aprende más Los ciudadanos votan para elegir a sus líderes. ¿Pero cómo hacen la elección? Los buenos ciudadanos prestan atención a los temas o asuntos que los líderes necesitan resolver. Pueden aprender cuál es el punto de vista de cada una de las personas que quieren ser elegidas para un cargo. Un *punto de vista* es lo que una persona piensa acerca de un tema. Fíjate en los temas que están a continuación, y también en el primer punto de vista. Luego completa el segundo punto de vista de cada tema. Encierra en un círculo el punto de vista con el que estás de acuerdo.

Inténtalo

Tema #1: ¿Se debería permitir votar a los niños de nueve años?

Primer punto de vista: No, a los niños de nueve años no se les debería permitir que voten porque no saben lo suficiente acerca de las personas que quieren ser elegidas.

Segundo punto de vista: Sí, a los niños de nueve años se les debe permitir votar porque

_____

_____

Tema #2: ¿Debería gastar nuestro gobierno más dinero en patios de recreo?

Primer punto de vista: No, nuestro gobierno no debería gastar más dinero en los patios de recreo porque ya hay suficientes.

Segundo punto de vista: Sí, nuestro gobierno debería gastar más dinero en patios de recreo porque

_____

_____

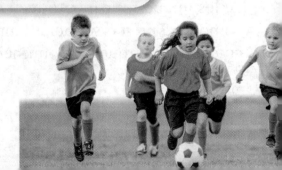

🐻 **H-CS 3.4.6** Describen la vida de los héroes estadounidenses que corrieron riesgos para asegurar nuestras libertades (Anne Hutchinson, Benjamin Franklin, Thomas Jefferson, Abraham Lincoln, Frederick Douglass, Harriet Tubman, Martin Luther King, Jr.).

¿Cómo han trabajado las personas por la libertad?

Vistazo previo

Vocabulario

riesgo *(s.)* posibilidad de que algo malo suceda

asegurar *(v.)* garantizar o proteger algo

derechos civiles *(s.)* derechos que las personas tienen porque son ciudadanos

Actividad de vocabulario

Completa la oración que está abajo con la palabra correcta del vocabulario.

A veces los héroes tienen que correr

_____ .

Personajes

Anne Hutchinson
Harriet Tubman
Frederick Douglass
Abraham Lincoln
Martin Luther King, Jr.

IMAGINA LA ESCENA

¿Alguna vez has ayudado a alguien? En el pasado, muchos estadounidenses ayudaron a otros a obtener nuevos derechos. ¿Cómo crees que alcanzaron sus objetivos?

🔊 Lectura: Causa y efecto

Destreza de lectura

Recuerda que una *causa* es la razón por la que algo sucede. Un *efecto* es lo que sucede como resultado. Subraya los detalles del primer párrafo de la página 108 que indican por qué Anne Hutchinson se mudó a Boston.

▷

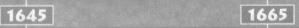
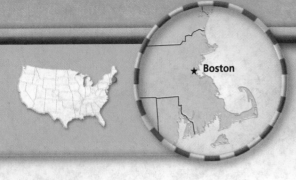

★ Boston

1637 Anne Hutchinson es expulsada por defender sus creencias religiosas.

Defender las creencias

Anne Hutchinson defendió sus creencias. En Inglaterra no se le permitía practicar su religión. Así que en 1634 se mudó a Boston, Massachussets, donde llegó con otras personas de su misma religión.

Sin embargo, las creencias de Hutchinson cambiaron. Creía que tener fe era más importante que obedecer las reglas de la Iglesia. Se tomó el riesgo de decirles sus creencias a otras personas. Un **riesgo** es la posibilidad de que pase algo malo. Algunos miembros de su grupo querían que dejara de hablar acerca de sus nuevas creencias. Finalmente fue expulsada del grupo en 1637. Hoy en día muchas personas reconocen a Hutchinson como una heroína, es decir, una mujer que actuó con valentía.

1. 🔄 Causa y efecto **¿Cuál fue la causa por la que Anne Hutchinson decidió mudarse a Boston?**

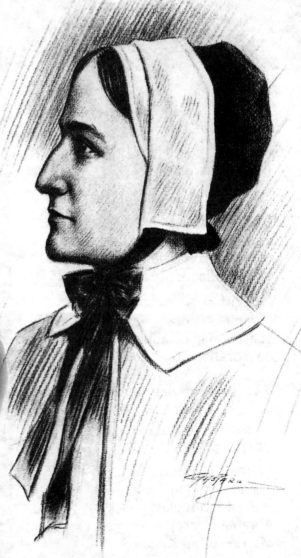

Anne Hutchinson defendió sus creencias religiosas.

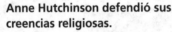

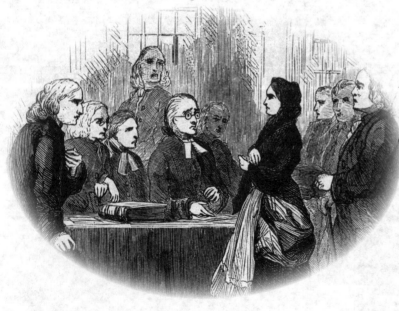

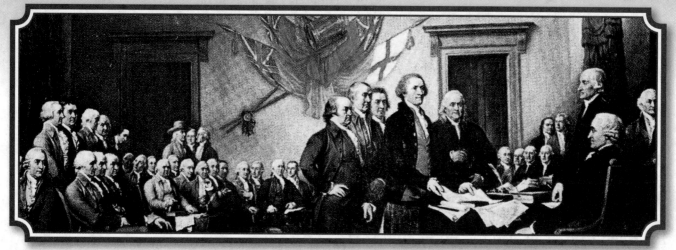

La Declaración de Independencia fue aprobada el 4 de julio de 1776.

Defender la libertad

Durante el siglo XVIII muchos de los residentes de lo que hoy llamamos los Estados Unidos querían tener un país que estuviera separado de Gran Bretaña. En aquel entonces, Gran Bretaña controlaba las primeras colonias de lo que hoy son los Estados Unidos. Muchas personas creían que lo mejor sería que tuvieran su propio país.

Mucha gente contribuyó a que los Estados Unidos se convirtieran en un país libre. Thomas Jefferson y Benjamin Franklin fueron dos de esos líderes. Jefferson era un rico granjero que después se convirtió en legislador. Franklin era científico e inventor. Los dos ayudaron a escribir la Declaración de Independencia en 1776. En ese documento se daban las razones por las que los Estados Unidos debían independizarse de Gran Bretaña. Jefferson y Franklin se arriesgaron para asegurar los derechos del pueblo estadounidense. **Asegurar** los derechos significa protegerlos o trabajar mucho por obtenerlos. Ambos arriesgaron su vida tratando de hacerlo.

2. Causa y efecto **¿Qué causó que la gente luchara contra Gran Bretaña?**

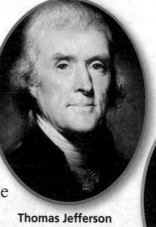

Thomas Jefferson

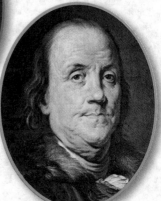

Benjamin Franklin

PENNSYLVANIA
Filadelfia
MARYLAND

1776 Jefferson, Franklin y otros escriben la Declaración de Independencia.

Defender a los demás

Durante parte del siglo XIX Harriet Tubman ayudó a muchas personas a obtener su libertad ayudándolas a escapar. Tubman nació en esclavitud alrededor de 1820, en Maryland. La esclavitud es el sistema en el cual una persona es propiedad de otra y es obligada a trabajar sin paga. De adulta, Tubman escapó a Filadelfia, Pennsylvania. Allí pudo haberse quedado a salvo, pero no lo hizo. Corrió el riesgo de perder su libertad y su vida para ayudar a otros afroamericanos a escapar de la esclavitud.

Tubman se convirtió en la líder del Tren Clandestino. El Tren Clandestino no era un tren. Era un grupo secreto que ayudaba a las personas esclavizadas a conseguir su libertad. Tubman ayudó a aproximadamente 300 esclavos a obtener su libertad. Nadie bajo su protección fue descubierto nunca.

3. ¿Qué sucedió después de que Harriet Tubman escapara de la esclavitud? *Secuencia*

_____

_____

_____

_____

Harriet Tubman ayudó a escapar a personas esclavizadas por medio del Tren Clandestino.

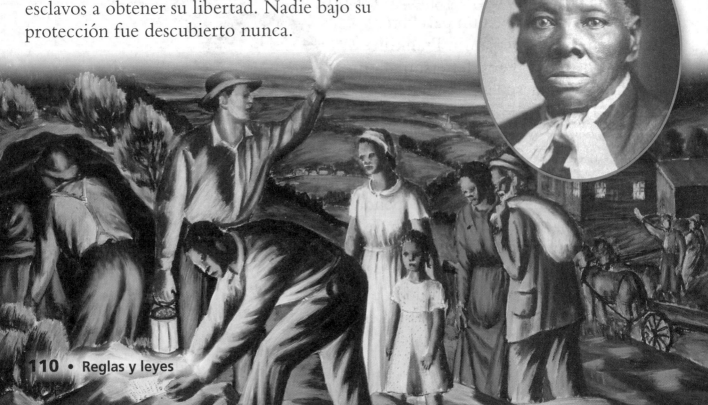

1847

1849 Harriet Tubman escapa de su esclavitud en Maryland.

"Le robé a mi amo esta cabeza, estas extremidades, este cuerpo y salí corriendo con ellos".

—Frederick Douglass

Frederick Douglass pronunció muchos discursos contra la esclavitud.

Frederick Douglass escapó de la esclavitud, al igual que Harriet Tubman. Él también usó sus talentos para ayudar a otras personas esclavizadas. Douglass era escritor y orador. Viajó a muchas ciudades y pronunció cientos de discursos contra la esclavitud.

Douglass también escribió artículos y tres autobiografías, o libros acerca de su propia vida. En 1847 fundó su propio periódico antiesclavista. Se llamaba *The North Star*. Los discursos y escritos de Douglass llegaron a oídos de mucha gente. Sus palabras llevaron a otros a unirse a la lucha contra la esclavitud.

4. **¿Por qué crees que Frederick Douglass fundó su propio periódico?** *Sacar conclusiones*

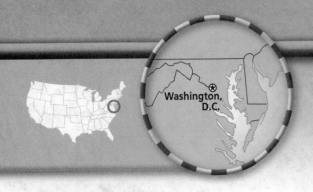

1863 El presidente Lincoln publica la Proclamación de Emancipación.

Defender nuestro país

El presidente Abraham Lincoln dirigió nuestro país durante un momento difícil de su historia. Ese momento fue la Guerra Civil, cuando los estados del Norte estaban en guerra con los estados del Sur. La Guerra Civil empezó en 1861, después que los estados del Sur se separaran de su propio país. Querían mantener la esclavitud y querían que les dieran más derechos a los estados. Los estados del Norte le declararon la guerra a los estados del Sur para evitar que eso sucediera.

El presidente Lincoln quería acabar con la esclavitud. En 1863, durante la guerra, publicó un documento llamado la Proclamación de Emancipación. El documento liberaba a las personas esclavizadas en muchos de los estados del Sur. Los estados del Norte ganaron la guerra en 1865, acabando así con la esclavitud.

5. Causa y efecto **¿Qué suceso liberó a las personas esclavizadas de los estados del Sur?**

_____

_____

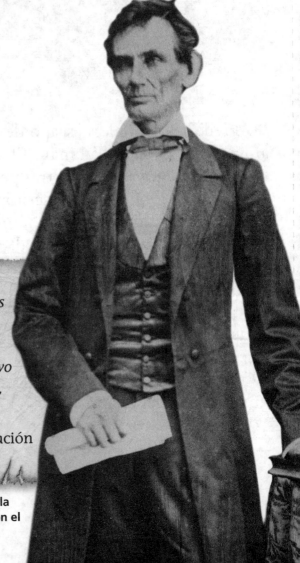

". . . todas las personas tenidas como esclavos en estados y partes de estados cuyos habitantes se encuentran al día de hoy en situación de rebelión contra los Estados Unidos, son, y en lo sucesivo deberán ser desde hoy, y para siempre, libres".

—de la Proclamación de Emancipación

El presidente Lincoln publicó la Proclamación de Emancipación el 1.º de enero de 1863.

1964

Defender los derechos

Durante las décadas de 1950 y 1960, el Dr. Martin Luther King, Jr., luchó por los derechos civiles de todas las personas. Los **derechos civiles** son aquellos derechos que las personas tienen porque son ciudadanos. A muchas personas negras no se les permitía votar, ni tampoco ir a las mismas escuelas que las personas blancas. El Dr. King encabezó muchas protestas y habló contra esa injusticia. A muchas personas blancas no les gustaba lo que el Dr. King estaba haciendo. Por eso enfrentó grandes peligros.

En 1963 el Dr. King pronunció uno de sus discursos más famosos en Washington, D.C. En él dijo que a los estadounidenses se les debía juzgar por sus palabras y sus acciones y no por el color de su piel. En 1964 finalmente se aprobó una ley de derechos civiles que decía que todos los estadounidenses tenían los mismos derechos.

6. Causa y efecto **¿Por qué el Dr. Martin Luther King, Jr., encabezó protestas?**

Resumen

Muchas personas corrieron riesgos para asegurar los derechos y las libertades de todos los estadounidenses. ¿Cuál de esas personas crees que fue un héroe? Explica por qué.

Kalpana Chawla (1961–2003)

Aprende más Kalpana Chawla fue astronauta de la Administración Nacional de Aeronáutica y el Espacio (NASA, por sus siglas en inglés). Nacida en la India, Chawla se mudó a los Estados Unidos para realizar sus estudios.

Chawla se hizo ciudadana de los Estados Unidos. Aproximadamente diez años después solicitó para ser astronauta y NASA la aceptó. Chawla recibió entrenamiento como especialista de misiones y para llevar a cabo experimentos en el espacio. En 1997 viajó en el transbordador espacial *Columbia*. Con ese vuelo, Chawla se convirtió en la primera mujer india en viajar al espacio. Cuando volvió a volar en el *Columbia,* en 2003, el transbordador sufrió un accidente en el que Chawla y el resto de la tripulación murieron.

Chawla llegó a viajar un total de más de treinta días en el espacio. Ayudó a NASA a saber cosas nuevas acerca del espacio y de los viajes espaciales. Recibió muchos premios por su trabajo, entre ellos la Medalla Congresional de Honor.

Contesta las siguientes preguntas.

1. **¿En qué fue Chawla la primera? Subraya tu respuesta en el texto.** *Identificar*

2. **¿Crees que Chawla merecía recibir la Medalla Congresional de Honor? ¿Por qué sí o por qué no?** *Analizar*

_____

_____

_____

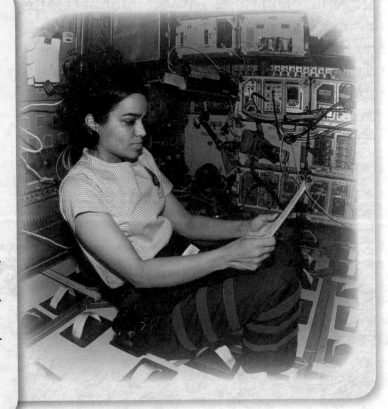

Diario de estudio

En esta unidad estudiarás distintos tipos de recursos y aprenderás cómo la cosas se compran y se venden. También aprenderás a tomar decisiones relacionadas con el dinero. Verás cómo la escuela te ayuda a tomar decisiones que afectarán tu futuro. Completa las actividades que aparecen en estas páginas a medida que leas la unidad.

Lo que sé sobre...

la economía de California:

Distintos tipos de recursos

Escribe un detalle que diga algo más sobre el tipo de recurso que se indica en cada cuadro.

Los productores usan tres tipos de recursos para producir bienes y prestar servicios.

Recursos naturales	Recursos humanos	Recursos de capital

Completa las siguientes oraciones. Luego escribe dos ejemplos de cada una.

Una necesidad es _____   **Un gusto es** _____

_____   _____

1. _____   **1.** _____

2. _____   **2.** _____

Escoge uno de los gustos que escribiste arriba. Escribe tres pasos que debes seguir en un plan de ahorro y así poder comprarlo.

Piensa en lo que quisieras hacer en el futuro. Escríbelo en el espacio titulado *Mi futuro*. En el espacio titulado *Ahora*, escribe dos decisiones que tendrás que tomar "ahora" en la escuela para prepararte para el futuro.

Mi futuro   **Ahora**

1. _____

_____

2. _____

¿Qué tipos de recursos usamos?

CONÉCTATE ¿Qué recursos usamos para satisfacer nuestras necesidades? Los árboles, la tierra, el viento y el agua son algunos de los recursos que utilizamos. ¿Pero sabías que las personas también pueden ser un recurso?

Vistazo previo
Vocabulario
productor *(s.)* persona o negocio que fabrica cosas

consumidor *(s.)* persona que usa o compra bienes y servicios

Actividad de vocabulario Un significado del sufijo *-or* es una persona que hace algo. Subraya las palabras en las definiciones de arriba que dicen lo que esa persona hace.

Personajes
César Chávez

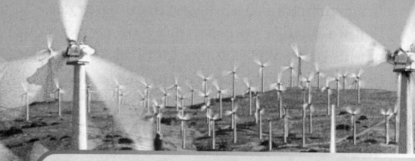

Lectura: Predecir

Predecir significa pensar en lo que podría suceder, antes de que suceda, basándote en lo que ya sabes. Fíjate en la fotografía y en los títulos de la página 118 antes de leerla. Encierra en un círculo el tema acerca del que tú predices que vas a leer.

gobierno   recursos naturales   exploradores

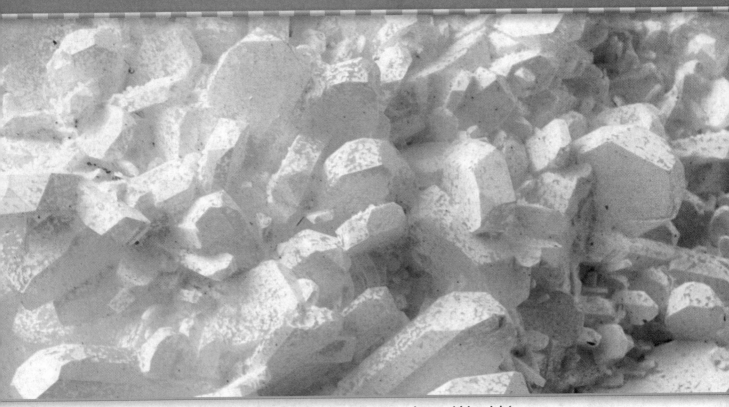

El boro es un mineral que se halla en el sureste de California. Sirve para hacer vidrio y jabón.

Recursos naturales de California

California es rica en recursos naturales. Algunos de estos recursos son la madera, las piedras preciosas, el petróleo y los minerales. Los productores usan los recursos naturales. Un **productor** es una persona o un negocio que fabrica cosas. Por ejemplo, los productores usan los árboles de los bosques para hacer madera y papel. Los productores también usan los minerales. Los minerales son sustancias naturales que se encuentran debajo de la tierra. Los minerales pueden ser sólidos o líquidos. El oro, el cobre y el tungsteno son algunos de los minerales que hay en nuestro estado. El tungsteno puede usarse para hacer bombillas.

Un negocio también puede ser un productor. Los negocios de los Estados Unidos producen bienes y los venden a otros países.

1. Predecir ¿Qué crees que sucedería si usáramos todos nuestros recursos naturales?

Otros recursos

Los recursos humanos y los recursos de capital son otros tipos de recursos. Los recursos humanos son los trabajadores que producen bienes y prestan servicios. Muchas personas de California trabajan en lugares que prestan servicios, tales como tiendas, oficinas, hospitales y otros lugares. Los recursos de capital son las máquinas, las herramientas y los edificios que se usan para producir bienes y prestar servicios. En el pasado, muchos productos se hacían a mano. Hoy en día las máquinas ayudan a que los productos se fabriquen con mayor rapidez.

Los consumidores usan la gran variedad de bienes que los trabajadores producen y de servicios que prestan. Un **consumidor** es una persona que usa o compra bienes y servicios.

2. ¿En qué se diferencian los recursos humanos de los recursos naturales?

Comparar y contrastar

_____

_____

_____

_____

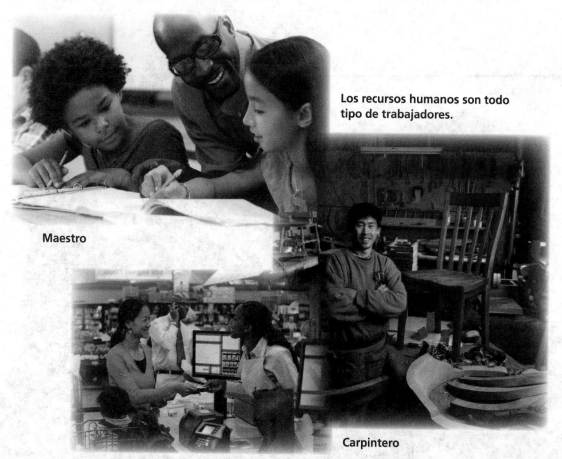

Los recursos humanos son todo tipo de trabajadores.

Maestro

Carpintero

Dependiente

Cuidar nuestros recursos

La Tierra tiene una cantidad limitada de recursos naturales. Los indígenas de California que vivían aquí antes de que llegaran los colonos, usaban sólo aquellos recursos que necesitaban. No cazaban ni pescaban más de lo que necesitaban.

Hoy en día usamos más recursos. Podemos conservar esos recursos naturales de modo que duren más tiempo. Conservamos los recursos cuando los usamos con cuidado. Una manera de conservar los recursos naturales es usándolos menos. Mucha gente conserva recursos replantando árboles, evitando usar la tierra demasiado y aprobando leyes que protejan los recursos. Además pueden reciclar papel y recipientes de vidrio, de plástico y de aluminio.

3. Escribe dos maneras en que podemos cuidar nuestros recursos naturales.

Idea principal y detalles

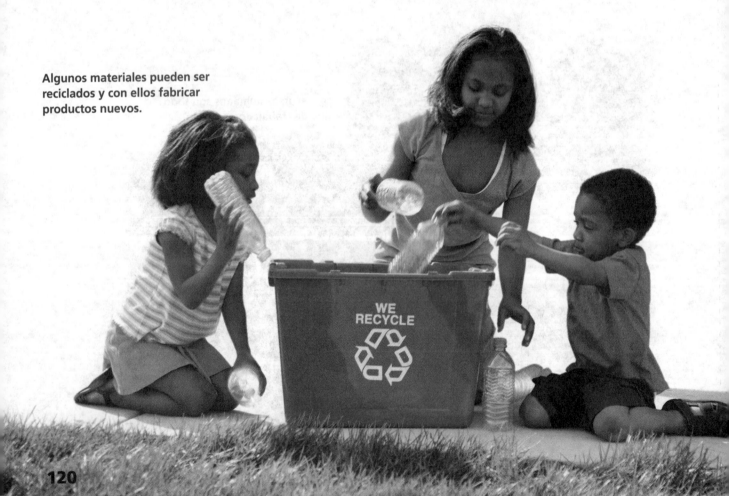

Algunos materiales pueden ser reciclados y con ellos fabricar productos nuevos.

Dar un trato justo a los trabajadores

También debemos cuidar nuestros recursos humanos. Un hombre llamado César Chávez se dio cuenta de que muchos de los dueños de las granjas de nuestro estado no pagaban justamente a sus trabajadores. Además los dueños a menudo obligaban a muchos de los trabajadores a hacer trabajos peligrosos. Durante las décadas de 1960 y 1970, Chávez y Dolores Huerta trabajaron y lograron organizar un sindicato de trabajadores de granjas. Un sindicato es un grupo que se asegura de que a los trabajadores se les dé un trato justo.

4. Subraya las razones por las que César Chávez y Dolores Huerta organizaron un sindicato de trabajadores de granjas. *Causa y efecto*

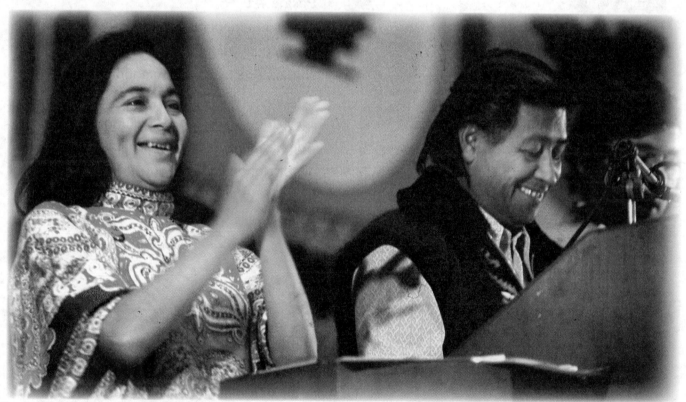

Dolores Huerta y César Chávez encabezan en Fresno la convención de los Trabajadores Agrícolas Unidos de 1973.

Resumen

Los productores han usado y continúan usando recursos para producir bienes y prestar servicios. Nombra los tres diferentes tipos de recursos y di cómo se usan.

Hechos y ficción

Aprende más Al momento de leer, es importante saber si lo que estás leyendo se basa en hechos o si es ficción. Un hecho es algo de la vida real o algo que de verdad sucede. Cuando un escritor escribe un hecho, los lectores generalmente creen que es cierto. La verdad de un hecho puede verificarse si se consulta una enciclopedia o un diccionario. La ficción es algo que ha sido inventado. Los personajes o los sucesos de un texto de ficción pueden parecer verdaderos, pero en realidad un escritor los ha creado para contar una historia.

El primero de los siguientes pasajes fue tomado de tu libro de texto. El segundo, no. Lee los dos pasajes y luego contesta las preguntas

Inténtalo

1. **Subraya las palabras que te indiquen cuál de los pasajes es de ficción.** *Identificar*

2. **En el otro pasaje, encierra en un círculo las oraciones que contengan hechos.** *Identificar*

3. **Escribe una oración que puedas añadir al final del pasaje #2.** *Aplicar*

_____

_____

4. **Explica la importancia de saber la diferencia entre hechos y ficción.** *Analizar*

_____

_____

_____

Pasaje #1

Una manera de conservar los recursos naturales es usándolos menos. Mucha gente conserva recursos replantando árboles, evitando usar la tierra demasiado y aprobando leyes que protejan los recursos. Además pueden reciclar papel y recipientes de vidrio, de plástico y de aluminio.

Pasaje #2

Antonio y Ana no querían que sus recursos se terminaran. Así que construyeron una caja especial. En ella guardaron los recursos que pudieron hallar. Esperaban que la caja no explotara con todos esos recursos que tenía adentro. Guardaban los recursos porque querían usarlos después.

H-SS 3.5.2 Entienden que algunos bienes se producen localmente, otros en otra parte de los Estados Unidos y otros fuera del país.

¿Dónde se hacen los bienes?

CONÉCTATE Piensa en lo que comiste de desayuno. ¿Comiste cereal, huevos o alguna otra cosa? Los alimentos y otros productos se pueden hacer aquí o en otros lugares.

Vistazo previo

Vocabulario

importación *(s.)* producto o recurso que se trae a un país desde otro país

exportación *(s.)* producto o recurso que se envía a otro país para venderlo

Actividad de vocabulario Subraya las palabras en las definiciones que diferencian *importación* y *exportación*.

Lectura: Idea principal y detalles

Recuerda que la *idea principal* es la idea más importante de un párrafo. Subraya la oración que dice la idea principal del primer párrafo de la página 124.

Bienes locales

En nuestro estado se produce todo tipo de bienes. Las uvas, el algodón, las almendras, los tomates, la leche y los huevos son algunos de los cultivos y alimentos que se producen aquí. Otros productos como aquellos hechos con minerales se producen mediante la minería.

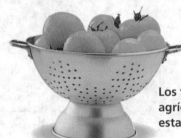

Los tomates son uno de los productos agrícolas más importantes de nuestro estado.

Bienes de otros lugares

Muchos de los bienes que usamos se producen aquí mismo en California. Pero también usamos bienes que vienen de otros lugares del país. Podemos comer papas de Idaho, miel de maple de Vermont o manzanas de Washington. También podemos disfrutar bienes de otras partes del mundo. Podemos comprar queso de Francia, bananos de Costa Rica o juguetes de la China. Muchos de los bienes que se producen en nuestro estado se envían a otros lugares del país y del mundo.

Los habitantes de California pueden disfrutar las manzanas de Washington.

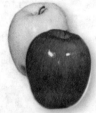

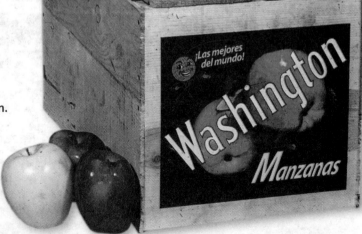

1. **¿Qué tipos de bienes se producen en nuestro estado?**

Idea principal y detalles

_____

_____

2. **¿Cuáles son algunos de los bienes que se producen en otros estados?**

Idea principal y detalles

_____

_____

_____

Producir bienes para vender

La mayoría de los lugares o regiones no pueden producir todos los bienes o prestar los servicios que necesitan sus habitantes. Por eso, la gente de distintas regiones comercia entre sí. Cuando los habitantes de distintas regiones comercian, eso quiere decir que compran o venden bienes y servicios. Hay razones importantes para comerciar. Tal vez una región no puede producir todo lo que necesita; o los bienes pueden ser más baratos en otro lugar.

El comercio con otros lugares

A menudo los habitantes de distintos países y estados comercian entre sí. Por ejemplo, las personas de los Estados Unidos comercian con las personas de países como Canadá, Japón y México. El producto o el recurso que un país trae desde otro país es una **importación**. Una **exportación** es el producto o el recurso que se envía a otro país para ser vendido. Los Estados Unidos importan carros, computadoras, ropa y petróleo. Nuestro país exporta carros, aviones y alimentos.

Muchos bienes enviados a California entran por barco por el puerto de San Francisco.

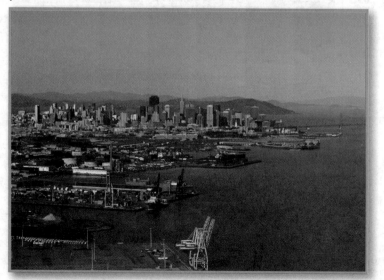

3. ¿Por qué necesitan intercambiar bienes los habitantes de distintas regiones?

Causa y efecto

4. Encierra en un círculo los productos que los Estados Unidos exportan a otros países. *Idea principal y detalles*

Resumen

Muchos de los bienes que usamos se producen en nuestra comunidad o en nuestro estado. Otros bienes se producen muy lejos. ¿Cómo intercambian bienes California y otros lugares?

Gráficas de barras

Aprende más Una gráfica de barras muestra cómo se puede comparar información. La gráfica de barras de abajo muestra algunos productos agrícolas que fueron exportados de California en 2001. La altura o longitud de cada barra representa un número. Ese número indica el valor, en millones de dólares, de la exportación de un producto agrícola.

Escoge una de las exportaciones agrícolas que aparecen en la gráfica de barras. Busca la línea que está encima de la barra y síguela hacia la izquierda hasta que llegues al número. Ese número te dirá el valor de esa exportación agrícola. Usa la gráfica de barras para contestar las preguntas.

Inténtalo

1. **¿Cuál de las exportaciones agrícolas de 2001 tenía el mayor valor?** *Identificar*

   _____

2. **¿Qué valor tuvieron las exportaciones de algodón en 2001?** *Aplicar*

   _____

3. **Encierra en un círculo la exportación agrícola que en 2001 tuvo un valor de aproximadamente $200 millones.** *Aplicar*

4. **Dibuja una estrella encima de las barras de las dos exportaciones que tenían más o menos el mismo valor.** *Interpretar*

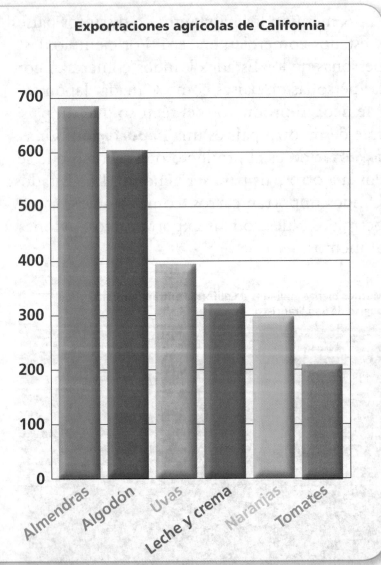

Exportaciones agrícolas de California

Fuente: Departamento de Alimentos y Agricultura de California, 2001

H-SS 3.5.3 Entienden que las elecciones económicas individuales implican soluciones de compromiso y la evaluación de los beneficios y costos.

¿Cómo decidimos lo que queremos?

CONÉCTATE ¿Alguna vez se te ha hecho difícil decidir qué hacer con tu dinero? Puedes gastártelo en algo que quieres, o puedes ahorrarlo para comprar algo más tarde. ¿Por qué crees que es importante aprender a gastar y a ahorrar el dinero con prudencia?

Vistazo previo

Vocabulario

ganar *(v.)* recibir dinero a cambio de hacer un trabajo

elección *(s.)* acción de escoger entre dos o más cosas

ahorros *(s.)* cantidad de dinero que se gana pero que no se gasta

ingresos *(s.)* todo el dinero que una persona recibe de su trabajo y de otras fuentes

presupuesto *(s.)* plan que muestra los ingresos, los gastos y los ahorros

Actividad de vocabulario Escribe una oración que describa cómo tú puedes ganar dinero.

_____

_____

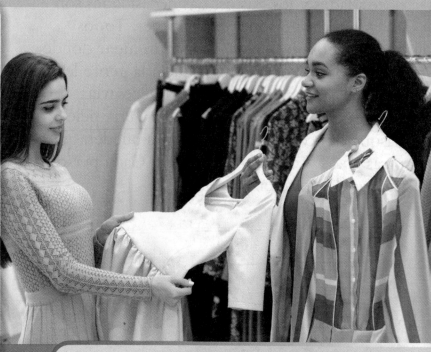

Lectura: Causa y efecto

A veces los escritores usan palabras de *causa* y *efecto* para ayudarte a entender qué sucedió y por qué sucedió. Una palabra clave que indica causa y efecto es *porque*. Subraya la palabra cuando la veas en la página 129.

Ganar, gastar y ahorrar el dinero

Es necesario ganar dinero para poder gastarlo. **Ganar** es recibir dinero a cambio de hacer un trabajo.

Usar dinero implica hacer una **elección,** es decir, escoger entre dos o más cosas. Puedes escoger, o elegir, gastar el dinero o ahorrarlo. Los **ahorros** son la cantidad de dinero que se gana pero que no se gasta. Si ahorras tu dinero, lo tendrás para comprar algo que verdaderamente quieras más tarde.

Necesidades y gustos

Cuando se gasta dinero se obtiene algo a cambio. A menudo tenemos que elegir entre las necesidades y los gustos. Las necesidades son cosas que las personas deben tener. Todos necesitamos alimentos, ropa y un lugar donde vivir. Los gustos son cosas que a la gente le gustaría tener pero que no son necesarias. Puedes querer un juego de video, una pelota de basquetbol o joyería. Tus amigos pueden querer otras cosas. Los gustos se eligen. Cada persona quiere algo diferente.

1. **¿Por qué ahorra dínero la gente?**
Causa y efecto

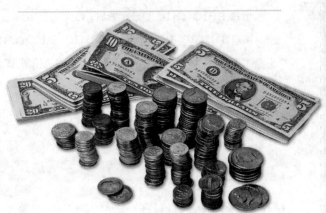

2. **¿Es una bicicleta una necesidad o un gusto? Explica tu respuesta.** *Sacar conclusiones*

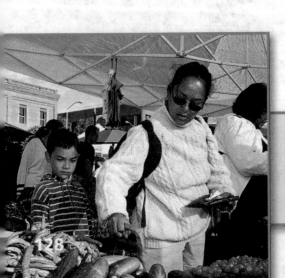

Elegimos entre necesidades y gustos. Los alimentos son una necesidad. Un juego de video es un gusto.

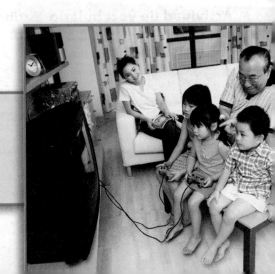

Llevar control de los gastos

La mayoría de la gente necesita tener cuidado con la manera en que gasta el dinero. Tiene que asegurarse de no gastar más de lo que recibe en ingresos. Los **ingresos** son todo el dinero que una persona recibe de su trabajo y de otras fuentes. La mayoría de las personas tienen un presupuesto para poder elegir la manera en que gastarán el dinero. Un **presupuesto** es un plan que muestra los ingresos, los gastos y los ahorros. Necesitas tener un presupuesto porque sin uno puedes gastar demasiado dinero.

Mi presupuesto

Semana	Ingresos	Gastos	Ahorros
Semana 1	$6.00	$1.00	$5.00
Semana 2	$6.00	$1.00	$5.00
Semana 3	$6.00	$1.00	$5.00
Semana 4	$6.00	$1.00	$5.00
Semana 5	$6.00	$1.00	$5.00
Semana 6	$6.00	$1.00	$5.00
Semana 7	$6.00	$1.00	$5.00
Total	$42.00	$7.00	$35.00

Pedro quiere comprar un juego de video, por lo que hace un presupuesto. Sus ingresos son de 6 dólares por semana, que los recibe por hacer tareas de casa. Si gasta 1 dólar a la semana, ahorrará 5 dólares a la semana. El juego de video cuesta 35 dólares. ¿Cuántas semanas le tomará a Pedro ahorrar el dinero para comprar el juego de video?

3. ¿Por qué necesitan tener las personas un presupuesto?

Comparar y contrastar

_____

_____

_____

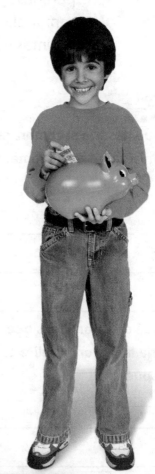

Resumen

Las personas toman decisiones con su dinero a la hora de elegir entre sus gustos y sus necesidades. ¿Cuál es la consecuencia de elegir gastar todo su dinero en una sola cosa?

Tomar decisiones

Aprende más Lo más seguro es que todos los días tomas decisiones, o sea que haces elecciones. Seguir paso a paso un plan te ayudará a tomar una buena decisión.

Supón que tienes muchas ganas de comprarte un casco de bicicleta nuevo. El casco cuesta 25 dólares. Tienes ahorrados 15 dólares. Necesitas 10 dólares más para comprarlo. Pero entonces ves una camiseta que has querido tener desde hace tiempo. Cuesta 15 dólares. ¿Gastarías tus ahorros en la camiseta o esperarías hasta que tuvieras suficiente dinero ahorrado para comprar el casco? Usa el diagrama de abajo para contestar las preguntas y para que te ayude a tomar una decisión.

Inténtalo

1. ¿Qué pasaría si compraras la camiseta en este momento? *Interpretar*

_____

_____

_____

2. ¿Qué decisión crees que sería la mejor? Explica tu respuesta. *Analizar*

_____

_____

_____

Diagrama de decisiones

1. Determina qué quieres decidir. **···**	_____ _____
2. Determina cuáles son tus opciones. **···**	a. Comprar la camiseta. b. Comprar el casco.
3. Determina las consecuencias que tiene cada opción. **···**	a. _____ _____ b. _____
4. Decide cuál de las opciones tiene el mejor resultado. **···**	a. Gastar el dinero que estaba ahorrando para comprar el casco. b. Ahorrar el dinero que necesito para comprar el casco.
5. Toma la decisión.	

H-SS 3.5.4 Discuten la relación del "trabajo" de los estudiantes en la escuela y su capital humano personal.

¿Cómo te ayuda tu trabajo en la escuela?

CONÉCTATE ¿Qué trabajo quieres hacer cuando seas grande? Puedes hacer prácticamente cualquier cosa. ¿Cómo te ayudará tu trabajo en la escuela a tomar buenas decisiones acerca de tu futuro?

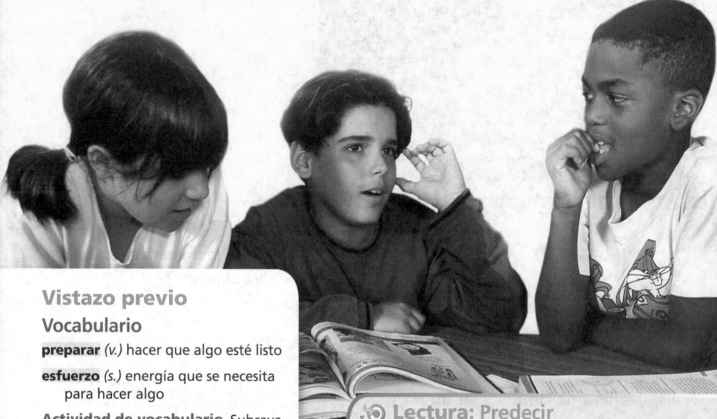

Vistazo previo

Vocabulario

preparar *(v.)* hacer que algo esté listo

esfuerzo *(s.)* energía que se necesita para hacer algo

Actividad de vocabulario Subraya la palabra del vocabulario que describa lo que harías antes de irte de viaje.

Personajes

Jaime Escalante

Lectura: Predecir

Destreza de lectura

Predecir significa pensar en lo que podría suceder, antes de que suceda, basándote en lo que ya sabes. Antes de leer la página 132, fíjate en la fotografía y en su leyenda para predecir por qué las opciones que tienes en la escuela son importantes para tu futuro.

Escoger entre distintas opciones

Con el tiempo decidirás lo que quieres hacer en tu vida. Decidirás dónde vivir, quiénes serán tus amigos y qué trabajo harás. Un buen modo de empezar a hacer estas elecciones es pensar en lo que te gusta hacer y en lo que haces bien. Saber cuáles son tus opciones también te ayudará. La escuela es un buen lugar para aprender acerca de las opciones.

1. 🎯 Predecir **¿Qué pasaría si la gente no tuviera opciones?**

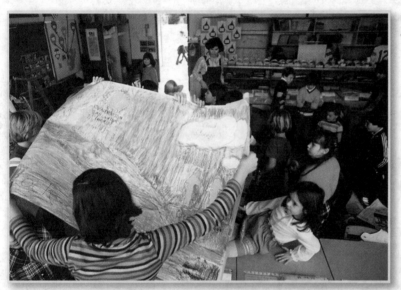

Lo que aprendemos en la escuela puede ayudarnos a tener éxito.

La educación es importante

La educación te ayuda a prepararte para el futuro. **Preparar** significa hacer que algo esté listo. Vas a la escuela con el fin de aprender las cosas que necesitas para tener éxito en la vida. Tener éxito puede significar conseguir un buen trabajo, tener una familia y ser un buen ciudadano. Los líderes de nuestro país quieren que la gente tenga una buena educación. Por eso todos los niños de California tienen derecho a una educación gratuita.

2. **¿Cómo te prepara la educación para el futuro?**

Idea principal y detalles

Trabajos para el futuro

Una elección importante que todos tenemos que hacer es lo que queremos para el futuro. Sea lo que sea que quieras hacer, puedes empezar a prepararte hoy mismo. Las materias que aprendas en la escuela te ayudarán a hacer diferentes trabajos. Por ejemplo, los doctores necesitan saber matemáticas para recetar la cantidad correcta de medicinas. Los padres de familia también necesitan saber matemáticas para mantener el presupuesto familiar. Los constructores necesitan saber matemáticas para construir casas.

Padre de familia

Trabajadora de construcción

3. Predecir **¿Qué materias de la escuela predices que te ayudarán en el futuro?**

_____

_____

_____

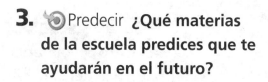

La lectura es una destreza importante para cualquier trabajo.

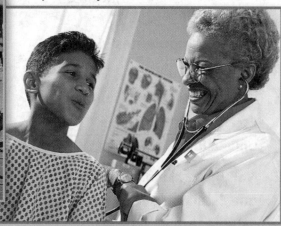

Doctora

4. Subraya los efectos futuros de hacer un esfuerzo por aprender hoy mismo.

Causa y efecto

Se necesita energía

El esfuerzo que hagas hoy por salir bien en la escuela te ayudará más tarde. Un **esfuerzo** es la energía que se necesita para hacer algo. Puede afectar el tipo de trabajo que tengas. También puede afectar la cantidad de dinero que ganes.

Resumen

La educación te puede ayudar a escoger las mejores opciones que tengas para prepararte para tu vida futura. ¿Cómo puede ayudarte en el futuro el trabajo que haces hoy en la escuela?

Jaime Escalante (n. 1930)

Aprende más A Jaime Escalante le gusta enseñar. Él fue maestro de matemáticas en Bolivia, un país que queda en América del Sur. Pero cuando se mudó a los Estados Unidos no sabía hablar inglés. Trabajó de conserje para poder ir a la universidad por la noche. Estudió ciencias y más matemáticas, y aprendió inglés. Después de graduarse de la universidad, trabajó de maestro de escuela secundaria en Los Ángeles.

Escalante contaba con que todos sus estudiantes trabajaran duro. ¿Por qué tuvo éxito? Porque creía en sus estudiantes. Sabía que aprenderían si se esforzaban. También hizo que las matemáticas fueran más divertidas comparándolas con cosas como el basquetbol.

La película *Stand and Deliver (Lecciones inolvidables)*, que se estrenó en 1988, relata el éxito que Escalante tuvo con sus estudiantes.

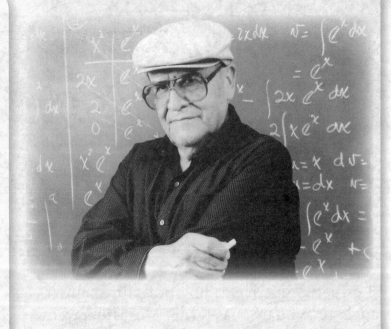

Contesta las siguientes preguntas.

1. **Subraya las materias que Escalante estudió en la universidad.** *Identificar*

2. **Nombra una manera en que Escalante ayudó a sus estudiantes.** *Interpretar*

_____

_____

_____

_____

Contenido

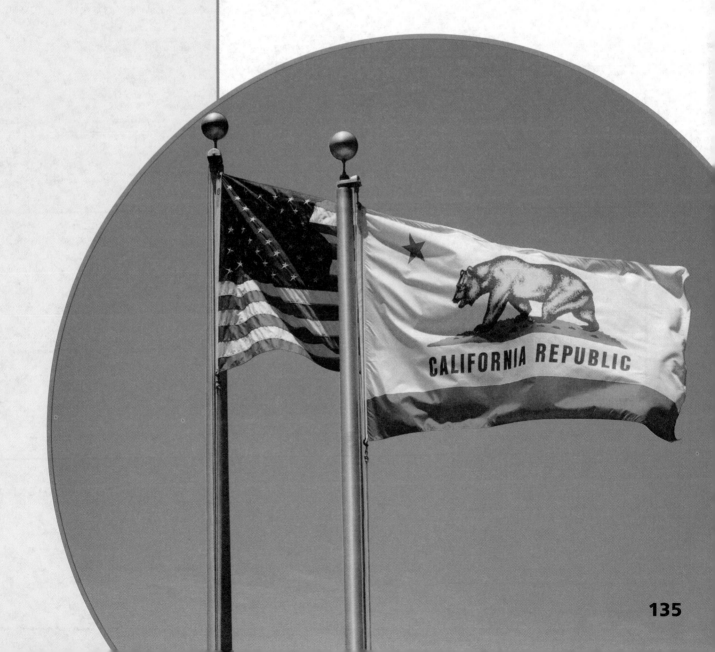

Atlas
Mapa político de nuestros cincuenta estados

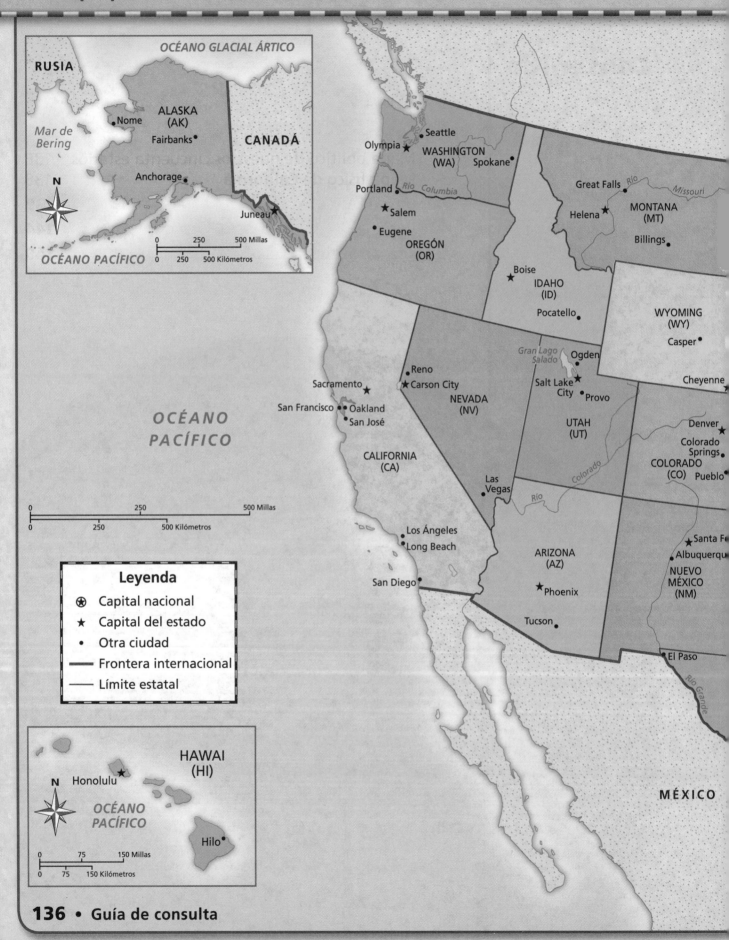

RUSIA

OCÉANO GLACIAL ÁRTICO

Mar de Bering

• Nome

ALASKA (AK)

Fairbanks •

CANADÁ

Anchorage •

N

Juneau ★

OCÉANO PACÍFICO

0   250   500 Millas
0   250   500 Kilómetros

OCÉANO PACÍFICO

0   250   500 Millas
0   250   500 Kilómetros

Leyenda
- ⊛ Capital nacional
- ★ Capital del estado
- • Otra ciudad
- ▬ Frontera internacional
- — Límite estatal

Seattle •
Olympia ★   WASHINGTON (WA)
Spokane •

Portland •   Río Columbia

★ Salem

• Eugene

OREGÓN (OR)

Great Falls •   Río

Helena ★   MONTANA (MT)

Billings •

Boise
★   IDAHO (ID)

Pocatello •

WYOMING (WY)

Casper •

• Reno
★ Carson City

Sacramento ★

San Francisco • • Oakland
• San José

NEVADA (NV)

Gran Lago Salado   Ogden •

Salt Lake City ★   • Provo

UTAH (UT)

Cheyenne

Denver ★

Colorado Springs •

COLORADO (CO)   Pueblo •

CALIFORNIA (CA)

Las Vegas •

Río   Colorado

Río

Los Ángeles •
Long Beach •

San Diego •

ARIZONA (AZ)

Phoenix ★

Tucson •

★ Santa Fe

• Albuquerque

NUEVO MÉXICO (NM)

• El Paso

Río Grande

MÉXICO

HAWAI (HI)

N

Honolulu ★

OCÉANO PACÍFICO

Hilo •

0   75   150 Millas
0   75   150 Kilómetros